The Nurses' Guide to Psychotherapy

Stacey Roles · Kamini Kalia
Editors

The Nurses' Guide to Psychotherapy

A Reference Book for Nurses Providing Psychotherapy

Springer

Editors
Stacey Roles
Roles & Associates Psychotherapy Services Inc. & CBT Training Centre of the North
Sudbury, ON, Canada

Kamini Kalia
Trillium Health Partners
Mississauga, ON, Canada

ISBN 978-981-97-4737-5 ISBN 978-981-97-4738-2 (eBook)
https://doi.org/10.1007/978-981-97-4738-2

This Springer imprint is published by the registered company Springer Nature Singapore Pte Ltd.
The registered company address is: 152 Beach Road, #21-01/04 Gateway East, Singapore 189721, Singapore

This book is dedicated to all of the nurses, who have been providing psychotherapy to their clients for many years without recognition or validation. This book is about formalizing this process to give confidence to what you have been doing all this time and to provide guidance in areas where it had not been provided before. It is also for those nurses who, more recently, might wish to pursue nurse psychotherapy as a career path. Thank you for all you do.

Foreword

In the landscape of nursing education, one essential cornerstone has long been absent: a comprehensive guide to psychotherapy tailored specifically for nurses. Now, with the advent of *The Nurse's Guide to Psychotherapy: A Reference Book for Nurses Providing Psychotherapy*, this void is admirably filled. Throughout modern history, nurses have been at the forefront of health care, pioneering advancements in clinical practices and therapeutic relationships. Nurses' tireless dedication spans the breadth of human experience, from bustling urban centers to remote rural outposts, from areas of affluence to regions of hardship, leaving virtually no corner untouched by their expert and compassionate care.

Central to our existence and functioning in the world is mental health—a foundation as vital as our physical well-being and interpersonal connections. Nurses have always been integral to their clients' mental health journey, whether in formal psychiatric settings or at the bedside of a patient grappling with anxiety over medical procedures or a new diagnosis. Therapeutic relationships and mental health training form the bedrock of interactions nurses engage in with clients necessitating care support and encouragement. Embracing a psychotherapeutic approach equips nurses to holistically address the complexities and pressing demands of individuals, communities and population health needs.

This seminal text arrives at a pivotal moment, offering guidance to nurses embarking on or enriching their psychotherapeutic practice. With meticulous attention to jurisdictional regulations and professional standards, this book opens the door for nurses to navigate the complexities of psychotherapeutic engagement. Whether novice or seasoned practitioner, readers will find within these pages a roadmap to develop the necessary insights, competencies and skills essential to this important specialty.

The editors, Stacey Roles RN, Ph.D., and Kamini Kalia RN, MScN, CPMHN(C), have curated a volume that traces the historical trajectory of psychotherapy and demystifies complex concepts. Through pragmatic tools, reflective inquiries, and vivid case vignettes, the book transforms learning into an inspiring and engaging journey. It is an indispensable addition to the library of any nurse committed to psychotherapeutic practice, offering practical wisdom alongside scholarly depth. The book also attends to policy and advocacy, acknowledging the indispensable role played by organizations like the Registered Nurses' Association of Ontario (RNAO) in advancing psychotherapy within the nursing profession and the health system.

As I reflect on the transformative potential of this text, I am honored to contribute this foreword, recognizing the immense value it brings to our profession. With this foundational work, authored by esteemed nurse leaders and experienced psychotherapists, I am optimistic about the exciting advancements that lie ahead for nursing psychotherapy.

Dr. Doris Grinspun
RN, BScN, MSN, Ph.D., LLD(hon),
Dr.(hc), DHC, DHC,
FAAN, FCAN, O.ONT.
Chief Executive Officer
Registered Nurses' Association
of Ontario (RNAO)
Toronto, ON, Canada

Preface

Nursing has evolved greatly since the days of Florence Nightingale (1820–1910) known as the founder of modern nursing. The title of her book *Notes on Nursing: What it is, and What it is Not* (1860) describes the confusion that has existed within the role of nursing for centuries passed. It is apparent that in each specialty of nursing, there are questions about what the role of nursing is and what it is not, and mental health, addictions, psychiatry and psychotherapy are no exception.

Nurses have been doing this work with clients living with mental health and addiction symptoms and challenges as far back as documented, from nurses in war helping those with shell shock, to the first psychiatric institutions and asylums that existed. Although Hildegard Peplau's theory on the nurse-patient relationship and advanced nurse psychotherapeutic interventions are taught, there has not been a foundational psychotherapy book for nursing, a reference book for nurses providing psychotherapy, to guide nurses and help them to distinguish 'what [nurse psychotherapy] is and what it is not.'

We wrote this book to provide understanding and clarity for nurses, with the intention to encourage more nurses to engage in the continuous learning of differing forms of psychotherapy. Learning can empower nurses to competently employ psychotherapy techniques and interventions with their clients, whether they work directly in the specialty of mental health and addictions, or if they work in the fields of oncology, medicine, diabetes, cardiology, or any other area where they are helping their clients through the struggles of physical illness, trauma, anxiety, or depression.

Nurses have the ability to touch many lives and to heal and support numerous individuals and communities. 'What nursing is' includes nurse psychotherapists. Nurses who are educated with these powerful interventions, who have the ability to ease suffering and to advocate for this very important role within the Canadian healthcare system and beyond.

I learned a long time ago the wisest thing I can do is be on my own side, be an advocate for myself and others like me.

—Maya Angelou

Sudbury, Canada Stacey Roles
Mississauga, Canada Kamini Kalia

Reference

Nightingale, F. (1860, reprinted 1969 Dover Publications, NY). Notes on Nursing: What it is, and what it is not.

Acknowledgements

First and foremost, we would like to acknowledge all of the chapter authors and contributors of this book. The knowledge and experience you have been willing to share within these pages for nurses who are currently practising and for nurses in the years to come will make a difference in their careers and in the lives of the clients they treat. Thank you for all of your hard work on this book. Sherry Price DDS, MSW, RSW thank you for all of the hours you have put in editing, formatting and supporting us. Lastly, we would like to thank all of the clients and families that we have personally had the privilege of working with, we have learned so much from all of you about strength, resilience and openness to change.

—Stacey Roles and Kamini Kalia

Personally, to my family, friends and support systems, I could not have evolved in the 20-plus years of my nursing career or have written this book without you. I am unable to prioritize the order of these names as there has been so much support in many different ways; so I am listing them alphabetically by first name: Alyssa Lamothe, Anilla Edwards, Billy Roles, Brent Edwards, Brian Joblin, Brian Roles, Brutus Roles, Bryson Van Heck, Carly Valiente, Chad Lamothe, Ellwood Edwards, Emelia Lamothe, Ethan Lamothe, Gwenne Roles, Hailey Dunn, Hercules Roles, Janna Tarini, Katherine Roles, Laurie Dunn, Lucy Roles, Nicholas Tarini, Stacey Tarini, Stephanie Paquette, Tammy Gill, Tryvge Janson, Vivian Oystrick, Walter Roles, Whiskers Roles, Xavier Martin, and Zoey Dunn. I cannot express how grateful I am for all of you.

Professionally, there are so many people who have helped to carve my career path and enhance my learning as a nurse and as a psychotherapist and collectively as a nurse psychotherapist. My mentors and supervisors both from the nursing profession and other disciplines have opened my practice to transdisciplinary approaches, doing similar work but from different foundational backgrounds. This interdisciplinary integration, which I was fortunate enough to complete within my Ph.D., enables the growth of each discipline to the benefit of one another and to the client. Of my mentors, there are a few that require special mention.

First, the late Dr. Albert P. Gouge, a brilliant man who specialized in PTSD treatment and who had all the confidence in the world in me to do new and difficult things, insisted, that because of my approach and experience in nursing and who I was as a person, that I needed to start learning psychotherapy. He not only advocated strongly to ensure that I was able to take an intensive Cognitive Behavioural Therapy (CBT) training program when nurses weren't being accepted into that particular program at that time, but also brought me into his private practice to teach me everything he could about different forms of psychotherapy and treating PTSD. He mentored me and changed my career path. Since then, the many multi-disciplinary therapists I have trained and supervised, and the clients I have treated throughout the years have all benefited because of his knowledge and guidance.

Dr. Ramamohan Veluri, who took me under his wing when I was a new psychiatric nurse working on the floor, educating me about assessing differing presentations and clinical symptoms in patients and who taught me and continues to teach me about psychopharmacology. Dr. Veluri mentored me throughout my clinical nursing training and in integrating multiple forms of psychotherapy into my practice and supported me throughout my Ph.D. work. I am extremely grateful for all of the guidance and support you have given me throughout the years.

I want to thank Dr. Michael Tompkins who supervised me in learning CBT and in becoming a trainer and consultant with the Academy of Cognitive Therapy, Dr. Denis Tirch and Dr. Laura Silberstein-Tirch who trained and supervised me in Compassion Focused Therapy (CFT) and Dr. Paul Gilbert, founder of CFT who mentored me as a trainer and supervisor in CFT. I want to acknowledge my Ph.D. supervisor Dr. Roberta Heale, who has done wonderful things for the expansion of the field of nursing and who has been a persistent and consistent role model in advocating for nursing by refusing to accept things as they are just because they've always been done that way.

I also want to thank my brilliant and compassionate team at Roles & Associates Psychotherapy Services Inc. and the CBT Training Centre of the North. The work you do has helped to ease the suffering of so many through psychotherapy sessions with individual clients, partners, groups and families and through the training, supervision and consultation that you provide to clinicians to support their practice.

Lastly, I want to thank my co-editor Kamini Kalia, thank you for keeping the momentum going on this book during the times when I had lost steam, it is always a pleasure working with you on all of our multiple endeavors. You are a true leader in the nursing profession.

—Stacey Roles, RN MScN Ph.D.

Stacey and I met many years ago at a continuous education event and over the years we kept in touch to talk about leading practices in the field of mental health nursing and our deep passion to improve access to those accessing the Canadian healthcare system. We've learned over the years how incredibly important it is to dedicate time to advocate for the profession of nursing and for our clients. We've also grown in the ways by which we do advocacy thanks to the support and guidance of leaders like

Dr. Irmajean Bajnok, Ph.D., MScN, BScN, RN and Dr. Doris Grinspin Ph.D., MSN, BScN, RN. When Stacey first asked me to join in co-editing this book, I was both honored and inspired. I was motivated by our authors and contributors, but also by how we could use our collective voice to validate our colleagues and additionally, mentor the future generation of nursing. I'm thankful that Stacey asked me to assist and for helping me to continue to find and use my voice.

I would like to extend my gratitude to my family who enabled me to be able to spend countless hours in my office to read, review, and write. Thank you Jeff Zagorac, our children (Sai and Ryker) and Raji Kalia for allowing me to work on this book as we could not have accomplished this without your love and support.

Lastly, I'm grateful for the mentorship I have received over the years from incredible mental health nurses including Dr. Cheryl Forchuk RN, Ph.D and Margaret Gehrs RN, MScN. Both have demonstrated excellence in nursing and pushed me to think critically about how I can influence healthcare systems. Thank you for your ongoing mentorship, and I promise to pay it forward.

—Kamini Kalia, RN MScN CPHMN(C)

Contents

Editors and Contributors

About the Editors

Stacey Roles RN MScN PhD Psychotherapist is an Academy of Cognitive and Behavioural Therapies (USA) Certified Trainer Consultant and Certified Cognitive Therapist and is also credentialed with the Canadian Association of Cognitive and Behavioural Therapies (CACBT). Stacey has advanced training and supervision in CBT, prolonged exposure therapy, brain spotting therapy, psychodynamic psychotherapies, solution-focused therapy, dialectical behavioural therapy and compassion-focused therapy. She is competent in treating clients across the lifespan from early childhood to older adults and works with individuals, couples and a variety of other forms of relationships. Stacey graduated from the RN program at Cambrian College in 2003 and has continued advancing her education throughout her over 20-year nursing career. She is an Adjunct Professor at Laurentian University with the School of Nursing and holds the rank of Assistant Professor at the Northern Ontario School of Medicine University. Stacey has extensive experience working with First Nations populations throughout Ontario specifically in the remote and rural areas of Northern Ontario. Stacey specializes in providing consulting services to those who work with complex mental health presentations, in both large and small organizations. She has extensive experience consulting with mental health clinicians and supportive staff in Indigenous communities and offers an assortment of other specialized and advanced learning and consulting options to meet the unique needs of individual organizations. Stacey is the owner and director of Roles & Associates Psychotherapy Services Inc. and CBT Training Centre of the North. e-mail: stacey@rolespsychotherapy.com

Kamini Kalia RN MScN CPHMN(C) completed her Bachelor of Science in Nursing from McMaster University (Hamilton, Ontario) and Masters of Science in Nursing from Western University (London, Ontario). Kamini is a systems leader who has extensive experience and education in psychiatric/mental health nursing, professional practice, clinical leadership and health informatics. Kamini has studied Cognitive Behavioural Therapy (CBT), as well as compassion-focused and mindfulness-based therapies, and is a CBT Diplomate with the Academy of Cognitive and Behavioral Therapies in the United States of America. She is currently employed as the Director, Health Information and Informatics Solutions at Trillium Health Partners in Mississauga, Ontario, Canada. She holds an Adjunct Assistant Professorship at the Arthur Labatt Family School of Nursing, Western University, as well as an Adjunct Lecturer Appointment at the Bloomberg Faculty of Nursing, University of Toronto. e-mail: kaminikalia@gmail.com

Contributors

Irmajean Bajnok RN MScN PhD FCAN FAAN Wounds Canada, North York, ON, Canada

Siobhan Bell NDP MN BScN RN Nursing@Heart Inc., Mono, ON, Canada; Nurse Psychotherapy Association of Ontario, Mono, ON, Canada

Nancy Brookes RN BN MSc(A) PhD Health Sciences, School of Nursing, University of Ottawa, Ottawa, ON, Canada

Kaitlin Marriner Brulotte RN RP MA DCP Chelsea, QC, Canada

Delaney Campbell Roles & Associates Psychotherapy Services Inc. & CBT Training Centre of the North, Sudbury, ON, Canada

Natalie Castonguay RN CPMHN(C) CpedN(C) BScInf DESP Roles & Associates Psychotherapy Services Inc. & CBT Training Centre of the North, Sudbury, ON, Canada

Cheryl Forchuk RN PhD O Ont FCAHS FRSC FCAN Nursing and Psychiatry, Lawson Research Institute, Western University, Parkwood Institute Research, St Joseph's Hospital, London, ON, Canada

Sheena Howard BScN MA RN Cavan, ON, Canada

Carmen Hust MScN PhD RN CPMHN(C) Chair, Algonquin College Chair of Nursing Studies, Kars, ON, Canada

Hoodo A. Ibrahim NP-PHC MSN BScN CPHMN(C) St Joseph's Healthcare Hamilton/Hamilton Health Sciences, Hamilton, ON, Canada

Myriam Innocent NP MScN Cobourg, ON, Canada

Kamini Kalia RN MScN CPMHN(C) Trillium Health Partners, Mississauga, ON, Canada

Alan Largo RN MScN CPMHN(C) Roles and Associates Psychotherapy Services Inc., Sunnybrook Health Science Center, Toronto, ON, Canada

Mary-Lou Martin RN MScN MEd St. Joseph's Healthcare Hamilton/McMaster University, Hamilton, ON, Canada

Sabrina Merali RN MN Registered Nurses' Association of Ontario (RNAO), Toronto, ON, Canada

Esther N. Monari RN MScN PhD Faculty of Nursing Health Sciences Centre, Memorial University of Newfoundland, St. John's, Newfoundland and Labrador, Canada

Madison Moxam BA Psychology Laurentian University, Sudbury, ON, Canada

Sheeba Narikuzhy MA RP CFRC Hopeful Minds Psychotherapy, Ajax, ON, Canada

Vivian Oystrick PhD MSW RSW Cambrian College, Sudbury, ON, Canada

Archna N. Patel RN MN Woodbridge, ON, Canada

Emma Quinn CD RN MC BNSc CPMHN(C) Wasaga Beach, ON, Canada

Ingrid Rijo RN Alliston, ON, Canada

Stacey Roles RN MScN PhD Roles & Associates Psychotherapy Services Inc. & CBT Training Centre of the North, Sudbury, ON, Canada

Carly Valiente BA(Hons) RSW Roles & Associates Psychotherapy Services Inc. & CBT Training Centre of the North, Sudbury, ON, Canada

Sophia Woloschuk Gassanova RN BScN MN CPMHN(C) Toronto, ON, Canada

Chapter 1
Introduction

Stacey Roles and Kamini Kalia

Abstract The profession of nursing is in a pivotal position to provide holistic care to the needs of Canadians across various settings. Nurses who possess the knowledge, skill, and judgment to independently practice psychotherapy can meet the demands of the population requiring psychotherapeutic treatment, thus extending access to equity-deserving populations, and enabling comprehensive care to be offered via the nurse-client therapeutic relationship. Enabling the full scope of nurses through supportive legislation, educational requirements, and regulation, ensures the safety of the public and is foundational to guiding nurses who wish to pursue this career trajectory. This chapter will provide context for this book by introducing the history of nursing and psychotherapy in North America and the ever-evolving landscape.

Keywords Nurse psychotherapy · History

Learning Objectives

After completing this chapter, the learner will:

1. Understand the need for guidance on nurse psychotherapy;
2. Have an understanding of the current Canadian landscape and standards of practice;
3. Demonstrate an awareness of nurse psychotherapy lived experiences and advocacy.

S. Roles (✉)
Roles & Associates Psychotherapy Services Inc. & CBT Training Centre of the North, Sudbury, ON, Canada
e-mail: stacey@rolespsychotherapy.com

K. Kalia
Mississauga, ON, Canada

S. Roles and K. Kalia (eds.), *The Nurses' Guide to Psychotherapy*,
https://doi.org/10.1007/978-981-97-4738-2_1

1 The Evolution of Nurse Psychotherapy

Nursing is an evolving profession that has historically been rooted in strong foundational knowledge and expertise from bio-psychosocial theories, models, and evidence-informed practices. Throughout the years, nursing has advanced in terms of scope of practice and care provision in response to changes in the environment, patient population trends, culture, and socio-economic shifts, established empirical evidence, and the integration of technology in care settings. Not only are individual nurses developing from novice to expert in their clinical practice (Benner, 1984), but the profession itself has emerged as "*an art and a science*" with advanced academic and pre-licensure requirements, growing autonomous and independent practices, established self-regulating bodies, as well as expanded expertise and scope within respective clinical specialties.

Nurse psychotherapy is one such example of a practice that has progressed over time, however, little is described in the literature about how an aspiring or licensed nurse can develop competencies or even set up an independent practice. This deficit has been reinforced through comparisons with other established health and social discipline training programs and professional practice standards. Although there is an abundance of expertise in those with an established practice within the profession of nursing, personal experiences coupled with the paucity of formal guidance for trying to sustain or initiate a nurse-led practice have led to the emergence of this text.

The Nurses' Guide to Psychotherapy: A Reference Book for Nurses Providing Psychotherapy is a foundational book for those looking to advance their own nursing practice in psychotherapy whether as a novice, advanced clinician, or an expert nurse. The chapters ahead describe the history of nursing and psychotherapy in North America, detail the current landscape of nurse-led psychotherapy, and identify how the profession can continue to evolve or progress into the future.

2 A Review of the Literature

Upon review of the literature surrounding mental health, psychiatric nursing, and the study and implementation of psychotherapy, it has become clear that there is limited guidance available for nurses in their study of psychotherapy, with nurses often having to refer to other professional disciplines for guidance or mentorship. Current literature surrounding undergraduate nursing baccalaureate curricula and nurses in practice in Canada have shown little evidence of introductions to psychotherapy and therapeutic techniques from a nursing perspective. While many current curricula do offer introductions to mental health nursing through essential texts (Austin et al., 2019; Townsend and Morgan, 2018), these reading materials only lightly touch on the aspect of psychotherapy and give sparse insight into how it can be implemented in clinical settings.

Other iterations of mental health and psychiatric nursing textbooks are designed for advanced nurses who regularly provide psychiatric/mental health care to patients and any mention of the use of psychotherapy is in an advanced capacity (Durham and Hardin, 1986; Wheeler, 2014; Tusaie and Fitzpatrick, 2017). While this knowledge is useful, it is not accessible to or geared towards entry-level nurses or nurses new to practicing psychotherapy who require foundational education on psychotherapeutic care.

Psychotherapy research and education run into a similar yet unique problem. The emergence and increased use of psychotherapy, such as cognitive behavioural therapy, has led to a plethora of research surrounding the uses and development of psychotherapy in clinical settings. While prolific amounts of psychotherapy texts exist to lay an educational framework (Yalom and Leszcz, 2005; Wampold, 2019), little to no information exists on psychotherapy in nursing. When academia does manage to mention nurses in psychotherapy, findings suggest that nurses offer a fresh and unique perspective on the intervention (Hurley et al., 2020), but that nurses are not able to provide such care in an effective manner due to limited training availability and the prioritizing of diagnosis and medication management over therapeutic techniques in the field (Delaney and Handrup, 2011; Gournay et al., 2000).

3 Review of Existing Standards of Practice

In Canada, psychotherapy is currently regulated in the provinces of Ontario, Quebec, Nova Scotia, New Brunswick, and Prince Edward Island. Alberta passed legislation to create a College of Counselling Therapy in 2021, and similarly, there is a great deal of activity ongoing in other provinces such as the involvement of regulatory colleges to aid in adhering to the psychotherapy regulations (Canadian Counselling and Psychotherapy Association, 2024).

In Ontario, members of six regulatory colleges (College of Nurses of Ontario, College of Psychologists of Ontario, College of Registered Psychotherapists, College of Social Workers and Social Service Workers, College of Occupational Therapists of Ontario and College of Physicians and Surgeons of Ontario) are authorized to provide the *Controlled Act of Psychotherapy* (Regulated Health Professions Act, 1991*)* provided these professional roles do so in compliance with the regulations and the bylaws established by their regulatory colleges. In other provinces where the act of psychotherapy is regulated (Quebec, Nova Scotia, New Brunswick, and Prince Edward Island) there are many different rules and some exclude nurses from practicing the act of psychotherapy unless they register with a second regulatory college that is acknowledged in that province (Table 1).

The legislation for psychotherapy would benefit from consistency across provinces in Canada including expected standards of practice from regulatory colleges within provinces. All three Canadian territories (Northwest Territories, Nunavut, and Yukon) do not show any activity toward the regulation of psychotherapy (Canadian Counselling and Psychotherapy Association [CCPA], 2024). In Ontario, where the regulated *Psychotherapy Act* (2007) allows differing colleges to regulate, there are inconsistencies as to how the guidelines and standards inform the professionals under their college regulations. See Table 1 for Canadian Provincial Regulations for Practicing Psychotherapy. For example, Ontario-based regulatory colleges of occupational therapists, social services workers and social workers, psychologists, and psychotherapists have well-defined standards and educational requirements, as compared to the College of Physicians and Surgeons and the College of Nurses of Ontario which have not defined requirements. In addition to regulations, the emphasis on clinical supervision and mentorship pre-licensure and post-licensure is well-defined within other colleges and across the country in relation to psychotherapy practices.

> Clinical supervision is a crucial component in the training of helping professionals. In the arena of supervised practice, nascent counsellors integrate theoretical and conceptual learning and apply skills and strategies in vivo. Clinical supervisors are simultaneously tasked with facilitating the professional growth and development of supervisees while safeguarding the wellbeing of clients and the public. (CCPA, 2021, para 1).

Nursing continues to provide limited guidance with psychotherapy mentorship and clinical supervision, leaving nursing lagging behind other regulated professions. These inconsistencies identify an opportunity for advancement and development within the practice of nurse psychotherapy to better access and care for clients not only in Ontario but across Canada.

Personal Experiences

As the practice of psychotherapy became more defined within the jurisdiction in consultation with regulated health professions in Ontario, it became increasingly important for nurses to speak up about their established clinical practice. S. Roles and K. Kalia, the editors of this book, have been involved since 2015 alongside many nurse psychotherapist colleagues, many of whom are chapter authors in this book. In 2015, the College of Nurses of Ontario (CNO), requested a content expert to engage in a roundtable discussion regarding the Ontario *Psychotherapy Act* (2007), to determine what would be considered within and outside of the controlled act of psychotherapy. Nurse leaders were included as panel members in the government facilitated discussion in 2017 and 2018 and since then, have been consulted as provincial members and as consultant leads within the structured psychotherapy project beginning in 2019. It was not until December 31st, 2017, whereby *Psychotherapy* was proclaimed a *Controlled Act* in the province of Ontario (Regulated Health Professions Act, 1991), thus framing ongoing discussions by specific health and social disciplines. This regulation served to place title protection regarding who would be able to initiate and

Table 1 Canadian provincial regulations for practicing psychotherapy

Regulation/regulatory bodies	Professional disciplines	Training/education requirements
Quebec		
The Quebec Counseling Association is an association and not an order, they cannot grant licenses or act upon protected terms	Psychologists and Medical Doctors may practice. Other disciplines must obtain a membership	Only psychologists and medical doctors are automatically granted the right to practice psychotherapy in Quebec
The Ordre des Psychologues du Québec (OPQ) is the governing body/college for psychotherapists in Quebec	The term "counsellor" is not a protected term in Quebec however, you may still belong to the Quebec Counselling Association (a joint membership that is granted through the CCPA membership)	If you wish to practice psychotherapy and do not belong to either of these colleges, you must complete the OPQs four-step process: A. Be a member of one of these professional orders: (1) Quebec Order of Guidance Counselors (2) Professional Order of Criminologists of Quebec (3) Quebec Order of Occupational Therapists (4) Quebec Order of Nurses (5) Order of Psychoeducators of Quebec (6) Professional Order of Sex therapists/Sexologists of Quebec (7) Quebec Order of Social Workers and Marriage and Family Therapists B. Have completed 600 h of internship in psychotherapy. Once again, the specifics of the internship are available at (https://www.ordrepsyqc.ca/resume-des-4-exigences) C. Hold a master's degree in mental health and human relations D. Have completed 765 h of theoretical training in psychotherapy at the university level. This training must have been acquired: As part of university studies or; As part of training in psychotherapy acquired: i. private establishment; ii. or with an independent trainer ii. or with an independent trainer

FAQ. QCA. (n.d.). http://www.quebeccounselling.ca/faq
Psychotherapeutes. Ordre des psycologues du Québec. (2024). https://www.ordrepsy.qc.ca/
Summary of the 4 requirements. Ordre des psycologues du Québec. (2024). https://www.ordrepsy.qc.ca/resume-des-4-exigences

(continued)

Table 1 (continued)

Regulation/regulatory bodies	Professional disciplines	Training/education requirements
New Brunswick		
College of Counselling Therapists of New Brunswick (CCTNB)	No professional designations are automatically granted license to practice therapy in N.B	Hold a master's degree from an accredited institution in a field of study prescribed by the CCTNB board of directors Complete counselling course requirements: 1. One course in counselling theory, practicum, skills, and ethics 2. Five courses (3 credit hours each) from a list available at: https://www.cctnb.ca/en/admissibilit%C3%A9 3. Have a minimum of 150 h of direct client contact during or after one's master's program 4. Pass a criminal record and vulnerable sector check 5. Submit a current resume 6. Possess or intend to possess professional liability insurance 7. Pay registration costs, sign an agreement with the CCTNB
Member Benefits. The College of Counselling Therapists of New Brunswick. (2022). https://www.cctnb.ca/en/avantages-pour-membres Eligibility. The College of Counselling Therapists of New Brunswick. (2022). https://www.cctnb.ca/en/admissibilit%C3%A9		
Nova Scotia		
Nova Scotia College of Counselling Therapists (NSCCT)	No professional designations are automatically granted license to practice therapy in N.S	Applicants must hold a counselling-related master's degree, which involves academic coursework and clinical practice training consisting of at least 120 h of direct client contact
		Following graduation, applicants are eligible to be licensed as a Registered Counselling Therapist—Candidate (RCT-C), which allows them to begin counselling independently under the oversight of an experienced and specifically trained Registered Counselling Therapist (RCT) supervisor. The required candidacy period (internship) involves 2,000 h of supervised practice with at least 800 h of direct counselling with individuals and groups, typically extending over a 2-to-5-year period

(continued)

Table 1 (continued)

Regulation/regulatory bodies	Professional disciplines	Training/education requirements
Register with the college. NSCCT. (2024). https://nscct.ca/graduate-of-a-canadian-counselling-therapy-masters-program/		
Ontario		
College of Registered Psychotherapists of Ontario	Registered Psychotherapists	Anyone whose practice involves the provision of the controlled act must be registered with one of the six colleges authorized to perform that act
College of Psychologists of Ontario	Psychologist	
Ontario College of Social Workers and Social Service Workers	Social Service Workers and Social Workers	Only those registered with the CRPO may use the title "registered psychotherapist". Those who are members of the five other regulatory colleges may only use the title "psychotherapist" with their professional designation
College of Nurses of Ontario	Registered Practical Nurses and Registered Nurses	
College of Occupational Therapists of Ontario	Occupational Therapists	If one's work falls within the scope of the practice of psychotherapy and they are not already registered with another Ontario regulatory college whose registrants can practise psychotherapy they should consider the CRPO
College of Physicians and Surgeons of Ontario	Physicians including specialists	
Controlled act of psychotherapy: Everything you need to know. College of Registered Psychotherapists of Ontario. (2024). https://www.crpo.ca/controlled-act-of-psychotherapy/ Controlled act of psychotherapy. College of Registered Psychotherapists of Ontario. (2018, June 29). https://www.cpca-rpc.ca/pub/docs/Controlled-Act-of-Psychotherapy-Final%20June%2029,%202018.pdf Applying to CRPO. College of Registered Psychotherapists of Ontario. (2024). https://www.crpo.ca/applying-to-crpo		
Prince Edward Island		
College of Counselling Therapy of PEI (CCTPEI)	No professional designations are automatically granted license to practice therapy in P.E.I	Only registrants with the CCTPEI may use the title "counselling therapist" or "CT" Have at least 450 direct client contact hours Have completed a master's degree program in counselling therapy approved by the Council or education and training that the Council considers substantially equivalent Pass the CCTPEI registration exam Pass a jurisprudence exam Obtain a record check, liability insurance, and pay annual dues
Required documents. College of Counselling Therapy PEI. (2024). https://www.cctpei.ca/required-documents Education requirements. College of Counselling Therapy PEI. (2024). https://www.cctpei.ca/education-requirements Welcome. College of Counselling Therapy PEI. (2024). https://www.cctpei.ca/		

(continued)

Table 1 (continued)

Regulation/regulatory bodies	Professional disciplines	Training/education requirements
Alberta		
Association of Counselling Therapy of Alberta (ACTA) to become: College of Counselling Therapy of Alberta (CCTA)	No professional designations are automatically granted license to practice therapy in Alberta as it is currently unregulated	
The Association of Counselling Therapy of Alberta. The Association of Counselling Therapy of Alberta. (2021). https://www.acta-alberta.ca/ Regulation in Alberta. Canadian Counselling and Psychotherapy Association. (2024). https://www.ccpa-accp.ca/regulation-in-alberta/		
British Columbia		
Federation of Associations for Counselling Therapists in British Columbia (FACT-BC) is currently working towards regulation	No professional designations are automatically granted license to practice therapy in B.C. as it is currently unregulated	
British Columbia Regulation. Canadian Counselling and Psychotherapy Association. (2024). https://www.ccpa-accp.ca/british-columbia-regulation/		
Manitoba		
Federation of Associations for Counselling Therapists in Manitoba (FACT-Manitoba) is currently working towards regulation	No professional designations are automatically granted license to practice therapy in Manitoba as it is currently unregulated	
Manitoba regulation. Canadian Counselling and Psychotherapy Association. (2024). https://www.ccpa-accp.ca/manitoba-regulation/		
Saskatchewan		
Federation of Associations for Counselling Therapists in Saskatchewan (FACT-SK) is currently working towards regulation	No professional designations are automatically granted license to practice therapy in Saskatchewan as it is currently unregulated	
Regulation in Saskatchewan. Canadian Counselling and Psychotherapy Association (2024). https://www.ccpa-accp.ca/regulation-in-saskatchewan/		
Newfoundland and Labrador		
Federation of Associations for Counselling Therapists in Newfoundland and Labrador (FACT-NL) is currently working towards regulation	No professional designations are automatically granted license to practice therapy in Newfoundland and Labrador as it is currently unregulated	

(continued)

Table 1 (continued)

Regulation/regulatory bodies	Professional disciplines	Training/education requirements
Regulation in Newfoundland and Labrador. Canadian Counselling and Psychotherapy Association. (2024). https://www.ccpa-accp.ca/regulation-in-newfoundland-and-labrador/		
N.W.T., Yukon, Nunavut		
All three territories are currently unregulated and show no activity towards regulation	No professional designations are automatically granted license to practice therapy in the territories as they are currently unregulated	
The Profession and Regulation. Canadian Counselling and Psychotherapy Association. (2024). https://www.ccpa-accp.ca/profession-and-regulation/#:~:text=Provinces%2FTerritories%20in%20RED%20currently,of%20Psychotherapy%3A%20Ontario%20and%20Quebec		

perform the controlled act of psychotherapy, as well as set protection of the activity of psychotherapy given the inherent risks in order to ensure patient safety. In Ontario it was decided that all psychotherapy falls under the controlled act should all five of the following criteria be met:

1. You are treating a [client]
2. You are applying a psychotherapy technique
3. You have a therapeutic relationship with the [client]
4. The client has a serious disorder of thought, cognition, mood, emotional regulation, perception, or memory
5. This disorder may seriously impair the [client's] judgment, insight, behaviour, communication, or social functioning. (CNO, 2023, para. 8)

However, as with any procedure, nurses continue to be accountable for having the knowledge, skill, and judgment to perform this controlled act safely. Even with this new regulation in place, some nurses in Ontario may still need an order due to workplace policies or requirements under the Public Hospitals Act (1990). Delegation of the controlled act of psychotherapy by NPs, RNs, and RPNs is also prohibited. Regrettably, during this time, many nurses left the profession joining other regulated professions often due to a lack of clear guidance from their regulatory body, nurse leaders, and employers as well as because of legitimate concerns about autonomy to initiate or perform the *Psychotherapy Act*. It was imperative for psychotherapy to have parameters to keep the public safe, but in doing so, new obstacles were established for nurses to self-initiate the therapy and differences emerged in how each profession was supported to perform psychotherapy. More specifically for the latter, a lack of insurance coverage for nurse-led psychotherapy existed and within hospital settings, the requirement of having a physician or nurse practitioner's order to initiate the *Act* created further barriers. These changes were disruptive to established therapeutic relationships, continuity of care, and interprofessional relations.

These realizations led to advocacy for the continued practice of psychotherapy on many levels. Examples of advocacy in partnership with the nursing professional body took place with the Ministry of Health and Long-Term Care, the regulatory body, employers, and insurance companies. This advocacy took form in providing education to nurses throughout the province of Ontario, which has had national exposure and implementation regarding the ability to engage in the role of nurse psychotherapy in a more in-depth way than they perhaps thought they ever could. Advocacy has taken the form of:

- Training and supervision of nurses implementing structured and unstructured psychotherapies such as cognitive behavioural therapy (CBT), psychodynamic psychotherapy, dialectical behavioural therapy (DBT), and compassion-focused therapy among others
- Nurses stepping into independent entrepreneur roles
- Interdisciplinary education on the role of the nurse to other health/social disciplines and insurance companies

Advocacy within the professional body highlighted that Registered Nurses had been providing "expert, safe, and compassionate psychotherapy services" over time (Registered Nurses' Association of Ontario, [RNAO], 2014). Preparation and continued learning for nurses as competent or to maintain competency were best described as nurses who had required theoretical knowledge, practicum experience, and clinical supervision (RNAO, 2014).

There was a 2-year transition period allotted from December 31st, 2017 before the *Controlled Act of Psychotherapy* came fully into effect on January 1st, 2020, enabling Registered Nurses in Ontario to continue to initiate psychotherapy without an order from a physician or a nurse practitioner in community-based settings. This transition period, which is now concluded and has become the continued regulation is a considerable milestone for nurses across the province as trained professionals. However, with this new legislation comes a need for standardized and improved educational requirements in psychotherapy within the nursing discipline, particularly as generalist requirements for licensure limit the opportunity for new nurses to gain confidence in performing psychotherapy. Further, the training and expertise required in order to become competent in psychotherapy is not standard or consistent in most undergraduate health and social discipline programs that can initiate and perform the *Act*. For example, the typical BScN curriculum is replete with praxis, pathologies, inpatient care, and some community work with little consistency of an in-depth understanding of mental health therapies. This is not uncommon for many of the disciplines enabled to initiate and implement the controlled act, and therefore, the purpose of this foundational textbook is to fill that particular gap within the undergraduate nursing curriculum.

4 Summary

- The literary gap on the subject of nurses in psychotherapy, coupled with personal experiences, as well as new legislation in the field of mental health nursing, presents the need for an original publication.
- This book aims to provide foundational knowledge for nurses to explore psychotherapeutic techniques and learn a foundational skill set for the application of these psychotherapies.

Acknowledgements to William Lawton BA MSc, Sudbury, ON, Canada for his contributions to this chapter.

References

Austin, W., Kunyk, D., Peternelj-Taylor, C., & Boyd, M. (2019). *Psychiatric & mental health nursing for Canadian practice*. Wolters Kluwer.

Benner, P. (1984). *From novice to expert: Excellence and power in clinical nursing practice*. Addison Wesley.

Canadian Counselling and Psychotherapy Association. (2021, September 27). *The Profession & Regulation*. Author. https://www.ccpa-accp.ca/profession-and-regulation/#:~:text=Provinces%2FTerritories%20in%20RED%20currently,of%20Psychotherapy%3A%20Ontario%20and%20Quebec.

College of Nurses of Ontario. (2023). *Nurses can now initiate psychotherapy without an order*. Author. https://www.cno.org/en/learn-about-standards-guidelines/magazines-newsletters/the-standard/January-2020/nurses-can-initiate-controlled-act-psychotherapy/.

Delaney, K. R., & Handrup, C. T. (2011). Psychiatric mental health nursing's psychotherapy role: Are we letting it slip away? *Archives of Psychiatric Nursing*, *25*(4), 303–305. https://doi.org/10.1016/j.apnu.2011.04.005

Durham, J., & Hardin, S. (1986). *The Nurse Psychotherapy in Private Practice*. Springer Publishing Company Inc.

Gournay, K., Denford, L., Parr, A.-M., & Newell, R. (2000). British nurses in behavioural psychotherapy: A 25-year follow-up. *Journal of Advanced Nursing, 32*(2), 343–351. https://doi.org/10.1046/j.1365-2648.2000.01482.x

Hurley, J., Lakeman, R., Cashin, A., & Ryan, T. (2020). The remarkable (disappearing act of the) mental health nurse psychotherapist. *International Journal of Mental Health Nursing, 29*(4), 652–660. https://doi.org/10.1111/inm.12698

Registered Nurses' Association of Ontario. (2014). Letter to CNO: Requiring an order to perform psychotherapy. Author. http://rnao.ca/policy/letters/cno-re-requiring-order-perform-psychotherapy

Regulated Health Professions Act (1991). SO 1991, c 18. Ontario. https://www.ontario.ca/laws/statute/91r18#BK24

Townsend, M. C., & Morgan, K. I. (2018). *Psychiatric mental health nursing: Concepts of care in evidence-based practice*. F.A. Davis Company.

Tusaie, K. R., & Fitzpatrick, J. J. (2017). *Advanced practice psychiatric nursing: Integrating psychotherapy, psychopharmacology, and complementary and alternative approaches across the life span*. Springer Publishing Company, LLC.

Wampold, B. E. (2019). *The basics of psychotherapy: An introduction to theory and practice* (2nd ed.). American Psychological Association.

Wheeler, K. (2014). *Psychotherapy for the advanced practice psychiatric nurse: A how-to guide for evidence-based practice*. Springer Publishing Company, LLC.

Yalom, I. D., & Leszcz, M. (2005). *The theory and practice of group psychotherapy* (5th ed.). Basic Books.

Part I
History of Nurse Psychotherapy—Becoming

Chapter 2
An Overview of Theories and Concepts

Nancy Brookes, Siobhan Bell, and Carmen Hust

Abstract This chapter is designed to introduce nurses and nursing students to the development of nursing knowledge and science upon which nursing psychotherapy practice is based. Nurses aspiring to have or, those with a psychotherapy practice may have had limited knowledge of the evolution of the theoretical base which enriches nursing psychotherapy practice. This may be in part because of an absence of a coherent compilation and integration of the extant theoretical works. An historical overview of some of the nursing theorists who have been integral to the evolution of nursing psychotherapy practice is provided. The grandmother of psychiatric nursing—Hildegard Peplau (1909–1999) and her psychodynamic model, and Joyce Travelbee (1926–1973) with her human-to-human theory, have been identified as early theorists of historical significance (Alligood, 2022). They provide foundational concepts for nurses' practice of psychotherapy. The Tidal Model® (Barker, 2000) expands the work of these two theorists. McAllister (2003) further develops solution-focused nursing which is particularly relevant for nursing psychotherapy practice and Leininger illuminates an important culture and diversity focus (McFarland, 2022). Foundational concepts for nurses' practice of psychotherapy have emerged and continue to develop in our historical evolution.

Keywords Nursing theory · Nursing psychotherapy · Foundational concepts · Tidal model

N. Brookes (✉)
Health Sciences, School of Nursing, University of Ottawa, Ottawa, ON, Canada
e-mail: nancy.brookes@sympatico.ca

S. Bell
Nurse Psychotherapy Association of Ontario, Mono, ON, Canada
e-mail: sbell@nursepsychotherapy.org

C. Hust
Algonquin College Chair of Nursing Studies, Kars, ON, Canada
e-mail: chustc@algonquincollege.com

S. Roles and K. Kalia (eds.), *The Nurses' Guide to Psychotherapy*,
https://doi.org/10.1007/978-981-97-4738-2_2

Learning Objectives

After completing this chapter, the learner will be able to:

1. Explain the historical significance of nursing theorists such as Peplau, Travelbee, Barker, and Leininger in the context of nursing psychotherapy.
2. Identify key foundational concepts derived from the historical evolution of nursing psychotherapy practice and describe how these concepts inform and enrich the practice of psychotherapy for nurses and nursing students.
3. Analyze and compare the psychodynamic model proposed by Peplau and the human-to-human theory by Travelbee, recognizing the unique elements and contributions of each theory to nursing psychotherapy practice.
4. Examine the importance of the integration of theoretical works in advancing the field of nursing psychotherapy.
5. Recognize the value of historical perspectives in shaping contemporary psychotherapy practices within nursing.

1 Introduction

The nurse psychotherapist sits with a person as they relate their challenges and feelings, grasping this information through their comprehensive nursing knowledge, inclusive of nursing theory, while taking stock of their personal and professional experience. One's curiosity around each encounter and continuous learning provides an expanding base to identify and find new ways to support the person toward enhanced growth, development, and health. Nurse psychotherapists use theoretical frameworks to facilitate assessment, organize findings, situate lived experiences, develop care plans, initiate therapy, and evaluate outcomes. Theoretical frameworks provide a lens for nurse psychotherapy practice.

2 Historical Significance

The practice of nursing psychotherapy has evolved significantly over the years, grounded in the work of early nursing theories by Peplau (1991) and Travelbee (1971). Nursing psychotherapy is a dynamic and evolving field where perspectives may differ, but foundational concepts are shared. The scope of nursing psychotherapy covers the lifespan and includes individual, couple, family, relationship, and group psychotherapy. Broadly, within psychotherapy, there are many schools, for example, psychoanalysis and psychodynamic therapies, behaviour therapy, cognitive therapy, humanistic therapy, solution-focused therapy, person-centred therapy, and integrative or holistic therapy, though therapists may not tie themselves to any one approach. Instead, therapists may blend elements from different approaches and tailor their treatment according to each person's needs. The more contemporary positive psychology also continues to contribute to the psychotherapy landscape. Neurobiology has informed and continues to inform our understanding of people. In addition to the multiplicity of psychotherapeutic approaches, our entry into the digital age with virtual care has influenced nursing practice, including nursing psychotherapy.

Hildegard Peplau (1909–1999) and Joyce Travelbee (1926–1973) are recognized as pioneers in nurse psychotherapy and their theories may be viewed as the initial work in the nursing psychotherapy journey. Each is a product of their time, and the context in which they worked and wrote. Both Peplau and Travelbee focused their theoretical foundation on the nurse-person relationship and therapeutic use of self. Their theories continue to be taught in many undergraduate nursing programs to this day and the concepts are integral in many curricula. Through their influence, the foundations that nursing psychotherapy has been built on continue to develop.

3 Psychodynamic Model and the Human-To-Human Theory

A brief overview situates Peplau in this introduction, see Chap. 3 for an indepth review. In the mid-twentieth century, Hildegard Peplau introduced, described, and clarified the grounding psychodynamic nursing theory, with the nurse-person relationship as central to nursing practice. The interpersonal interactional process and relationship-centred therapy became an important part of nursing psychotherapy. Peplau described nursing as a "...human relationship between an individual who is sick, or in need of health services [with}a nurse especially educated to recognize and to respond to the need for help" (Peplau, 1991, pp. 5–6). This brought a new perspective, a new approach and a theoretical foundation for nursing practice with the emphasis being on the nurse-person relationship. Nurse-person relationships emphasize this relationship as a powerful therapeutic tool, where trust, empathy, and open communication foster a safe and supportive personal environment. This concept enriches nursing psychotherapy practice by highlighting the importance of building rapport and collaboration, allowing nurses to engage more effectively with persons in addressing their psychological and emotional needs (Alligood, 2022).

Peplau made a point of exhorting nurses not to limit themselves to her writing and provided myriad references for nurses to explore. She noted that the social science and psychiatry disciplines would continue to explore new ideas of importance in solving common nursing problems that recur in varied nursing situations (Peplau, 1991). Peplau revolutionized the psychotherapy field as she placed the nurse-patient/person relationship as central in psychiatric nursing. She identified nursing as "a significant, therapeutic, interpersonal process. It functions cooperatively with other human processes that make health possible for individuals in communities...Nursing is an educative instrument, a maturing force, which aims to promote forward movement of personality in the direction of creative, constructive, productive, personal and community settings" (Peplau, 1991, p. 16). This ground-breaking work situating the nurse-person relationship as central to nursing, is perhaps her most significant contribution to psychiatric nursing and nursing in general. This is clearly foundational in nursing practice, education, and research.

Peplau noted that the kind of nursing she advocated for was not new, as nursing had long been practicing within interpersonal relations. Rather her work explicated some concepts and principles underlying interpersonal relations and transformed nursing situations into learning experiences (Peplau, 1991). Two guiding assumptions underpin her work, Interpersonal Relations in Nursing and Fostering Personality Development:

> The kind of person each nurse becomes makes a substantial difference to what each patient will learn as he is nursed throughout his experience with illness… Fostering personality development in the direction of maturity is a function of nursing and nursing education; it requires the use of principles and methods that permit and guide the process of grappling with everyday interpersonal problems and difficulties. (Peplau, 1991, p. x)

Clearly, within interpersonal relations, the nurse's personality and self-awareness are important. The expectation is that the interpersonal experience may at times be problematic but also provides the opportunity for growth and development for both the nurse and the person.

Peplau's seven nursing roles

1. Stranger role: Receives the person the same way one meets a stranger in other life situations; provides an accepting climate that builds trust.
2. Resource role: Answers questions, interprets clinical treatment data, provides information.
3. Teaching role: Gives instructions and provides training; involves analysis and synthesis of the learner's experience and reflection on what the nurse has learned.
4. Counselling role: Helps clients understand and integrate the meaning of current life circumstances; provides guidance and encouragement to make changes.
5. Surrogate role: Helps client clarify domains of dependence, interdependence, and independence and acts on client's behalf as an advocate.
6. Active leadership: Helps clients assume maximum responsibility for meeting treatment goals in a mutually satisfying way.
7. Technical expert role: Provides physical care by displaying clinical skills; operates equipment. (Peplau, 1991, pp. 43–69)

Peplau identifies four phases of the nurse–person relationship, which may be viewed as interlocking. Each phase also defines the roles and tasks required of the nurse in that situation:

1. Orientation: "initial reaction between the nurse and the patient".
2. Identification: "explores the experience and the needs of the patient".
3. Exploitation: "the patient derives the full value of the relationship"
4. Resolution: "in the final stage, the patient earns independence over his care" (Peplau, 1991, p. 17).

> Nursing is a significant, therapeutic, interpersonal process. It functions cooperatively with other human processes that make health possible for individuals and communities ... Nursing is an educative instrument, a maturing force, aims to promote forward movement of the personality in the direction of creative, constructive, productive, personal and community living (Peplau, 1991, p. 16).

Joyce Travelbee introduced the human-to-human theory (Travelbee, 1971). Through the process of interaction or relating to each other, everything the nurse (a human) did with an ill person (a human) helped to fulfill the purpose of nursing. The nurse and the person are humans relating to one another, and the nurse psychotherapist promotes human-to-human connections (Travelbee, 1971). Travelbee highlights the importance of mutual understanding of the person's emotional and existential needs, working with empathy, and developing mutual understanding and rapport. The human conditions and life experiences encountered by all humans include suffering, hope, pain, and illness (Tomey, 2006). This facilitates a better understanding of both the person in care and the nurse. Of note, Travelbee clarified and elaborated on the therapeutic use of self where "the therapeutic use of self is the ability to use one's personality consciously and in full awareness in an attempt to establish relatedness and to structure nursing intervention." (Tomey, 2006, p. 420). It "requires self-insight, self-understanding, an understanding of the dynamics of human behaviour as well as the behaviour of others, and the ability to intervene effectively in nursing situations" (Tomey, 2006, p. 418). This has been particularly significant for nursing psychotherapy practice.

Travelbee contends that "there are no patients, there are only human beings in need of care, services and assistance of other human beings" (Travelbee, 1971, p. 32). "The human being is a unique, irreplaceable individual—a one-time being in this world, yet unlike any person who ever lived or will ever live" (Travelbee, 1971, p. 26). "Nursing is an interpersonal process whereby the professional nurse practitioner assists an individual or family to prevent, or cope with, the experience of illness and suffering and, if necessary, assists the individual or family to find meaning in these experiences" (Travelbee, 1971 p. 1).

Within the human-to-human relationships theory seven concepts are defined:

1. Establishing, maintaining and terminating a one-to-one relationship are activities that fall within the province of nursing practice. She notes that other health professionals have neither the education nor experience to direct nursing activities.
2. Nurses have but one dependent function, that of executing legal medical orders. In the same way that a nurse cannot give medical orders, a physician cannot "order" nursing care.
3. A relationship is established only when each participant perceives the other as a unique human being. She notes that the term nurse-patient relationship is a misnomer used in the text for communicative economy.
4. Only qualified psychiatric nurses are prepared to supervise nurses in psychiatric nursing.

5. The major learning experience provided in the psychiatric nursing course is to provide students with the opportunity to establish, maintain and terminate one-to-one relationships.
6. Nurses must know how to use library facilities and search the literature for needed information.
7. The knowledge, understanding and abilities needed to plan, structure, give and evaluate care during the one-to-one relationship are necessary prerequisites for developing competency in group work.

4 Several Assumptions Underpin Travelbee's Human to Human Theory

Suffering—An experience that varies in intensity, duration and depth, ranging from a feeling of unease to mild and extreme pain.
Meaning—The reason attributed to a person.
Nursing—Helps a person find meaning in the experience of illness and suffering.
Hope—Faith that there can and will be a chance that would bring something better with it. There are six characteristics of hope.
Communication—"A strict necessity for good nursing care".
Self-Therapy—The ability to use one's own personality consciously and in full awareness; refers to the nurse's presence physically and psychologically (Travelbee, 1971, pp. 55–56).

There are interactional phases within the Human-to-Human Relationship model. Nursing is accomplished through human relationships that begin with the original encounter, the first impression of the nurse. As the relationship begins, it progresses, and empathy and sympathy develop. Finally, mutual understanding and rapport are established (Tomey, 2006).

Travelbee discusses the goals of the nurse: the nurse helps/assists the ill person; to cope with present problems; conceptualize his problems; perceive his participation in an experience; face emerging problems realistically; envision alternatives; test new patterns of behaviour; communicate; socialize; find meaning in illness (Travelbee, 1971).

> The practice of psychiatric nursing is a searching, tiring, sometimes tedious but always interesting process. It involves disciplined observation, a skill derived by applying theory to practice – a skill most difficult to learn. Observation of behavior must be based on knowledge – not intuition – and must be validated, whenever possible, with the ill person. Nursing intervention is based on this application of theory and observation of the human being in his totality. (Travelbee, 1971, p. 23)

Peplau and Travelbee's work has influenced the evolution of nurse psychotherapy and their theories continue to provide strong anchors in nurse psychotherapy practice today.

5 Foundational Concepts Derived from the Historical Evolution of Nursing Theory

Aside from the concepts of Hildegard Peplau's therapeutic nurse-person relationship and Travelbee's therapeutic use of self-described above, there were many other contributors of concepts and foundations that paved the way for the path of nurse psychotherapists today. The Tidal Model® of Mental Health Recovery and Reclamation (initially, the Tidal Model of Psychiatric and Mental Health Nursing) elaborates on Peplau and Travelbee. Vives, Linkes and Soucy (2023) studied select core competencies in nursing psychotherapy practice. They identified five domains for the competencies: professionalism, cultural diversity, ethical/legal standards of care, reflective practices and application of knowledge and skill. Madeleine Leininger's Culture Care Diversity and Universality Theory (McFarland, 2022) addresses cultural diversity. Leininger's theory focuses on describing, explaining and predicting nursing similarities and differences focused primarily on human care and caring in human cultures. Care always occurs in a cultural context, and this is important for nursing psychotherapists.

The Tidal Model® of Mental Health Recovery and Reclamation, a more contemporary model, was created by Phil Barker, Poppy Buchanan-Barker and colleagues. Barker was, at the time, a professor of psychiatric nursing who also maintained a private psychotherapy practice. "Water is the core metaphor for both the lived experience of the person…and the care system that attempts to mold itself around a person's need for nursing" (Barker, 2000, p. 10; Barker et al., 1999, 2000). The theory developed from a series of research studies directed at "the proper focus of nursing" and toward understanding and explaining the human condition (Barker et al., 1999) as well as the Empowering Interactions study (Barker et al., 2000). This work clarified the discrete roles, functions and focus of mental health nursing within the interprofessional care and treatment process (Brookes et al., 2008, p. 24). Barker worked with several nursing colleagues, but the team also included people with lived experience, particularly Dr. Irene Whitehall, reflecting his interest in the possibilities of genuine collaborative relationships with those who use mental health services (Brookes, 2022, p. 504). While Barker had several influences, those of Travelbee and Peplau, who was also a friend and colleague, contributed to this nursing theory and Tidal practice. The Tidal Model® may be considered radical because it conceptualizes mental health problems as human rather than psychological, social, or physical. Here, Travelbee (1971) is relevant and even more so as her therapeutic use of self flows through the Tidal Model®. Within the Tidal Model®, mental health problems are seen as problems in living. Peplau is echoed in the "emphasis on the central importance of developing an understanding of the person's needs through collaborative working, developing a therapeutic relationship through discrete methods of active empowerment, establishing nursing as an educative element at the heart of interdisciplinary interventions" (Brookes, 2022, p. 504).

Two major assumptions underlie the Tidal Model: change is the only constant, nothing lasts, and people are their stories. These stories, of course, are framed in the first person and provide an account of how they came to be here with their problem(s) in living (Brookes, 2022, p. 510). Like Travelbee, Barker uses people and person(s) rather than patient and client, which is significant as we move towards a more person-centred care approach. Nursing is seen as an enduring interpersonal activity and involves a focus on the promotion of growth and development (Barker & Whitehill, 1999, p. 17). The model of the person is represented in three domains: the self-domain, the world domain, and the others domain.

The proper focus of nursing studies found universal acceptance of special interpersonal relationships between nurses and persons, echoing Peplau's (1952/1991) work. Three roles were illuminated: the ordinary me, the pseudo-ordinary or engineered me and the professional me. "Knowing you, knowing me" emerged as the core concept in these studies (Barker et al., 1999). Another study looked at empowerment within nurse-person relationships through the Empowering Interaction Model (Barker et al., 2000). This study developed Peplau's assumptions about the importance of specific interpersonal transactions:

- Being respectful of people's knowledge and expertise about their own health and illness;
- Putting the person in the driver's seat in relation to the interaction;
- Seeking permission to explore the person's experience;
- Valuing the person's contribution;
- Being curious is a way of validating the person's experience;
- Finding a common language to describe the situation;
- Taking stock;
- Reviewing collaboratively and inspiring hope through designing a realistic future together (Brookes, 2022, p. 508).

Within the Tidal Model®, the primary therapeutic focus of mental health care lies in the community as wherever the person might be, they would return to their "ocean of experience." Change is a constant ongoing process. Empowerment is at the heart of the caring process. The nursing encounter is like the nurse and the person are united temporarily like dancers in a dance, reminding nurses that genuine caring encounters involve "caring with" (Brookes, 2022, p. 508).

The essential values of the Tidal Model® are expressed through 10 commitments. Value the voice, respect the language, develop genuine curiosity, become the apprentice, reveal personal wisdom, be transparent, use the available toolkit, craft the step beyond, give the gift of time and know that change is constant (Brookes, 2022, pp. 506–507). The Tidal Model® provides an orientation to practice that is research-based, holistic, collaborative and person-centred. The Tidal Model® is not a reified work nor a recipe for practice but a practical and evolving guide for delivering collaborative, person-centred, solution-focused and empowering care through relationships and respecting culture and creed (Brookes, 2022, p. 515).

Additional theorists such as Jean Watson, Patricia Benner, Madeleine Leininger and Helen Erickson, among others, have contributed significantly to developing nursing knowledge and its application in psychotherapy practice. Their work has enriched the field by emphasizing holistic care, the importance of experiential learning, transcultural nursing and exploring nursing as an art, and modeling and role-modeling. Collectively, these theorists form the historical tapestry that continues to guide and shape the practice of nursing psychotherapy, emphasizing the holistic and humanistic dimensions of person care (Alligood, 2022).

Another foundational concept emerging from the historical evolution of nursing psychotherapy is holistic care. This has been championed by nursing theorists such as Jean Watson, Patricia Benner, and Phil Barker. This concept recognizes the interconnectedness of physical, psychological, social, and spiritual dimensions of health and well-being. It enriches psychotherapy practice by encouraging nurses to consider many dimensions when assessing, planning, and providing care interventions to and with persons. By addressing the whole person, nurses can better support persons in their psychotherapeutic journey, fostering a more comprehensive and person-centred approach to mental health and overall well-being (Alligood, 2022).

The concept of cultural competence and/or transcultural nursing was first espoused by nursing theorist Madeleine Leininger and has since become integral to nursing psychotherapy practice. This concept underscores the importance of understanding and respecting diverse cultural beliefs, values, and practices when providing psychotherapy care. It enriches nursing practice by promoting cultural sensitivity and inclusivity, enabling nurses to deliver more culturally competent and effective psychotherapy interventions. By recognizing the impact of culture on mental health, nurses can tailor their approaches better to meet the unique needs of diverse persons and populations (McFarland, 2022). These foundational concepts derived from historical evolution serve as guiding principles for nurses enhancing the quality and effectiveness of psychotherapy.

McAllister (2003) provides an evolution of the solution focus dimension for nursing psychotherapy, Solution Focused Nursing. She addresses the concern that nursing tends to be quite problem-focused, which is an uncontested idea and is taken for granted, but this is insufficient for nursing. A solution focus acknowledges problem-solving as part of nursing work, whereas this orientation foregrounds both problems and solutions, which are forms of clinical reasoning (McAllister, 2003). She argues that nursing needs to move beyond problem-solving as nurses address such issues as health, health promotion and well-being, and focus on strengths. Also, in this way, we are differentiated from but complementary to medicine.

Within a solution-focus, there are five characteristics of people likely to adapt to stressful situations: hardiness, internal locus of control, resilience, hope and social support (McAllister, 2003). McAllister notes that in using a solution focus, one works alongside, that is, with and for a person. This involves significant reframing where both people in a relationship have expertise. People are competent, resilient and resourceful (McAllister, 2003). Like Barker, she suggests getting to know the person, not the label, and using the person's words. McAllister advocates reclaiming human-to-human relationships. McAllister et al. (2005) evaluated Solution-Focused Nursing (SFN) as a new philosophy of care that underpins their Bachelor of Nursing program. Echoes of Peplau in the different and complementary role of nursing from the biomedical psychiatric model, Travelbee in human-to-human relationships and

Barker (Tidal) in working with and using the person's own words are evident in McAllister's work.

While Peplau's psychodynamic model delves into the intricacies of the psyche and unconscious processes, Travelbee's human-to-human theory prioritizes the emotional and existential dimensions of the nurse-person relationship. Both models recognize the importance of the nurse-person connection, with different focal points. In contemporary nursing psychotherapy practice, nurses may draw from elements each to create a comprehensive and person-centred approach that addresses the dimensions of personhood and persons' needs, offering a more holistic and nuanced approach to mental health care.

6 Understanding and Examining Theoretical Works and Their Value

The importance of the integration of theoretical works in advancing the field of nursing psychotherapy cannot be overstated. Theoretical works serve as a knowledge repository, allowing nurses to access and build upon rich theoretical frameworks. When theories from various nursing theorists are considered, it provides a broader perspective on the multifaceted nature of nursing psychotherapy. The understanding and examination of theories help practitioners not only learn the historical context, and evolution of nurse psychotherapy but also allow the nurse an opportunity to discover the diverse range of approaches that have and will continue to contribute to the field (Alligood, 2022).

Integration of these theoretical works is equally vital as it promotes synergy and cross-fertilization of ideas. Through integration, nurses can identify common themes, principles, and core concepts that transcend individual theories. This process fosters the development of a broader theoretical framework, enhancing the coherence and effectiveness of nursing psychotherapy practice. It allows nurses to synthesize knowledge from various sources, creating a holistic and person-centred approach to mental health care that draws from the strengths of different theoretical perspectives (Alligood, 2022).

The compilation and integration of theoretical works can further facilitate the ongoing evolution of nurse psychotherapy by providing a solid foundation upon which new theories and approaches can be developed and refined and studied. When nursing scholars and practitioners have access to a well-organized body of theoretical knowledge, they can identify gaps and areas for further exploration encouraging research and innovation. Continuous improvement of nursing psychotherapy practice is necessary to ensure that it remains responsive to the changing needs of our persons-in-care/population and our ever-changing healthcare landscape (Alligood, 2022). The compilation and integration of theoretical works are essential for the growth and adaptability of nursing psychotherapy, ultimately leading to better (person) outcomes and the advancement of nursing as a profession.

7 Reflective Questions

1. If nursing theory is like one leg on a three-legged stool, the other two legs being practice and research, how do you see psychotherapy nursing practice as being influenced by nursing theory?
2. How has nursing research driven or contributed to the development of nursing psychotherapy?

8 Summary

- Nursing theorists such as Peplau, Travelbee, Barker, McAllister and Leininger have been integral to the evolution of nursing psychotherapy practice.
- Key foundational concepts, such as the psychodynamic model proposed by Peplau and the human-to-human theory by Travelbee contributed to the historical evolution of nursing psychotherapy practice.
- The Tidal Model® by Barker expands the work of Peplau and Travelbee.
- McAllister further developed Solution Focused Nursing which is particularly relevant for nursing psychotherapy practice.
- Leininger illuminated an important culture and diversity focus.
- It is of importance to integrate these theoretical works in advancing the field of nursing psychotherapy as historical perspectives continue to shape contemporary psychotherapy practices within nursing.

References

Alligood, M. Ed. (2022). *Nursing theorists and their work* (10th Ed.). Elsevier.

Barker, P., Jackson, S., & Stevenson, C. (1999). What are psychiatric nurses needed for? Developing a theory of essential practice. *Journal of Psychiatric and Mental Health Nursing, 6*(4), 273-282.

Barker, P., Stevenson, C., & Leamy, M. (2000). The philosophy of empowerment. *Mental Health Practice, 20*(9), 8-12.

Barker, P. & Whitehill, (1997). The craft of care: Towards collaborative caring in nursing. In S. Tilley (Ed.), *The mental health nurse. Views of practice and education* (pp. 15–27). Blackwell Science.

Barker, P. (2000). *The Tidal Model: Theory and practice.* University of Newcastle.

Brookes, N. (2006). The tidal model® of mental health recovery. In A. M. Tomey & M. R. Alligood (Eds.), *Nursing theorists and their work* (6th ed., pp. 696–725). Mosby.

Brookes, N., Murata, L., & Tansey, M. (2008). Tidal waves: Implementing a new model of mental health recovery and reclamation. *Canadian Nurse, 104*(8), 22-27.

Brookes, N. (2022). The tidal model® of mental health recovery. In M. R. Alligood (Ed.), *Nursing theorists and their work* (10th ed., pp. 503–525). Mosby.

McAllister, M. (2003). Doing practice differently: Solution-focused nursing. *Journal of Advanced Nursing, 41*(6), 528-535.

McAllister, M., Moyle, W., & Iselin, G. (2005). Solution focused nursing: An evaluation of current practice. *Nurse Education Today, 26*(5), 439–447. https://doi.org/10.1016/j.nedt.2005.12.004
McFarland, M. R. (2022). Madeleine M. Leininger: Theory of culture care diversity and universality. In M. R. Alligood (Ed.), *Nursing theorists and their work* (10th ed., pp. 334–353). Mosby.
Peplau, H. (1991). *Interpersonal relations in nursing: A conceptual frame of reference for psychodynamic nursing.* Springer.
Tomey, A. (2006). Human to human relationship model. In A. M. Tomey & M. R. Alligood (Eds). *Nursing theorists and their work* (6th ed.). Mosby.
Travelbee, J. (1971). *Interpersonal aspects of nursing* (2nd ed). F.A. Davis Company.
Vives, M., Linkes, C., & Soucy, M. (2023). Teaching psychotherapy to psychiatric/mental health nurse practitioner students in the virtual classroom. *Issues in Mental Health Nursing, 44*(6), 551–561. https://doi.org/10.1080/01612840.2023.2212769

Chapter 3
Peplau and Therapeutic Relationships

Cheryl Forchuk

Abstract Hildegard Peplau's theory of therapeutic relationships is foundational to nursing psychotherapy. Historically, Dr. Peplau has been considered the mother of modern psychiatric-mental health nursing. A key part of the theory is the phases of the developing relationship: Orientation, Working (subdivided into Identification and Exploitation), and Resolution. Forchuk and colleagues later expanded on the phases to also consider phases of the non-therapeutic relationship: Orientation, Grappling and Struggling, and Mutual withdrawal. Other key concepts of the theory include communication (verbal, non-verbal, and empathic linkages) and pattern integration (i.e. how the pattern of the nurse interfaces with the pattern of the client). Common examples of patterns include complementary, mutual, and antagonistic. Antagonistic patterns are used to promote change. Peplau's theory has been supported by research evidence and has influenced other nurse theorists.

Keywords Therapeutic relationships · Relationship phases · Communication · Pattern integration

Learning Objectives

After completing this chapter, the learner will be able to

1. Summarize the historical context and significance of Peplau's work.
2. Identify and describe the phases of the therapeutic relationship.
3. Identify and describe the phases of the non-therapeutic relationship.
4. Give examples of pattern interactions between nurse and client.

C. Forchuk (✉)
Nursing and Psychiatry, Lawson Research Institute, Western University, Parkwood Institute Research, St Joseph's Hospital, London, ON, Canada
e-mail: cforchuk@uwo.ca

S. Roles and K. Kalia (eds.), *The Nurses' Guide to Psychotherapy*,
https://doi.org/10.1007/978-981-97-4738-2_3

1 Introduction

History is often important to understanding a current situation. In understanding nurse psychotherapy, Hildegard Peplau is an important part of our history. This chapter will contextualize and describe Peplau's theory of interpersonal relationships, which is the essence of her work. Peplau's phases of therapeutic relationships have been widely adopted in nursing and therapeutic work generally. This chapter will discuss the origins of the approach, major concepts of the theory, and give examples to illustrate implementation. The chapter will also briefly highlight some of the research evidence related to this approach.

1.1 Who Was Hildegard Peplau—What Was Her Role in Nurse Psychotherapy?

Hildegard Peplau (1909–1999) has been described as the mother of modern psychiatric-mental health nursing (Forchuk 2021) and is similarly the mother of nurse psychotherapy (Field 1979). She was also foundational to my own development as a nurse. I had the privilege of meeting Dr. Peplau in 1984 when we brought her in as a guest speaker to what was then Hamilton Psychiatric Hospital. I was a clinical nurse specialist at the time and provided consultation and clinical supervision to nurses, while maintaining a caseload of patients with complex needs. Although the hospital was the first in Canada to require nursing practice to be based on nursing theory, the choice of theory was up to the nurse (theoretical pluralism). Dr. Peplau's work was the most common theory used by staff, so we were thrilled to host her for three days of education sessions and discussions on difficult therapeutic situations. After this visit, she asked me to write to her, and we maintained correspondence until her death in 1999. She encouraged me to pursue a doctorate in nursing, however, at the time there was no doctorate in nursing in Canada (she asked how we would get one without some nurses leaving the country for PhDs so we could establish our own programs). I explained I had two preschoolers, and she suggested that it would be easier to do a PhD once they were in school. My PhD at Wayne State tested her theory.

To understand the importance of her foundational work, it is important to understand the historical context of its development. When Dr. Peplau started her psychiatric nursing career, that specialty was in a very primitive state. She recounted that there were often only two registered nurses (RNs) and often thousands of patients. One RN was typically the director of nursing and the other the director of the school of nursing. There was similarly just one psychiatrist. The major nursing labour force was student nurses. The care was quite custodial and what Dr. Peplau called the "parent surrogate" role, which ensured people were fed, dressed, etc. … There were also few pharmacological options other than opioids to assist sleep. Dr. Peplau was an Army nurse during the Second World War. This was a period where psychiatric issues became quite a national concern in the United States (US) and elsewhere. Mental health issues influenced people's ability to serve during the war as well as impacted integration back into civilian life. Funding for psychiatric and mental health services therefore became more prominent. There were similar issues in Canada. For example, Nora Harris who was head of the graduate program at the University of Toronto in the 1980s spoke of the shift where new resources became available. She had trained at the former Hamilton Psychiatric Hospital, and with the increased funding post-World War II, there was now an RN for each ward, rather than two for the hospital. There were approximately 4000 patients. Nora, during an education session at Hamilton Psychiatric Hospital years later, said she remembered the day a second nurse was also available in each ward and wondered what to do with so much help.

There was an urgent need for advanced psychiatric-mental health practice. Also prominent after the war was the importance of nursing generally, and the need for higher education. The nursing scholar program in the US had nurses receiving PhDs in related fields so that a PhD in Nursing could be possible. Dr. Peplau was one of these pioneers. She studied interpersonal psychology, became certified in psychoanalysis in the 1950s, and then went on with an education focus for her doctorate. She wanted to develop an interpersonal approach to nursing education and practice, and to develop advanced practice nursing. Nursing needed to shift from doing to, to doing with. She studied the therapeutic relationships that nurses and patients developed which then became the cornerstone of her approach (Peplau 1952). She lobbied, with varied success in different states, for nurses' right to practice psychotherapy. Her second book used the phrase "counselling" rather than "psychotherapy" to sidestep some of the legislative battles (Peplau 1964).

Peplau also had important roles in nursing leadership generally. She, at different times, was both the president of the American Nurses Association and the executive director of that organization. She was also the vice-president for the International Council of Nurses which had her visit countries and promote psychiatric nursing practice around the world. For decades, she spent her summers visiting psychiatric hospitals and providing education for the nurses to shift the focus of their work to therapeutic relationships (Sills 1978). When she started the first program for advanced practice nursing, a master's program for psychiatric nurses in 1953 at Rutgers University, the first antipsychotics were just being developed. It would be another decade for antidepressants to emerge. Dr. Peplau emphasized that it was the relationship that was the treatment. As new treatments emerged, they allowed more therapeutic progress through the therapeutic relationship. For her to have an emphasis on therapeutic relationships, psychotherapy, and counselling as a nursing focus during this period of history is truly visionary. Peplau (1964) quotes, from a time when the interdisciplinary team was still only nurses and physicians, "if [nurses] are unable to contribute in a truly corrective manner to the care of mental patients, the traditional nurse-patient relationship will be usurped by those who can; and nurses will be shunted into the role of glorified custodian or superclerk" (p. 7).

2 Peplau's Theory of Interpersonal Relationships

Peplau first laid out her theory in her 1952 book, *Interpersonal Relations in Nursing*. In the introduction, she describes the guiding principles of her theory: "[t]he kind of nurse each person becomes makes a substantial difference in what clients will learn as they are nursed through their experience with illness" (p. xi), and "fostering personality development in the direction of maturity is a function of nursing and nursing education; it requires the use of principles and methods that permit and guide the process of grappling with everyday interpersonal problems or difficulties" (p. xi). This theory clearly identifies the importance of the development of the nurse as well as the development of the client. The nurse must use self-reflection with each client encounter to promote this growth and development. Peplau often said if people put more emphasis on the assessment of the client than self-assessment, they are not using her theory. This is in sharp contrast to other theories or models which focus, sometimes exclusively, on the client. The primary focus is not simply on the client or the nurse in this model, but on the processes that include both the client and nurse. This includes the nurse-client relationship, communication, pattern integration and roles (Forchuk 2021).

It was difficult that Dr. Peplau had not developed a picture to summarize her theory, so I attempted to develop one. Through correspondence with Dr. Peplau, and a few iterations, we agreed on Fig. 1.

The interpersonal processes are at the centre. There is equal attention to the nurse and client. All are encompassed by the context of the relationship. In looking at the layers for the nurse and client closest to the centre, you can see that the nurse brings the concepts and processes to the relationship, employs specific roles, and develops one's own self-understanding and competencies with each relationship. The client also develops competencies and self-understanding. Looking at the centre layer of both people, you can see both bring prior learning, other relationships, thinking, preconceptions and anxiety to the new relationship. The outer layer for the nurse is the development of further self-understanding which may also improve the nurse's own health. The main goal in this layer for the client is to improve their health, but with this generally also comes increased self-understanding. The environment/context of the relationship relates to parameters. Is the relationship part of a therapeutic team or a sole practitioner? Is this part of crisis management/emergency care, in-patient care, community care, clinic care? These different contexts have different implications for things such as the length of service, payment, and with whom information will be shared. The relationships between these concepts are described in more detail in Forchuk (1991).

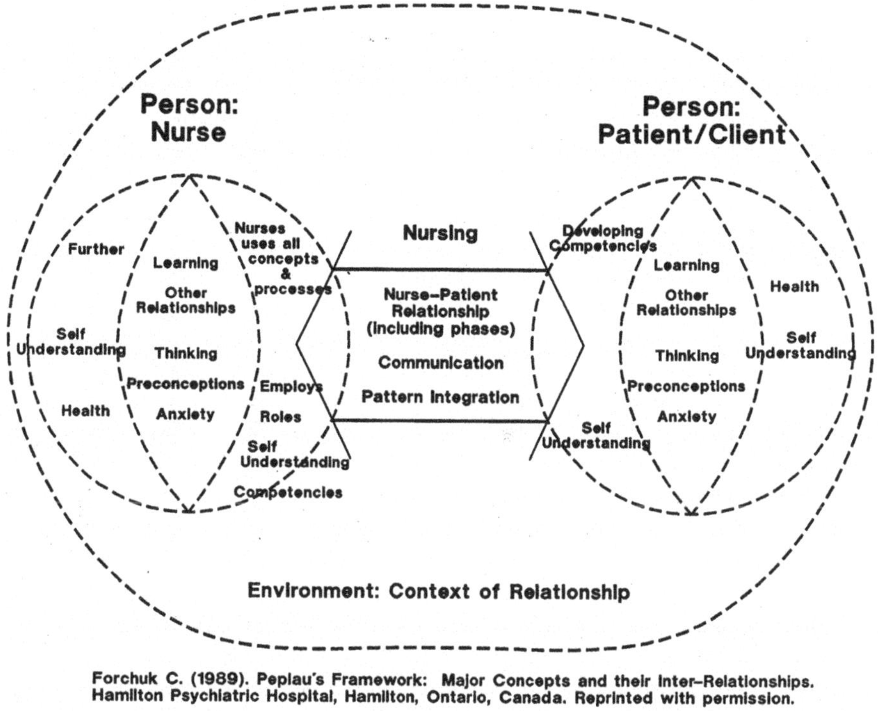

Fig. 1 Forchuk, C. (1989). Peplau's framework: major concepts and their inter-relationships. Hamilton Psychiatric Hospital, Hamilton, Ontario, Canada. Reprinted with permission

2.1 Interpersonal Concepts with Nurse-Client Relationship

2.1.1 Phases of Relationship

In her 1952 book, Dr. Peplau described the phases of the relationship as *orientation, identification, exploitation* and *resolution.* The identification and exploitation phases were later combined to form the subphases of the working phase. Peplau has described these phases as interlocked and overlapping.

The orientation phase is about first getting to know each other and establishing trust with each other. For the nurse this is about being clear about the parameters of the relationship: how often will you be meeting? How long? Where? Who would information be shared with, and under what circumstances? What is the purpose of the interaction? Who is the "client"? (e.g. individual, couple, family, group). The parameters are related to the role of the nurse. The nurse works on establishing a consistent process. The content of the meetings (i.e. what is to be discussed within those parameters) is then related to the role of the client. Consistency is very important for establishing trust. The job of the client, in order to establish trust, is to test those parameters. Common examples include testing the timing by identifying a major area of concern as the session is closing or arriving late, talking/asking about others rather than oneself, or starting with more trivial/safe issues to see how they are addressed before moving to more serious matters. As an example, when starting a community group within a long-term psychiatric unit, the initial area of concern that arose (with full consensus yet) was the importance of moving the public phone to the opposite wall within the same room. By responding seriously to this, and a couple of similar requests, it was possible to move on to the highly emotional topic of issues related to leaving the hospital and the losses and conflicts that would come with this change.

Peplau speaks of us all having "preconceptions". Preconceptions are ideas of who the other person is before we actually know them. These preconceptions are often rooted in the past. As a nurse, how well things worked out (or did not) with similar people can influence how they assess the current person. Similarly, past relationships, particularly with other nurses, can influence how the client perceives the current nurse. Getting past these preconceptions to know the person as a person is part of the work of the orientation phase for both parties.

The first subphase of the working phase is identification. The idea of identification builds on the trust established in the orientation phase. The identification subphase includes identifying the nurse as a helping person as well as the identification of the issues to be worked on in the context of the relationship. It is not uncommon during the orientation phase for a generic role term to be used rather than the nurse's name (the nurse, case manager, therapist) and to have this shift as the identification phase is entered. In my example given in the orientation phase of the community group meeting, oftentimes issues closer to the heart of matters arise at this point. People identify the actual work they want to do with the relationship. The nurse provides unconditional acceptance and will often ask questions to help the client focus on identifying the work to be done. The testing decreases and the client increases focal attention (since anxiety is reduced with trust). There becomes an increasing continuity between sessions.

Exploitation is the second subphase of the working phase. Exploitation today is often a negative word for taking advantage of others in the context of a power dynamic, however, earlier connotations simply meant to make full use of. During this subphase, it is the client that is able to make full use of the services of the nurse, allowing the client to go beyond identifying problems to identifying and testing solutions. The results of this are discussed together with the nurse. Much of this testing of solutions happens between sessions. A common example is that the client will try out new behaviours with a particular person, such as listening more. The client takes more of a lead role during the nurse-client interactions, while the nurse continues to provide support with questions and clarifications. At times, additional community support will be identified. The reason that the working phase contains two subphases is that as issues are resolved the client often identifies further underlying issues. It is like peeling back the layers of an onion. It is not "going backward" to go "back" to identification. It is going deeper.

It is important to work on the client's goals. This may seem obvious in the abstract but less so in the implementation. An example was when working with a homebound client in a group home. She had not been out of bed for 2 years and had meals and a bedpan brought to her, although there was no physical disability. Her medication had not been reviewed in decades and she was on high levels of central nervous system depressants. As a nurse, there were many things I was concerned about. In discussing goals, she said she wanted her watch fixed as her primary goal. There was a jewelry store down the street, so a series of plans were made to get there. In implementing this plan over the next few weeks, she had several things improve. She identified she was dizzy which was why she couldn't go there (and why she was afraid to get out of bed), so we had her medications reviewed by a psychiatrist. She took increasingly longer walks and eventually the bus to be able to get to the jewelry store. These activities got her out of the room and out of the boarding home for practice walks, including joining a small group that went out regularly to a coffee shop. By the time she got the watch fixed, she had identified further goals including reconnecting with family. This all circled around discussions related to her fear of risk-taking. She later explained this underlying fear was why she wanted a concrete "easy" goal to work towards.

The final stage of the therapeutic relationship is the resolution phase. This is the phase where the client frees themselves of the need of the nurse. During this phase, the client reflects and integrates what has been learned. The nurse includes a discussion on preventive measures, community resources and self-care. This is the phase from when the last issue has been worked through until the therapeutic relationship is ended. This can be a difficult period. During this phase, discussions on the topic of death or other loss frequently arise. Talking about these issues in the context of the therapeutic relationship is important to resolve this relationship.

As mentioned earlier, these phases are interacting and overlapping. The example of a hologram vs. a photograph can be used to help describe it. If you cut a photograph in half, the two halves look different—but fit together. If you cut a holographic image in half, both are identical, but smaller than the original. A nurse might work with someone for a year and spend a month in orientation, ten in the *working phase* and a month in resolution. However, an observer for an individual session would see reflections of all phases. A nurse might open with "this is your time. What would you like to talk about today?" reflecting the *orientation* phase. The client identifies topics and potential related issues/solutions are discussed. At the end of the session, there is a summary reflecting the resolution. For an even smaller slice, a nurse may pass an in-patient they are working within the hallway. They would approach, acknowledge each other, and separate.

Another frequently asked question is—how long does it take to establish a therapeutic relationship? It varies a lot. When working with people with schizophrenia who had not responded to medication, we could take months in the orientation phase. I can remember examples where it took 6 meetings for the person to respond verbally to me at all. A study (Forchuk 1992) found the length of time in *orientation* was very related to the length of hospitalization. It makes sense that if it takes longer to identify underlying issues it is harder to resolve them. It can be circular, though, since longer and more frequent hospitalizations can also erode trust in "helping" professionals. On the shorter end of things, in public health, colleagues doing first baby visits often joked that they got through the first couple phases in under a minute (hello I'm...

Thank goodness you're here! My nipples are killing me/baby won't stop crying etc.). The amount of time spent per session, however, also generally relates to the time it takes to get to the working phase (Forchuk 1995a). For example, one hour per week is better than two 30-min sessions, which is better than three 20-min sessions even though all take an hour. It is related to the depth you can reach in a short interaction. A common practice of short, frequent interactions in many in-patient units does not support the depth needed for therapeutic relationships. Where attention span is an issue, longer meetings may be more difficult. However, even when the nurse has had to start with shorter meetings, the goal is to increase to at least 30 min so they can discuss issues in depth.

The phases of relationships apply not only to formal psychotherapy but all nurse-patient relationships. Sometimes nurses have commented that they do not have the necessary time to get to a therapeutic relationship. For example, they may be working on a crisis team and are meeting for the first and possibly final time. Crises must be treated as crises. However, issues raised will more likely be at a more surface and immediate level.

3 Non-therapeutic Relationships

Peplau's theory focuses on therapeutic relationships. Unfortunately, not all nurse-client relationships are therapeutic. Concurrent with the earlier quantitative testing of Peplau's Theory (Forchuk 1994a), I also did a qualitative test (Forchuk et al. 1998). I did a longitudinal qualitative study with 10 nurse-patient dyads. It was in some ways a replication of Dr. Peplau's original work developing her theory. In my doctoral program, I was fortunate to have Madeline Leininger (1985a, b, 1987) teach me qualitative methods. Dr. Leininger is also a nurse theorist (transcultural nursing) and was also one of the early nurse scholars. Her PhD was in anthropology. Dr. Leininger was a consultant on this study to review the transcripts as a person who does not employ Dr. Peplau's theory. The research team interviewed both the nurse and client separately a minimum of monthly over a year and also recorded videotapes of their interactions. Seven of the dyads looked like they had read Peplau thoroughly. These clients all used phrases such as going to a new phase, level, or step when they went to the *working* phase.

Unfortunately, the other three dyads did not get into a therapeutic relationship. Interestingly, in the quantitative study testing Dr. Peplau's theory, it appears as though a third had been "stuck" in orientation. This qualitative study on inpatient units sheds more light. They were not remaining in the orientation phase, they moved to a new phase called *grappling and struggling*. This was a very frustrating phase for both the nurses and clients. When discussed with nurses they would say, "maybe I should try longer sessions, shorter sessions, focus on the here and now, focus on the past", etc. The interesting thing is they did not maintain strategies but would constantly change them. Similarly, when discussing with clients they would say, "maybe I need to talk more about me, more about my family, more about the past," etc., but also did not sustain efforts. Eventually, they colluded to avoid each other in a phase called *mutual withdrawal*. The nurse would schedule the meeting near the end of shift and be "surprised" to run out of time for anything but a quick meeting. The client would "forget" and be off the unit, in the shower or with another meeting. When the nurses were asked what happened when they did meet, they all suggested they might as well keep it short since nothing changes anyway. When clients were spoken with they said if they did meet, they tried to keep it superficial since it does no good anyway. An example of how to keep it superficial was to ask about their medications and side effects ("Nurses love to health teach"). Fortunately, with therapeutic transfers, therapeutic relationships could be formed. This was not about "difficult patients" or "incompetent nurses," this was about a combination that didn't work. Nurses were generally reluctant to transfer to another nurse; however, since they assumed the same problems would develop with another nurse, "It is only fair that we all get our share of difficult patients." I thought I should subtitle this study "we would rather fight than switch". In Forchuk (1995b), it was demonstrated that one difficult or good relationship did not predict the same outcome with the next combination for nurse or client.

4 Communication and Pattern Integration

Dr. Peplau describes three types of communication: verbal, non-verbal and empathic linkages. Verbal and non-verbal communication are commonly understood as essentially what you say and how you say it. The non-verbal is not only the tone and speed of words but also the body gestures. Dr. Peplau puts great emphasis on the importance of language as a tool in nursing. We cannot directly understand thoughts or feelings except through language. This tool is important not only for assessment but by making thoughts more explicit allowing change to occur. Dr. Peplau refers to this as the corrective use of language. For example, when working with people with addiction, there can be noted a preference for using the second person. "You know how when you get home and don't know how you got there so you have to check the car for bumps and scrapes …" to which you can respond, "are you talking about me doing this or you?" and would encourage the client to use first person. Similarly, someone experiencing paranoia may use third-person language such as, "they always give me a hard time". A clarifying question would be "who are they?" Other examples Dr. Peplau used, such as overgeneralization (this always happens), are very similar to the later work of Aaron Beck (1979) on cognitive therapy. The importance of understanding the power of words remains today. For example, acknowledging a person by using preferred pronouns is also consistent with this understanding (Braybrook et al. 2023).

Empathic linkages are the communication of feelings from one person to another. For example, one could be talking with someone who is highly anxious or depressed and becomes aware of a similar feeling within oneself. Empathic linkages are important to self-assess and provide clues to how the other person is feeling. They are tricky though, since sometimes what another says can also trigger past memories or feelings of one's own rather than the client's. It is important to use self-assessment and self-awareness as well as validation with the client about the feeling. For example, "in discussing this with you, I get a sense of sadness. Is that what you are saying to me?" Another suggestion Dr. Peplau often makes is to ask the client to label the feelings they are experiencing.

Pattern integrations are about how the pattern of each individual fits together as a dyad. Dr. Peplau describes three types of pattern integrations. The first is a mutual pattern which means the nurse and client do the same thing. Examples include mutual respect, mutual avoidance, mutual anger, or mutual courtesy. This pattern means the behaviour of each person is reinforced by the other. The second pattern is complementary. These are patterns that fit together like a hand and glove. A common example could be someone who always wants to help do for others, with someone who prefers others do for them. Another example would be anger and withdrawal. This pattern also tends to be reinforced for both people. The third pattern is antagonistic. These are two behaviours/reactions that don't reinforce each other, but rather move things in a different direction. An example that Dr. Peplau would often use is an angry patient with an inquisitive nurse. Generally, you would use mutual and complementary patterns where you want to reinforce the pattern and be antagonistic to change.

5 Relationship to Other Theories and Approaches

Dr. Peplau studied interpersonal psychology, so it is not surprising to find overlaps with that field. In particular, she found the work of Vygotsky (1930, 1978) useful. Vygotsky was a social psychologist who believed internal processes are first developed externally through social processes before being internalized. Cognitions are first formed through social interactions. Dr. Peplau saw the therapeutic relationship as an external social process that could provide the scaffolding so clients could make internal changes. Like a scaffold, the relationship provides a safe structure on the outside for change on the inside.

Dr. Peplau worked with Harry Stacks Sullivan at the Chestnut Lodge, a private psychiatric facility. Also, at this facility were theorists Erich Fromm, and Frieda Fromm-Reichmann. Sullivan (1953) is best known for his work on interpersonal psychiatry. Some of the concepts, such as those related to self-concept and anxiety are similar in both works since they are derived from similar sources. Dr. Peplau told me it took her 3 years to publish her 1952 book, the main reason being that she did not have a physician co-author, as was common for nursing texts of that period. She could have asked Sullivan or others to co-author given their collaborative relationships. However, since this was to be a theory for nursing she held out until a publisher was willing to publish without a co-author.

Dr. Peplau was very strong in mentoring other nurses, particularly in relation to theory development and testing. While corresponding with me, she would regularly connect me with other psychiatric nurses with similar interests. For example, Bill

Reynolds' (2000) work on empathy extends some of Peplau's work on empathic linkages. Barker and Buchanan-Barker's (2005) work on the Tidal Model is also grounded in Peplau's work on therapeutic relationships with an emphasis on the client reclaiming their story and respect for the client's wishes. The transitional discharge model (Forchuk et al. 2005, 2012, 2019) extends the therapeutic relationship to also include peer support as well as professional support to provide a safety net of relationships, particularly over the discharge process. Peplau's work has also been extended to group therapy (Lego 1998), family therapy (Forchuk and Park Dorsey 1995), peer support (Coatsworth-Puspoky et al. 2006), and case management (Forchuk et al. 1989).

6 Does Peplau's Theory Actually Work?

In my doctoral work, I successfully tested the concepts within the theory to predict the time to establish a therapeutic relationship as well as the strength of the therapeutic alliance (Forchuk 1994a). The preconceptions the nurse and client had of each other at the beginning were most predictive of the relationship even 6 months later (Forchuk 1994b). Similarly, qualitative work was consistent with the theory but added phases of the non-therapeutic relationship (Forchuk et al. 1998, 2000). The work on the transitional discharge model/transitional care model has demonstrated positive outcomes, such as earlier discharge and reduced readmissions, that saved millions of dollars in multi-site studies (Forchuk et al. 2005, 2012, 2019).

7 Conclusion

Peplau's work has been an important foundation for nurse psychotherapy specifically as well as psychiatric and mental health nursing generally. Her work has stood the test of time and concepts such as the therapeutic relationship are indeed foundational to care.

8 Reflective Questions

1. Consider your last interaction with a client. How did Peplau's work influence your work and interaction?
2. Think of an example where also assessing your own reaction changed the interpretation of the client's situation. What are common situations where your own history could interfere with client assessment?
3. What examples can you think of where preconceptions of your own and your clients interfered with the developing relationship?

9 Summary

- Dr. Peplau has been considered the mother of modern psychiatric-mental health nursing.
- Hildegard Peplau's theory of therapeutic relationships is foundational to nursing psychotherapy.
- The phases of the therapeutic relationship include: Orientation, Working (subdivided into Identification and Exploitation) and Resolution.
- The phases of the non-therapeutic relationship include: Orientation, Grappling and Struggling and Mutual withdrawal.
- Pattern interactions between nurse and client include how the nurse interfaces with the pattern of the client. Common examples of patterns include complementary, mutual, and antagonistic. Antagonistic patterns are used to promote change.
- Concepts such as the therapeutic relationship are foundational to all forms of nursing including psychotherapy.

References

Barker, P., & Buchanan-Barker, P. (2005). *The tidal model: a guide for mental health professionals* (1st ed.). Brunner-Routledge.

Beck, A. T. (1979). *Cognitive therapy and the emotional disorders*. New American Library.

Braybrook, D., Bristowe, K., Timmins, L., Roach. A., Day, E., Clift, P., Rose, R., Marshall, S., Johnson, K, Sleeman, K. & Harding, R. (2023). Communication about sexual orientation and gender between clinicians, LGBT+ people facing serious illness and their significant others: a qualitative interview study of experiences, preferences and recommendations. *BMJ Quality & Safety, 32*(2), 109–120. https://doi.org/10.1136/bmjqs-2022-014792

Coatsworth-Puspoky, R., Forchuk, C., & Ward-Griffin, C. (2006). Peer support relationships: An unexplored interpersonal process in mental health. *Journal of Psychiatric and Mental Health Nursing 13*(5), 490–497. https://doi.org/10.1111/j.1365-2850.2006.00970.x.

Field, W. E., Jr. (1979) *The Psychotherapy of Hildegard E. Peplau*. PSF Productions.

Forchuk, C. (1991). Peplau's theory: Concepts and their relations. *Nursing Science Quarterly, 4*(2), 54–60. https://doi.org/10.1177/089431849100400205

Forchuk, C. (1992). The orientation phase of the nurse-client relationship: How long does it take? *Perspectives in Psychiatric Care, 28*(4), 7–10. https://doi.org/10.1111/j.1744-6163.1992.tb00384.x

Forchuk, C. (1994a). The orientation phase of the nurse-client relationship: Testing Peplau's theory. *Journal of Advanced Nursing Practice, 20*(3), 532–537. https://doi.org/10.1111/j.1365-2648.1994.tb02392.x

Forchuk, C. (1994b). Preconceptions in the nurse-client relationship. *Journal of Psychiatric and Mental Health Nursing, 1*(3), 145–149. https://doi.org/10.1111/j.1365-2850.1994.tb00037.x

Forchuk, C. (1995a). Development of nurse-client relationships: What helps? *Journal of American Psychiatric Nurses Association, 1*(5), 146–153. https://doi.org/10.1177/107839039500100503

Forchuk, C. (1995b). Uniqueness within the nurse-client relationship. *Archives of Psychiatric Nursing, 9*(1), 34–39. https://doi.org/10.1016/s0883-9417(95)80015-8

Forchuk, C. (Ed.). (2021). *From therapeutic relationships to transitional care: A theoretical and practical roadmap* (1st ed.). Routledge. https://doi.org/10.4324/9781003000853

Forchuk, C., Beaton, S., Crawford, L., Ide, L., Voorberg, N., & Bethune, J. (1989). Incorporating Peplau's theory and case management. *Journal of Psychosocial Nursing, 27*(2), 35-38. https://doi.org/10.3928/0279-3695-19890201-11

Forchuk, C., & Park Dorsay, J. (1995). Hildegard Peplau meets family systems nursing: Innovation in theory-based practice. *Journal of Advanced Nursing Practice, 21*(1), 110–115. https://doi.org/10.1046/j.1365-2648.1995.21010110.x

Forchuk, C., Martin, M. L., Chan, L., & Jensen, E. (2005). Therapeutic relationships: From Hospital to Community. *Journal of Psychiatric and Mental Health Nursing, 12*(5), 556–564. https://doi.org/10.1111/j.1365-2850.2005.00873.x

Forchuk, C., Martin, M., Sherman, D., Corring, D., Srivastava, R., O'Regan, T., Gyamfi, S., Harerimana, B. (2019). Healthcare professionals' perception of the implementation of the transitional discharge model for the community integration of psychiatric clients. *International Journal of Mental Health Nursing 29*(3), 495–507. https://doi.org/10.3138/jmvfh-2019-0042

Forchuk, C., Martin, M. L., Ouseley, S., Sealy, P., Jensen, E., Beal, G., Reynolds, W., & Sharkey, S. (2012). Integrating the transitional relationship model into clinical practice. *Archives of Psychiatric Nursing. 26*(5), 374–381. https://doi.org/10.1016/j.apnu.2011.12.002

Forchuk, C., Westwell, J., Martin, M. L., BamberAzzapardi, W., Kosterewa, Tolman, D., & Hux, M. (1998). Factors influencing movement of chronic psychiatric patients from the orientation to the working phase of the nurse client relationship on an inpatient unit. *Perspectives in Psychiatric Care, 34*(1), 3644. https://doi.org/10.1111/j.1744-6163.1998.tb00998.x

Forchuk, C., Westwell, J., Martin, M. L., Bamber-Azzapardi, W., Kosterewa-Tolman, D., & Hux, M. (2000). The developing nurse-client relationship: Nurses' perspectives. *Journal of the American Psychiatric Nurses Association, 6*(1), 3–10. https://doi.org/10.1177/107839030000600102

Lego, S. (1998). The application of Peplau's theory to group psychotherapy. *Journal of Psychiatric and Mental Health Nursing, 5*(3), 193–196. https://doi.org/10.1046/j.1365-2850.1998.00129.x

Leininger, M. M. (1985a). Ethnography and ethnonursing: Models and modes of qualitative data analysis. In M. M. Leininger (Ed.), *Qualitative research methods in nursing.* (pp. 33–72). Grune & Stratton, Inc.

Leininger, M. M. (1985b). Transcultural care diversity and universality: A theory of nursing. *Nursing and Health Care, 6*(4), 209–212.

Leininger, M. M. (1987). Importance and use of ethnomethods: Ethnography and ethnonursing methods. In. M. Cahoon (Ed.), *Recent Advances in Nursing.* (pp. 12–15). Churchill Livingstone of Edinburgh.

Peplau, H. (1952). *Interpersonal relations in nursing: A conceptual frame of reference for psychodynamic nursing.* Putnam.

Peplau, H. (1964). *Basic principles of patient counseling.* Smith, Kline and French Laboratories.

Reynolds, W. (2000). *The measurement and development of empathy in nursing.* Routledge. https://doi.org/10.4324/9781315192499

Sills, G. M. (1978). Hildegard E. Peplau: Leader, practitioner, academician, scholar, and theorist. *Perspectives in Psychiatric Care, 16*(3), 122–128. https://doi.org/10.1111/j.1744-6163.1978.tb00928.x

Sullivan, H. S. (1953). *The interpersonal theory of psychiatry.* W. W. Norton & Co.

Vygotsky, L. S. (1930). *Mind and society.* Harvard University Press. http://www.cles.mlc.edu.tw/~cerntcu/099-curriculum/Edu_Psy/EP_03_New.pdf

Vygotsky, L. S. (1978). *Mind in society: Development of higher psychological processes* (M. Cole, V. Jolm-Steiner, S. Scribner, & E. Souberman, Eds.). Harvard University Press. https://doi.org/10.2307/j.ctvjf9vz4

Chapter 4
Foundational Concepts

Sheena Howard and Ingrid Rijo

Abstract The provision of psychotherapy as a successful intervention relies on quality therapeutic nurse-client relationships. This chapter outlines the foundational concepts of the nurse psychotherapist's role in creating rapport and building trust and highlights the importance of self-awareness, boundaries, and self-disclosure. This chapter will cover advanced therapeutic communication techniques needed for an effective therapeutic nurse-client alliance to help attain psychotherapy treatment goals. Advanced therapeutic communication techniques discussed will include verbal and non-verbal therapeutic communication techniques, communication blocks, defense mechanisms, empathy, and listening. Consideration will be given in this chapter to the effect on rapport, trust, and communication by the provision of psychotherapy virtually.

Keywords Communication techniques · Trust · Empathy · Nurse psychotherapy · Rapport

Learning Objectives

After completing this chapter, the learner will:

1. Understand the importance and role of the nurse psychotherapist in building therapeutic relationships with clients.
2. Explain the concepts of rapport, trust, boundaries, and self-disclosure in the context of psychotherapy.
3. Demonstrate advanced therapeutic communication techniques including verbal and non-verbal cues, handling communication blocks, recognizing defense mechanisms, and implementing empathy, and active listening.

S. Howard (✉)
Cavan, ON, Canada
e-mail: sheena@acceptanceclinic.ca

I. Rijo
Alliston, ON, Canada

S. Roles and K. Kalia (eds.), *The Nurses' Guide to Psychotherapy*,
https://doi.org/10.1007/978-981-97-4738-2_4

1 Introduction

The nurse psychotherapist plays a critical role in the delivery of psychotherapy, functioning as both a caregiver and a counsellor. This role requires deep insight, emotional intelligence, advanced communication skills, and a strong understanding of ethical considerations. This chapter delves into the nuances of the therapeutic nurse-client relationship, highlighting the importance of rapport, trust, boundaries, and self-disclosure in effective psychotherapy.

2 The Importance of Empathy and Communication Skills

Nursing is a profession deeply rooted in empathy, communication, and interpersonal connection. These qualities are essential for providing holistic care to clients. When nurses extend their role to include psychotherapy, they leverage these inherent skills to facilitate healing and growth in clients dealing with mental health challenges. Understanding the foundational concepts of psychotherapy and therapeutic communication is crucial for nurse psychotherapists to ensure success in this expanded role. Empathy, defined as the ability to understand and share the emotions of another person, is a core characteristic of nursing practice. Moudatsou, Stavropoulou, Philalithis, and Koukouli (2020) demonstrated that empathetic nursing care contributes to increased client satisfaction and improved treatment outcomes. Empathy enables nurses to connect with their clients on an emotional level, providing support and understanding, which is particularly valuable when addressing mental health challenges in psychotherapeutic contexts.

Effective communication is a fundamental skill in nursing that becomes even more crucial in nurse psychotherapy. Kourkouta and Papathanasiou (2014) emphasize that effective communication is vital in building trust, promoting understanding, and facilitating therapeutic relationships. Through clear and compassionate communication, nurse psychotherapists establish a safe and non-judgmental environment, allowing clients to openly express their thoughts, feelings, and concerns. This process fosters therapeutic engagement, enables accurate assessment, and enhances the delivery of person-centered care. Expanding the role of nurses to include psychotherapy requires a solid understanding of the foundational concepts of psychotherapy and therapeutic communication. Stuart (2013) supports the integration of psychotherapeutic approaches within nursing practice, emphasizing the importance of theoretical knowledge and practical skills. Understanding theories, therapeutic modalities, and evidence-based practices equips nurse psychotherapists to tailor interventions to individual client needs, promoting effective treatment outcomes and facilitating client growth and healing.

Therapeutic communication is a key aspect of nurse psychotherapy, enabling effective collaboration with clients. Arnold and Boggs (2022) highlight the value of therapeutic communication techniques, including active listening, reflection, and empathy. These techniques allow nurse psychotherapists to create a therapeutic alliance, encouraging clients to explore their emotions, thoughts, and experiences. By facilitating open dialogue and offering genuine support, nurse psychotherapists can empower clients to develop insight, resilience, and self-efficacy.

Nursing is inherently a profession steeped in empathy, communication, and interpersonal connection. When nurses expand their role to include psychotherapy, these skills become essential in facilitating healing and growth in clients facing mental health challenges. Understanding the foundational concepts of psychotherapy and therapeutic communication is crucial for nurse psychotherapists to ensure success in this expanded role.

3 Foundations of the Therapeutic Nurse-Client Relationship

The therapeutic nurse-client relationship, a keystone in nursing practice, and notably in the domain of psychotherapy, provides an essential foundation for efficacious mental health care. Rooted deeply in professional intimacy, this relationship is a structured and deliberate interaction founded on trust, respect, empathy, and open communication.

Hildegard Peplau's pioneering theory on the therapeutic nurse-client relationship, as outlined in her (1952) work *Interpersonal Relations in Nursing*, emphasizes the profound significance of interpersonal dynamics in nursing. Her theory unfolds through four crucial phases. In the orientation phase, clients initially seek help, with the nurse guiding them to comprehend their issues and the ensuing treatment, laying the groundwork for trust. The identification phase sees clients recognizing helpers, especially the nurse, leading to mutual understanding and a sense of client validation. During the exploitation phase, clients actively engage with and maximize available services, while the nurse nurtures their knowledge, skills, and independence. The relationship culminates in the resolution phase, where clients, having their needs met, gradually transition from reliance on the nurse to autonomous healthcare decision-making. Ideally, throughout the nurse-client relationship, both engage collaboratively, fostering a climate of mutual respect and open communication. This interaction also reflects Bordin's (1979) concept of the working alliance that underscores the emotional bond and shared agreement on therapeutic goals and tasks.

Through the therapeutic nurse-client relationship, nurse psychotherapists gain a profound understanding of clients' mental and emotional landscapes. This rich insight is fundamental in cultivating a healing environment, thereby amplifying the efficacy of psychotherapeutic interventions (Cormack, 2004). Empathetic understanding, nurtured within this alliance, empowers nurse psychotherapists to navigate clients on their recovery path, significantly influencing mental health outcomes (Shattell et al., 2007). The depth of the therapeutic nurse-client relationship can introduce complexity, possibly blurring the boundaries between professional responsibilities and personal involvement (Austin et al., 2006). Herein lies the challenge and necessity to maintain a delicate equilibrium between empathetic care and professional boundaries. The College of Nurses of Ontario (2019) emphasizes the importance of this balance, considering it integral to preserving the integrity of the therapeutic relationship and averting potential harm or exploitation.

Canada's diverse and multicultural landscape necessitates that the therapeutic nurse-client relationship embraces cultural competence. The approach of acknowledging, respecting, and valuing each client's unique cultural heritage can augment client satisfaction and overall health outcomes (Campinha-Bacote, 2002). Consequently, nurse psychotherapists must prioritize culturally sensitive care within the therapeutic alliance, ensuring that their interactions are responsive and respectful of cultural differences.

The therapeutic nurse-client relationship embodies a symbiotic process, in which shared decision-making is a significant contributor. Active collaboration between the nurse and the client in devising care plans and treatment decisions enhances the therapeutic relationship (Charles et al., 1997). When clients are actively involved in their care, it leads to improved health outcomes and higher client satisfaction.

Confidentiality and privacy are of paramount importance in the therapeutic nurse-client relationship. Clients entrust nurse psychotherapists with highly personal and sensitive information, necessitating the protection of this data to maintain trust (Canadian Nurses Association, 2017). Breaches in confidentiality can destabilize the therapeutic relationship and invoke legal and ethical implications, thereby significantly undermining the therapeutic process.

With the rise of digital health technologies, virtual psychotherapy is becoming increasingly prevalent (see Chap. 8). While virtual offerings improve access and convenience, the transition from in-person to virtual interactions could present unique challenges to the therapeutic nurse-client relationship (Richardson et al., 2009). This medium could potentially affect the depth of emotional connection, as some subtle cues of empathy, such as physical presence or non-verbal communication, may be less perceivable (Agha et al., 2009).

The transition to virtual psychotherapy has raised substantial concerns about client safety, particularly in relation to maintaining privacy in their own homes. Especially in instances of domestic violence, the home environment may not always be conducive to open communication, as victims may be under surveillance or at risk of retaliation from their abusers (Mishna et al., 2017). Furthermore, the challenge of ensuring a confidential environment falls to clients who might have to use their cars as a makeshift therapy space to find privacy (Reay et al., 2020). Yet, the nurse may not know exactly where the client is located and is advised to ask for confirmation of location and address at the beginning of a virtual psychotherapy session in the case of a potential threat to themselves, from others, or if they pose a risk to someone else.

Nurse psychotherapists should adapt their therapeutic approach to maintaining the integrity of the therapeutic relationship in the virtual setting, including the use of enhanced verbal communication and active listening skills (Simpson et al., 2020).

It is also essential to address technical issues and privacy concerns promptly to prevent disruptions in therapeutic interactions and maintain trust in the therapeutic relationship (Békés & Aafjes-van Doorn, 2020). Despite these challenges, research suggests that with adequate adjustments, therapeutic engagement can be maintained in virtual psychotherapy, contributing to effective treatment outcomes (Berrouiguet et al., 2016).

The Registered Nurses' Association of Ontario (RNAO) (2020) echoes the significance of the therapeutic nurse-client relationship by presenting comprehensive best practice guidelines. These guidelines emphasize client-centered care, advocating for individualized care plans that respect clients' unique needs and values. They highlight the importance of therapeutic communication, underscoring the need for nurses to skillfully use verbal and non-verbal communication to establish and maintain the therapeutic relationship. Furthermore, they address the necessity of ensuring privacy and confidentiality, acknowledging the impact of these elements on fostering trust within the therapeutic nurse-client relationship.

The therapeutic nurse-client relationship, a multifaceted and dynamic interaction, is critical to the role of nurse psychotherapists. Upholding professional boundaries, endorsing culturally sensitive practices, championing shared decision-making, and ensuring confidentiality are fundamental elements of this relationship. By adhering to these principles nurse psychotherapists can offer high-quality, client-centered care, thereby contributing significantly to improved client outcomes. The continuous evolution and expansion of these practices reflect the ongoing commitment of nursing professionals to enhance therapeutic engagement and mental health care delivery. By embracing the inherent complexity of the therapeutic nurse-client relationship, nurse psychotherapists can create a safe and supportive environment for their clients. Through active listening, empathetic understanding, and effective communication, nurse psychotherapists foster trust and collaboration with their clients. Nurses adapt their approach to respect cultural differences, ensuring that care is tailored to meet the unique needs and values of each individual.

The therapeutic nurse-client relationship is an ever-evolving process that requires ongoing self-reflection, continuous learning, and ethical practice. Nurse psychotherapists must take care in maintaining professional boundaries and safeguarding confidentiality to uphold the trust placed in them by their clients. As technology advances, nurse psychotherapists should embrace virtual platforms while being mindful of the potential challenges and adapt their therapeutic strategies accordingly. The therapeutic nurse-client relationship is at the core of effective mental health care. It serves as a foundation for compassionate, client-centered care, and enables nurse psychotherapists to support their clients on their journey toward improved mental well-being. By fostering a strong therapeutic alliance, nurse psychotherapists can make a meaningful difference in the lives of their clients, promoting healing, growth, and positive mental health outcomes.

4 Advanced Therapeutic Communication Techniques

Communication, a dynamic interpersonal process, may be considered therapeutically effective when the meaning, information, message, emotions, and beliefs are fully expressed and understood by both the receiver and sender in this interactive exchange (Burke, 2023). Communication may be verbal or oral, written, and nonverbal including gestures, facial expressions, body language, tone of voice, and pace of the conversation. Nurses learn to assess the client's unique communication needs related to age, level of development, language, culture, individual values, beliefs, and perceptions, to accommodate and remove any barriers to communication.

Nurses meet the therapeutic communication standard when they provide a supportive environment that empowers the client to speak freely and openly without judgment, assumptions, or jumping to advice-giving, as these can serve as detrimental communication blocks that may interfere with achieving successful therapeutic outcomes (CNO, 2006). The intent of communication should be to seek an understanding of the client's unique lived experience through careful empathy and mindful inquiry (Settani et al., 2022). Empathy connects with what the client is saying by using their own words to paraphrase what they are thinking and feeling (Burns, 2006). Inquiry demonstrates a genuine curiosity in the client's truth and invites the client to expand further on what they are sharing by asking gentle, probing questions to deepen understanding of how the client is thinking and feeling.

Active listening is a vital psychotherapy core skill. It requires mastery in the ability to hear what the client is sharing, both verbally and non-verbally, directly and indirectly (Goldberg & Plakun, 2013). As the name suggests, active listening is not a passive attempt to listen to the client's words in silence. It is an interactive exchange where the nurse not only actively pays attention to what the client is verbalizing but also repeats what they heard and asks open-ended clarifying questions to process and purposefully comprehend the meaning behind the client's words and nonverbal communication (Burke, 2023). Nurse psychotherapists attune to the unique intellectual, emotional, physical, and behavioural expressions of the client. Nurses may pay close attention to content, thought processes, and patterns that may drive emotions or behaviours, as well as observe for cues around tonality, expression, and response to therapy, such as resistance and avoidance. The nurse identifies and helps remove potential communication and therapy barriers such as language, literacy, developmental, cognitive, or individual vulnerabilities such as past traumatic events, triggers, or any factor that can cause the client additional distress. Addressing potential barriers is vital to strengthen the therapeutic alliance, and ultimately, help the client achieve their therapeutic goals. Using clear, simple language free of medical jargon, slang, or complicated terminology, and providing a calm, supportive environment with proper lighting and minimized noise or other distractions are a few examples of how a nurse helps to nurture therapeutic communication. The nurse demonstrates respect and creates a climate of acceptance and understanding by addressing the client by their preferred name, title, and pronouns, modifying communication to meet client needs, exploring the client's values, beliefs, preferences, wishes, needs, and opinions, as well as providing adequate information to promote client's own informed therapeutic care choice. Communication can be greatly impaired when the client is adversely affected by stress and other emotional states such as anxiety, fear, distress, and confusion. For this reason, the nurse will attempt to alleviate these symptoms to be able to overcome this barrier to effective communication (Burke, 2023).

Self-reflection on the nurse's own attitude, behaviour, beliefs, thoughts, and feelings during each client interaction is also an important way to identify and address any potential contributions to communication barriers. Some communication errors include giving personal opinions, asking irrelevant personal questions, providing false reassurance, arguing, defensive responses, changing the subject, imposing personal values or beliefs, and offering judgment or criticism. Nurses must be aware of potential barriers that may impair communication and try to reduce their impact by continually seeking feedback and checking understanding (Open RN, 2021). Defense mechanisms exhibited by either nurse or client may indicate a rupture in the therapeutic alliance, however, if identified and addressed skillfully, these may solidify the relationship and strengthen the therapeutic process and effectiveness. Changes in affect, attitude, feelings or behaviour towards the nurse or therapy may indicate anxiety, confusion, distrust, discomfort, or offense around communication, interventions, or progress in the therapeutic relationship or process (Settani et al., 2022). The nurse learns to identify and address instances where the client may seem angry, defensive, or withdrawn instead of taking it personally, in an attempt to repair the therapeutic bond and process (Kourkouta & Papathanasiou, 2014).

5 The Role of Self-awareness, Boundaries, and Self-disclosure in Psychotherapy

The role of a nurse psychotherapist extends beyond traditional nursing responsibilities, encompassing a profound understanding and application of psychotherapeutic techniques within the nurse-client relationship. This multifaceted role requires a comprehensive skill set that integrates medical expertise, psychological knowledge, and compassionate care.

One crucial aspect of the nurse psychotherapist's role is self-awareness. Self-awareness involves a deep understanding of one's thoughts, emotions, and behaviors, which inevitably impact interactions with clients. It requires continuous introspection and reflection to examine personal biases, values, and attitudes that might influence therapeutic interventions (Görgens-Ekermans & Brand, 2012). Self-awareness is not only about recognizing one's strengths but also acknowledging vulnerabilities and limitations. By cultivating self-awareness, nurse psychotherapists can enhance their ability to provide client-centered care.

Self-awareness is not a static state but an ongoing, dynamic process. It requires active engagement in self-reflection, seeking feedback from colleagues and supervisors, and participating in continuing education and professional development activities. By engaging in these practices, nurse psychotherapists can continually refine their skills, deepen their self-understanding, and adapt their approach to meet the evolving needs of their clients. Moreover, self-awareness assists in maintaining the objective stance necessary for the nurse psychotherapist's role, promoting a supportive environment conducive to the client's healing and growth (Freshwater & Stickley, 2004). It enables nurse psychotherapists to separate their own experiences and emotions from those of their clients, allowing them to provide unbiased support and guidance. Another facet of self-awareness is recognizing personal triggers that can elicit emotional responses. Through self-awareness, nurse psychotherapists can better manage their reactions, thereby maintaining the therapeutic alliance. By understanding their emotional triggers, nurse psychotherapists can respond to challenging situations with empathy and composure, preventing potential harm to the therapeutic relationship (Aasan et al., 2022). Furthermore, self-awareness enables nurse psychotherapists to appreciate the impact of their cultural background, beliefs, and experiences on their interactions with clients. It helps them recognize and address potential cultural biases, allowing for culturally sensitive and inclusive care. By understanding their cultural lens, nurse psychotherapists can adapt their approach to meet the diverse needs of clients from various cultural backgrounds.

The delineation of boundaries within the nurse-client relationship is another pivotal aspect of the nurse psychotherapist's role. Boundaries ensure a safe, ethical framework that enables clients to delve into their issues without fear of exploitation. These boundaries involve a clear understanding of roles and responsibilities, respect for the client's autonomy, and a mindful avoidance of dual relationships that could lead to conflicts of interest (Pettifor et al., 2002). Establishing and maintaining boundaries requires careful navigation. Nurse psychotherapists must be able to assert themselves while also remaining empathetic and compassionate. It involves setting limits on the therapeutic relationship, such as appropriate physical contact, time boundaries, and maintaining professional confidentiality. Clear and consistent communication of these boundaries helps foster trust and respect between the nurse psychotherapist and the client. The lack of appropriate boundaries can lead to boundary violations, often linked to ethical dilemmas and malpractice in healthcare. Such violations can severely damage the therapeutic relationship and compromise the quality of client care (Austin et al., 2017). Nurse psychotherapists must recognize and address boundary issues promptly, seeking supervision or consultation when necessary. The nurse psychotherapist must diligently uphold and enforce these boundaries to maintain the integrity of the therapeutic relationship and provide effective client-centered care.

Self-disclosure, the act of revealing personal information to the client within a therapeutic context, is another critical element within the nurse psychotherapist's role. Used judiciously, self-disclosure can enhance the client's trust, foster rapport, and help normalize their experiences, thereby serving as a therapeutic tool (Ziv-Beiman, 2013). However, self-disclosure must be carefully controlled to maintain the focus on the client. Overuse or inappropriate self-disclosure can shift the focus from the client to the nurse, undermining the therapeutic alliance (Unhjem et al., 2018). The nurse psychotherapist must carefully weigh the potential benefits and risks of self-disclosure, ensuring it aligns with and promotes therapeutic goals. Effective self-disclosure involves considering factors such as the relevance of the information shared, the timing and context in which it is shared, and the potential impact on the therapeutic relationship. It should always prioritize the client's needs and therapeutic progress. By sharing appropriately, nurse psychotherapists can create a sense of shared humanity and validate the client's experiences, while still maintaining professional boundaries.

The role of the nurse psychotherapist is multifaceted, necessitating an astute awareness of self, others, and the dynamic interplay between them. Self-awareness, the careful delineation of boundaries, and thoughtful self-disclosure are fundamental to this role. These elements serve as guiding principles for nurse psychotherapists, shaping their professional interactions, and ultimately influencing the trajectory of the therapeutic process. By integrating these concepts into their practice, nurse psychotherapists can provide holistic and effective care to clients, promoting their healing and growth. Through ongoing self-reflection, continuous learning, and ethical practice, nurse psychotherapists can navigate the complexities of their role and make a meaningful difference in the lives of their clients. Expanding on these concepts ensures that nurse psychotherapists can continuously improve their skills, adapt to changing client needs, and provide compassionate and effective care. By embodying self-awareness, establishing and maintaining appropriate boundaries, and utilizing self-disclosure judiciously nurse psychotherapists can create a therapeutic environment where clients feel safe, understood, and supported. The success of the therapeutic process hinges on the nurse psychotherapist's ability to navigate these essential elements and foster a collaborative and healing relationship with their clients.

6 Reflective Activity

Each day, you will record and analyze an interaction considering the following aspects:

- Your self-awareness before, during, and after the interaction.
- Boundaries and self-disclosure involved in the interaction.
- The communication techniques used, including active listening and empathy.
- If virtual, how the medium affected rapport and communication.

You can choose interactions from your personal life or professional settings, ensuring you respect confidentiality where necessary:

1. Each day, record at least one interaction you've had, preferably in a virtual setting. If not available, any interaction will do.

2. Analyze the interaction in terms of the therapeutic nurse-client relationship. Though you may not be in a nurse-client situation, try to extrapolate the concepts to your scenario.
3. Focus on the role of self-awareness during the interaction. Reflect on your thoughts and emotions before, during, and after the interaction.
4. Consider the boundaries within this interaction. Did you or the other person disclose any personal information? Was it appropriate? How did it impact the interaction?
5. Reflect on the communication techniques used in the interaction. Did you use active listening, empathy, and verbal/non-verbal cues effectively? Were there any communication blocks, and if so, how were they handled?
6. If the interaction was virtual, how did this impact the rapport and communication? Were there any unique challenges or advantages presented by the virtual medium?
7. At the end of the week, review your journal entries. Reflect on your growth and any patterns that emerge from your entries. Identify areas where you feel you could improve and create an action plan for implementing changes based on your reflections.

7 Case Vignette

Sofia, a nurse psychotherapist, began working with Rajesh, a 38-year-old client diagnosed with chronic depression. Rajesh had a history of mistrust in healthcare professionals due to previous negative experiences. He exhibited reluctance during the initial sessions, often responding with one-word answers and displaying defensive body language.

7.1 Application of Concepts

7.1.1 Rapport and Trust

Understanding the importance of rapport and trust in therapeutic relationships, Sofia made an effort to show consistency and reliability. She ensured she was always punctual, actively listened to Rajesh, and validated his feelings without rushing to offer solutions. Over time, Rajesh started to trust Sofia and opened up more during their sessions.

7.1.2 Self-awareness and Boundaries

Sofia recognized her initial feelings of frustration when Rajesh was not responsive. Utilizing self-awareness, she acknowledged these feelings and refrained from letting them influence her professional role. She maintained boundaries by keeping their interactions professional and focused on Rajesh's therapeutic needs.

7.1.3 Advanced Therapeutic Communication Techniques

Sofia used both verbal and non-verbal communication techniques to engage Rajesh. She employed open-ended questions to encourage Rajesh to express himself more and maintained eye contact to show her attentiveness. When Rajesh displayed defensive body language, Sofia noted it and gently inquired about his comfort level, demonstrating her observation and concern.

7.1.4 Handling Communication Blocks and Defense Mechanisms

Sofia noticed that Rajesh would often change the subject whenever his childhood was mentioned. Recognizing this as a potential communication block and defense mechanism, Sofia did not force the conversation. Instead, she allowed Rajesh to take the lead while subtly guiding him towards confronting these difficult topics when he was ready.

7.1.5 Empathy and Active Listening

Sofia showed genuine empathy and understanding of Rajesh's experiences. She demonstrated active listening by reflecting on Rajesh's feelings, which helped him feel understood and supported.

7.1.6 Virtual Psychotherapy

Sessions recently shifted to a virtual platform to support waitlists. Sofia acknowledged the potential challenges of this setup, including the potential impact on their rapport and communication. To mitigate these, Sofia ensured she created a safe and private space for her sessions, used clear and empathic verbal communication, and regularly checked in with Rajesh about how he was finding the online therapy experience.

The case of Sofia and Rajesh illustrates how a nurse psychotherapist can apply the concepts discussed in this chapter to establish a therapeutic relationship and effectively facilitate a client's therapeutic journey.

7.2 Reflective Questions Related to Case Vignette

Consider Sofia's approach when Rajesh exhibited defensive body language and communication blocks. How did her actions facilitate trust and openness in their therapeutic relationship?
Sofia had to adapt to the shift to virtual therapy due to the clinic demands. How do you think this change might have affected their therapeutic relationship? What strategies did Sofia use to maintain rapport and effective communication?
How might you ensure you establish and maintain a positive client-centric therapeutic alliance throughout the psychotherapeutic process to help achieve successful therapeutic outcomes?

8 Summary

Understanding the role of the nurse psychotherapist is crucial to delivering effective psychotherapy.
The therapeutic nurse-client relationship is built on rapport, trust, boundaries, and self-disclosure.
Advanced therapeutic communication techniques can significantly enhance the efficacy of psychotherapy.
The virtual delivery of psychotherapy presents unique challenges and opportunities for building rapport, trust, and effective communication.

References

Aasan, O. J., Brataas, H. V., & Nordtug, B. (2022). Experience of managing countertransference through self-guided imagery in meditation among healthcare professionals. *Frontiers in psychiatry, 13*, 793784. https://doi.org/10.3389/fpsyt.2022.793784

Agha, Z., Roter, D. L., & Schapira, R. M. (2009). An evaluation of patient-physician communication style during telemedicine consultations. *Journal of Medical Internet Research, 1*(3), e36. https://doi.org/10.2196/jmir.1193

Arnold, E. C., & Boggs, K. U. (2022). *Interpersonal relationships: Professional communication skills for nurses*. Elsevier Health Sciences.

Austin, C. L., Saylor, R., & Finley, P. J. (2017). Moral distress in physicians and nurses: Impact on professional quality of life and turnover. *Psychological Trauma: Theory, Research, Practice and Policy, 9*(4), 399–406. https://doi.org/10.1037/tra0000201

Austin, W., Bergum, V., Nuttgens, S., & Peternelj-Taylor, C. (2006). A re-visioning of boundaries in professional helping relationships: Exploring other metaphors. *Ethics & Behavior, 16*(2), 77–94. https://doi.org/10.1207/s15327019eb1602_02

Békés, V., & Aafjes-van Doorn, K. (2020). Psychotherapists' attitudes toward online therapy during the COVID-19 pandemic. *Journal of Psychotherapy Integration, 30*(2), 238–247. https://doi.org/10.1037/int0000214

Berrouiguet, S., Baca-García, E., Brandt, S., Walter, M., & Courtet, P. (2016). Fundamentals for future mobile-health (mHealth): A systematic review of mobile phone and web-based text messaging in mental health. *Journal of Medical Internet Research, 18*(6), e135. https://doi.org/10.2196/jmir.5066

Bordin, E. S. (1979). The generalizability of the psychoanalytic concept of the working alliance. *Psychotherapy: Theory, Research & Practice, 16*(3), 252–260. https://doi.org/10.1037/h0085885

Burke, A. (2023). *Therapeutic Communication: NCLEX-RN.* Registered Nursing.org https://www.registerednursing.org/nclex/therapeutic-communication/

Burns, D. (2006). *Feeling great: The revolutionary new treatment for depression and anxiety.* PESI Publishing and Media.

Campinha-Bacote, J. (2002). The process of cultural competence in the delivery of healthcare services: A model of care. *Journal of Transcultural Nursing, 13(*3), 181–184. https://doi.org/10.1177/10459602013003005

Canadian Nurses Association. (2017). Code of Ethics for Registered Nurses. Author.

Charles, C., Gafni, A., & Whelan, T. (1997). Shared decision-making in the medical encounter: What does it mean? (Or it takes at least two to tango). *Social Science & Medicine, 44*(5), 681–692. https://doi.org/10.1016/S0277-9536(96)00221-3

College of Nurses of Ontario. (2006) *Practice Standard.* Author. https://www.cno.org/globalassets/docs/prac/41033_therapeutic.pdf

College of Nurses of Ontario. (2019). *Therapeutic Nurse-Client Relationship.* Author.

Cormack, D. F. (2004). *The Research Process in Nursing* (4th ed.). Blackwell Publishing.

Freshwater, D., & Stickley, T. (2004). The heart of the art: emotional intelligence in nurse education. *Nursing inquiry, 11*(2), 91–98. https://doi.org/10.1111/j.1440-1800.2004.00198.x

Goldberg, D. A., & Plakun, E. M. (2013). Teaching psychodynamic psychotherapy with the Y model. *Journal of the American Academy of Psychoanalysis & Dynamic Psychiatry, 41*(1), 111–126.

Görgens-Ekermans, G., & Brand, T. (2012). Emotional intelligence as a moderator in the stress-burnout relationship: A questionnaire study on nurses. *Journal of Clinical Nursing, 21*(15–16), 2275–2285. https://doi.org/10.1111/j.1365-2702.2012.04171.x

Kourkouta, L., & Papathanasiou, I. V. (2014). Communication in nursing practice. *Materia socio-medica, 26*(1), 65–67. https://doi.org/10.5455/msm.2014.26.65-67

Mishna, F., Fantus, S., & McInroy, L. B. (2017). Informal use of information and communication technology: Adjunct to traditional face-to-face social work practice. *Clinical Social Work Journal, 45*, 49–55. https://doi.org/10.1007/s10615-016-0576-3

Moudatsou, M., Stavropoulou, A., Philalithis, A., & Koukouli, S. (2020). The role of empathy in health and social care professionals. *Healthcare (Basel, Switzerland), 8*(1), 26. https://doi.org/10.3390/healthcare8010026

Open Resources for Nursing (Open RN); Ernstmeyer, K., & Christman, E., (Eds.) (2021). Nursing Fundamentals [Internet]. Eau Claire (WI): Chippewa Valley Technical College.

Peplau, H. (1952). *Interpersonal relations in nursing: A conceptual frame of reference for psychodynamic nursing.* G. P. Putnam's Sons.

Pettifor, J. L., Estay, I., & Paquet, S. (2002). Preferred strategies for learning ethics in the practice of a discipline. *Canadian Psychology/Psychologie canadienne, 43*(4), 260–269. https://doi.org/10.1037/h0086922

Reay, R. E., Looi, J. C., & Keightley, P. (2020). Telehealth mental health services during COVID-19: Summary of evidence and clinical practice. *Australasian Psychiatry: bulletin of Royal Australian and New Zealand College of Psychiatrists, 28*(5), 514–516. https://doi.org/10.1177/1039856220943032

Registered Nurses' Association of Ontario. (2020). *Establishing therapeutic relationships.* Author.

Richardson, L. K., Frueh, B. C., Grubaugh, A. L., Egede, L., & Elhai, J. D. (2009). Current directions in videoconferencing tele-mental health research. *Clinical Psychology: Science and Practice, 16*(3), 323–338. https://doi.org/10.1111/j.1468-2850.2009.01170.x

Settanni, M., Bronzini, M., Carzedda, G., Godino, G., Manca, M. L., Martini, L., Provvedi, G., Quilghini, F., Zucconi, A., & Francesetti, G. (2022). Introducing the QACP: Development and preliminary validation of an instrument to measure psychotherapist's core competencies. *Research in Psychotherapy (Milano), 25*(2), 599. https://doi.org/10.4081/ripppo.2022.599

Simpson, S. G., & Reid, C. L. (2014). Therapeutic alliance in videoconferencing psychotherapy: A review. *Australian Journal of Rural Health, 22*(6), 280–299. https://doi.org/10.1111/ajr.12149

Shattell, M. M., Starr, S. S., & Thomas, S. P. (2007). 'Take my hand, help me out': Mental health service recipients' experience of the therapeutic relationship. *International Journal of Mental Health Nursing, 16*(4), 274–284. https://doi.org/10.1111/j.1447-0349.2007.00477.x

Stuart, G. W. (2013). *Principles and practice of psychiatric nursing* (10th ed.). Mosby Elsevier.

Unhjem, J. V., Vatne, S., & Hem, M. H. (2018). Transforming nurse-patient relationships – A qualitative study of nurse self-disclosure in mental health care. *Journal of Clinical Nursing, 27*(5–6), e798–e807. https://doi.org/10.1111/jocn.14191

Ziv-Beiman, S. (2013). Therapist self-disclosure as an integrative intervention. *Journal of Psychotherapy Integration, 23*(1), 59–74. https://doi.org/10.1037/a0031783

Chapter 5
Trauma-Informed Approaches

Archna N. Patel and Mary-Lou Martin

Abstract Recognition of the significance of psychological trauma and its impact on individuals, families, communities, and society at large has greatly expanded over the past 20 years, calling for the need to develop both trauma-sensitive and trauma-responsive healthcare services. Nurses, as direct care providers who practice within a holistic perspective, are positioned to play an integral role in the advancement of both trauma-informed care (TIC) and trauma-specific services (TSS). This chapter will provide an overview of the concept of trauma, as defined by three complex interrelated elements; the event, the experience, and the effects. Neurophysiological effects of unpredictable, severe, and/or prolonged stress as they relate to our stress-response systems and the ability to relate within the intrapersonal and interpersonal will be reviewed. The concepts of TIC, an approach based on principles that are sensitive to the needs of those with histories of trauma to be delivered universally to all that engage with the system, as well as TSS, services designed to treat trauma, will be explored within the implications for nursing practice. Issues raised in the current literature related to operationalizing and implementing TIC and TSS care will be presented and offer insights for future directions.

Keywords Trauma · Trauma-informed care · Trauma-specific care · Vicarious trauma

Learning Objectives

After completing this chapter, the learner will:

1. Describe trauma and trauma-informed care.
2. Discuss the prevalence and impact of trauma.

A. N. Patel (✉)
Woodbridge, ON, Canada
e-mail: archnap@gmail.com

M.-L. Martin
St Joseph's Healthcare Hamilton/McMaster University, Hamilton, ON, Canada

S. Roles and K. Kalia (eds.), *The Nurses' Guide to Psychotherapy*,
https://doi.org/10.1007/978-981-97-4738-2_5

3. Describe examples of specific tests/tools.
4. Describe vicarious trauma and its impact.

1 What is Trauma

Trauma is described as "an event, series of events, or set of circumstances that is experienced by an individual as physically or emotionally harmful or life-threatening and that has lasting adverse effects of an individual's functioning and mental, physical, social, emotional, or spiritual well-being" (Substance Abuse and Mental Health Services Administration, [SAMHSA], 2014, p. 7). Trauma occurs when an external threat overwhelms the person's coping resources and affects their life (Van Der Kolk 2014). The underlying premise of trauma-informed care (TIC) is for healthcare providers to understand and assume that many of their clients have been affected by trauma.

The prevalence of trauma in Canadians is high: 76% of Canadian adults report some form of trauma exposure in their lifetime, 9.2% meet the criteria for PTSD and an estimated 50% of all Canadian women and 33% of Canadian men have survived at least one incidence of sexual or physical violence (Arthur et al. 2013; Cowling & MacDougall 2019). In the United States of America, 13,494 adults completed a questionnaire about adverse childhood events which revealed that 75% of the population had experienced at least one traumatic event in their lifetime (Felitti et al. 1998) and another study by Meusar and colleagues (1998) reported that 90% of mental health clients have been exposed and most have had multiple experiences of trauma.

Despite the prevalence of traumatic experiences, the experience of trauma is unique to each person. Experiences of trauma and violence are associated with the social determinants of health (Wathen & Varcoe 2021) and matters beyond our control such as natural disasters. Individuals will respond differently to trauma based on genetics, history, internal (biological, psychological), and external factors. The length of trauma, frequency of trauma, and intensity of trauma may also have an impact.

Trauma has been defined as experiences that overwhelm an individual's capacity to cope (Arthur et al. 2013). Examples of trauma early in life can include child abuse, neglect, witnessing violence, and disrupted attachment (Arthur et al. 2013). Later-stage traumatic experiences can include violence, accidents, natural disasters, war, sudden unexpected loss, and other life events that are out of one's control (Arthur et al. 2013). When understanding trauma there are several domains to consider; these include the magnitude, complexity, frequency, duration, and whether it occurs from an interpersonal, or external source (Arthur et al. 2013).

Trauma has been identified to have many dimensions (Arthur et al. 2013; Malchiodo 2020):

1. Single incident,
2. Complex or repetitive trauma,
3. Developmental trauma,

4. Intergenerational trauma,
5. Historical trauma,
6. Relational, and
7. Vicarious Trauma.

Single-incident trauma can include those involving an accident, single episode of assault/abuse, sudden loss, violence, or natural disaster (Arthur et al. 2013). Complex or repetitive trauma can include ongoing emotional, physical, or sexual abuse, or war (Arthur et al. 2013). Developmental trauma occurs during the early stages of life (infant, child, youth) and can involve neglect, abandonment, physical, sexual, or emotional abuse or witnessing violence or death as well as coercion or betrayal (Arthur et al. 2013). Trauma at birth, early childhood, or in youth can have significant effects on the person. Infants and children are especially vulnerable, being completely dependent on caregivers, and some adolescents are partially dependent on adults. Trauma can have an impact on the development of identity and beliefs about the self and the external world. Studies indicate that the environment of children; family, community, and culture, impacts the brain development as well as the health and genetics (Earls 2018) of these children. Attachment patterns form early in life and the ways in which you learn how to feel, think, behave, and communicate will be affected by life experiences as the brain continues to grow and develop (Van Der Kolk 2014). Trauma can result in many difficulties including the inability or difficulty in coping with stress or adversity and continues through all of the development stages of the lifespan (Van Der Kolk 2014). Intergenerational trauma comprises trauma experienced by people who live with or are born from trauma survivors. Coping and adaptation patterns developed in response to trauma can be passed between generations (Arthur et al. 2013; Framo, 1981). Historical trauma is a cumulative emotional and psychological wounding over the lifespan and across generations and can include genocide, or colonialism such as in situations including residential schools, slavery, and war (Arthur et al. 2013; Sotero 2006). Relational and vicarious trauma can happen in response to others' traumas. Relational trauma is the interpersonal trauma that can help to clarify the complex traumas resulting from abuse and neglect from other individuals (Malchiodo, 2020). Vicarious trauma can impact professionals who experience compassion overload and can develop negative symptoms that can be serious and life-altering (Van Der Kolk 2014).

The effects of trauma are many and varied and may be an individual or collective experience. Two individuals can have a similar trauma but be impacted in completely different ways pointing to the complexities of trauma. Trauma impacts the individual's response neurobiologically, physically, emotionally, cognitively, behaviorally, spiritually, and relationally, and may cause short and long-term physical and mental health outcomes. How the individual experiences trauma is connected to the way they feel, think, and act all in relation to their previous life experiences. People who experience trauma may identify a myriad of issues including helplessness, anxiety, emotional dysregulation, depression, rage, nightmares, insomnia, flashbacks, binge eating, and self-injury or suicide attempts (Gutierres & Van Puymbroeck 2006; Nadew 2012; Ponic et al. 2016; Schafer 2009; Van Der Kolk & Fisher 1995;

Van der Kolk 2014). It may also lead to the use of alcohol and/or drugs, hypersexuality, overeating, and self-harming behaviours (Gutierres & Van Puymbroeck 2006; Haskell 2018; Nadew 2012; Schafer 2009) as ways to escape or self-medicate to mitigate the effects of trauma, which more often than not cause worse outcomes for the individual. Some individuals may not even be aware of the trauma that occurred earlier in their life and yet still experience complex negative effects.

2 Impact of Trauma

All humans are susceptible to trauma and no one is immune to it. It is widespread throughout the world and it can affect individuals from all population groups and every socioeconomic status. Trauma can impact individuals, families, communities, cultures, generations, services, and organizations. Trauma can be pervasive in an individual's life, impacting the entire person. Trauma can influence how a person thinks, feels, the way they learn, how they remember things, how they feel about themselves, and how they view other people and the world around them (SAMHSA, 2014).

3 Neurobiological Impacts of Trauma

The brain responds to trauma with changes in function and structure (Bellis & Zisk 2014; Kozlowska et al. 2015; Van Der Kolk, 2014). Alterations in the brain can include changes to the sensory systems, gray-matter volume, and neural architecture and circuits (Read et al. 2014). With trauma, the stress response is activated, and its effects are complex (Evans & Coccoma 2014). The amygdala is the defensive part of the brain (Evans & Coccoma 2014; Van Der Kolk 2014) and has a primary purpose of keeping us alive. The amygdala is activated when trauma occurs and responds by activating the fight, flight, freeze, or fawn hyperarousal response (Walker 2013) to the threat of danger. The fight response occurs when the individual is ready to fight off a threat and occurs when the individual takes flight from the threat or danger (Kozlowska et al. 2015), and the freeze response occurs when fight and flight are not workable (Haskell 2018) and the individual freezes to avoid a threat, (this may also be a dissociative response as some trauma can become overwhelming for some individuals who may disconnect) (Howell 2020; McHugh & Egan 2023; Van Der Kolk & Fisher 1995) and the fawn response occurs when the individual neutralizes the threat by being overly helpful, and attempts to make someone else happy to avoid conflict (Walker 2013) and lessen the hyperarousal response.

It is here that sights, sounds, smells, tastes, and body sensations are encoded and the amygdala prepares individuals to act quickly and without thought (Haskell 2018; Treleaven 2018). The amygdala recognizes threats and previous traumas and activates the defense response triggering the adrenal glands to release a cascade of neurochemicals which initiates the adrenal stress response (Friedman 2015; Haskell 2018). When these neurochemicals such as cortisol and epinephrine are released, the body prepares for action with increased heart rate, respiration, sweat, oxygen, and a multitude of other physical reactions (Haskell 2018).

Studies have also shown that trauma may contribute to changes not only in the amygdala but also in the hippocampus which impacts the memory centers of the brain (Heningberg et al. 2019). Emotions, physical symptoms, and thinking may become fragmented as people attempt to disconnect from these sensations and experiences (Boyer et al. 2022; Fisher 2017; Freiven & Lanius 2015; Lanius 2015), this may result in nightmares, flashbacks, or thoughts of the memory when they were not deliberately recalled. Triggers are reminders of past threats whether real or imagined and they raise the alarm response and are protective. A trigger is something that can elicit re-traumatization, a trauma response, and/or distress at the moment and can occur as a result of environment, sounds, smells, colours, movements, objects, or events (Jean Tweed Centre 2013). When this happens, the individual may feel and act as though they are re-living the danger or are currently in danger (Van Der Kolk 2014). For example, when someone touches another person without their permission a flight or fight response may occur whether or not the threat might be real or imagined (Ponic et al. 2016). Understanding these effects of trauma on the brain response can help us to provide responsive interventions and treatment and be aware of the risk of triggers and re-traumatization. This will enable the psychotherapist to cultivate a safe space for the client.

4 Assessment of Trauma

Priority tasks of assessment of trauma include safety of the individual, connection with the client, and an intervention plan that includes a path towards healing, recovery, and resilience (Herman 1992). Clients are the experts in their own trauma experience(s) and the therapist must be willing to hear their stories and learn from them. It is important for clients to feel respected and accepted as collaborators in the therapeutic relationship, development of the plan of care, and the evaluation of outcomes. For individuals who have experienced trauma, it is important to work from a strength-based perspective as this can help to build trust and therapeutic alliance. It is also important that the language used is trauma-sensitive, for example, identifying the individual as a survivor, not a trauma victim. Further, understanding the meaning that the client gives to a traumatic incident from their cultural perspective is of importance. Providing the client with choices and involving them in the decision-making process can create a collaborative partnership in their healing and the therapeutic plan. The safety of the individual is paramount and is important to discuss considering past or recent trauma.

5 Recovery

Recovery does not necessarily mean complete freedom from post-traumatic effects but generally includes the ability to live in the present without being overwhelmed by the thoughts, feelings, and experiences of the past. Trauma recovery is a non-linear process that is worked on over time and in intentional stages. One can promote recovery by emphasizing hope and optimism in order to foster and support the client's personal journey. Clients with trauma can learn to feel safe, trust other people, learn new strategies for relating to individuals, and develop self-compassion (Van Der Kolk 2014). Principles of TIC including creating safety and trust are paramount in supporting those with traumatic histories and are pertinent in the discussion or trauma recovery.

6 Components of Trauma-Informed Care

TIC integration is a framework that is interwoven into the practices, policies, and culture of an individual practitioner or an entire organization so that clinicians have awareness, knowledge, and the skills needed to support trauma survivors. TIC is a strengths-based framework grounded in an understanding of and responsiveness to, the impact of trauma (Elliot et al. 2005; SAMHSA 2014; Sweeney et al. 2018; Jean Tweed Centre, 2013). TIC emphasizes physical, psychological, and emotional safety for clients, and creates opportunities for survivors to rebuild a sense of control and empowerment (Elliot et al. 2005; SAMHSA, 2014; Sweeney et al. 2018; Jean Tweed Centre 2013). TIC does not always require the need to treat symptoms or syndromes related to any specific type of trauma, rather, the care or services provided are to be informed, and be sensitive to, the intersection of care and the trauma-related issues that can be present (SAMHSA 2014; Jean Tweed Centre 2013). Assumptions held for TIC during care, when relating with clients, assume that all have experienced some form of trauma and use this perspective when interacting with the clients during psychotherapy for all types of clients in any type of service (SAMHSA, 2014; Jean Tweed Centre 2013).

TIC might include services for those who have known trauma(s) and those whereby it is unknown to the care provider and/or the client. TIC also involves being attentive in anticipating possible responses and thus avoiding institutional or systemic processes in practice that may re-traumatize individuals who already have a history of trauma (Elliot et al. 2005; SAMHSA, 2014; Sweeney et. al 2018; Jean Tweed Centre 2013). In order to mitigate the possible risk of re-traumatization, the client is involved in the treatment plan and can provide feedback on the care they are receiving. Overall, integrating TIC involves understanding how to design services to accommodate the vulnerabilities of trauma survivors and allows services to be delivered in a way that will avoid unintentionally re-traumatizing the clients, and instead will facilitate a person-centered, strength-based approach to treatment.

7 Implementing TIC for Nurse Psychotherapists

The TIC process includes acknowledging that trauma can pervasively affect an individual's well-being, in all domains of life (SAMHSA, 2014). It reinforces the importance of acquiring trauma-specific knowledge and skills to meet the specific needs of clients; it recognizes that individuals may be affected by trauma regardless of its acknowledgment; it understands that trauma likely affects many clients who are seeking behavioral health services; and acknowledges that providers can retraumatize clients through standard or unexamined policies and practices (SAMHSA, 2014). TIC stresses the importance of addressing the client individually rather than applying general treatment approaches and provides clients with opportunities to engage in services that reflect a compassionate perspective of their presenting problems. TIC can potentially provide a greater sense of safety for clients who have histories of trauma and a platform for preventing more serious consequences of traumatic stress (Harris & Fallot 2001). Trauma-informed services (TSS) offer clients a chance to explore the impact of trauma, their own individual strengths, and their personal creative adaptations in managing traumatic histories, including their resilience and the relationships among trauma, substance use, and psychological symptoms.

8 Components of Trauma-Specific Services

TSS are clinical interventions, models of care, and treatments that are created to address trauma-related symptoms and Post-Traumatic Stress Disorder (PTSD) directly through individual sessions and/or groups (Authur et al. 2013; Bloom 2006). These services directly treat specific trauma, and its impact on daily living, and work to facilitate trauma recovery for the specific trauma(s) that the client is seeking treatment for (Elliot et al. 2005; SAMHSA, 2014; Sweeney et al. 2018; Jean Tweed Centre 2013). There are gold standard treatments used to treat specific types of trauma, as well as PTSD in which the first line of treatment is often a specific form of psychotherapy.

Many psychotherapists do not have formal training in treating trauma or an understanding of the integration of trauma-informed services, and at the same time, each client with a history of trauma presents with various clinical presentations. As a result, the psychotherapist may not be confident in how to therapeutically respond to a client's trauma-related reactions or symptoms. Coupled with this challenge is the prevalence of experiencing traumatic events, including that some psychotherapists may have their own trauma patterns that could be triggered by clients' reports of their trauma. Furthermore, psychotherapists may be triggered by their clients' coping strategies, responses, and reactions, due to the impact of the trauma that they have experienced. Although nurses should always be assessing trauma, it is imperative to self-assess one's own competence in the delivery of trauma-informed approaches. If the nurse psychotherapist identifies that the trauma is outside of their ability to treat, they should know when and how to refer the client to a competent nurse psychotherapist or another provider who has training in gold-standard treatments for different types of trauma.

Without a deeper understanding of how trauma manifests into a client's daily life and training on how to manage traumas and triggers, those interested in helping clients with trauma can unknowingly cause harm by pushing too quickly into the clients' trauma history and or by inadvertently downplaying, dismissing or disregarding a client's personal account of their trauma (Elliot et al. 2005; SAMHSA, 2014). Before trying to help clients who struggle with trauma histories, and/or delving too quickly into understanding past traumas, psychotherapists must be aware of (SAMHSA, 2014):

1. Trauma-related symptoms,
2. Assessing and recognizing trauma-related reactions,
3. Incorporating care plans for managing trauma-related symptoms,
4. Knowing how to help clients build a safety net to manage and prevent being re-traumatized,
5. Knowing how and when to provide psychoeducation as the appropriate intervention,
6. Knowing when to seek help through clinical supervision or psychotherapy, and
7. Knowing when to make treatment referrals for specialized consultation and trauma-specific treatment services if it is out of their scope of practice.

Implementing trauma-informed approaches requires the therapist to intentionally and regularly engage in self-awareness, self-reflection, training, and clinical supervision to better understand their responses to clients and their therapeutic effectiveness. Active self-study can help to manage or mitigate transference and countertransference to avoid unintentionally harming their clients further (see Chap. 19 on Supervision and Consultation). Therapists must also bring to the forefront the consistent practice of compassion into their interactions with clients by intentionally practicing self-compassion. To foster this practice, it's important for nurses to assess their own compassion fatigue, vicarious trauma, and Adverse Child Events (ACE) score (See Appendix A for assessments for Compassion Fatigue and ACE), and then work towards goals to address or build one's own strengths, skills, recovery, and healing.

Questions about experiences of trauma can open the space to start helping a person understand and deal with the impacts of trauma, however, asking about experiences of trauma can also trigger trauma-related responses. Questions about experiences of trauma must be asked with skills of sensitivity and flexibility (Sweeney et al. 2018). Questions should be well-paced to give the client space to share and feel safe, and should include grounding practices, such as breath work or engaging the senses (Sweeney et al. 2018). The therapist should be able to astutely assess if the client is ready or not ready, and should have a sense of when to stop asking questions to avoid harm. If the client becomes triggered, is in crisis, or dissociates, the therapist should pivot from gathering this information to instead using grounding strategies. Further to this, the psychotherapist can normalize seeking an understanding of the trauma history as part of building the therapeutic relationship and by supporting the client to achieve their goals (Sweeney et al. 2018).

9 Outcomes of Integrating TIC in Your Practice

Clinical outcomes for those clients who have TIC-integrated therapy interventions report having reductions in symptoms of mental health concerns and substance use, increased knowledge in managing triggers and coping strategies, improvement in learning how to feel safe and trust others; and also report improved trust and confidence in mental health care providers and therapists (SAMHSA, 2014). This shift in practice has reframed common ways of responding and thinking about client' behaviours from "what is wrong with the person" to "what happened to this person" (Bloom 1999) and has advanced the state of TIC. Trauma survivors often do not see their own capabilities and strengths without support from others who can connect their experiences as evidence of strength and skills for how they managed the events and challenges in their life (Jean Tweed Centre 2013). To promote recovery, and to help the client achieve their goals in therapy, the psychotherapist can incorporate into the session(s); skills strengthening and building through psychoeducation, practicing new skills with the client during the psychotherapy session(s), and giving learning activities for the client to practice at home.

10 Standardized Screening and Assessment Tools

Standardized screening and assessment tools are helpful during the assessment phase and throughout ongoing evaluation. The tools vary in length and purpose. Some tools are clinician rated and others are self-reported by the client. Some tools may require formal training. Examples of some common tools can be found in Appendix B.

11 Trauma-Informed Interventions Applied in Structured Psychotherapy

Trauma-informed interventions reflect a diversity of approaches that acknowledge and accept the uniqueness of the individual. This type of intervention requires courage from the individual with trauma experience(s). The therapeutic relationship is foundational and treatment plans are individualized to ensure the best outcomes. Generally, a therapist requires training in trauma-specific interventions with clinical supervision. Differing types of psychotherapy interventions can be found in Chap. 16.

12 Vicarious Trauma and Its Impact on Psychotherapy

Vicarious trauma is an occupational hazard. Psychotherapists may have experienced trauma in the past and they may be triggered by client behaviours (Canadian Centre On Substance Abuse, 2014). Psychotherapists who work with clients who have experienced trauma are often repeatedly exposed to scenarios of violence and other forms of trauma and these experiences can lead to vicarious trauma with negative outcomes similar to those experienced by their own clients with trauma (Bartoskova 2015; Middleton & Potter 2015; van Mol et al. 2015). Vicarious traumatization can include the feelings, personal distress, and symptoms that are sometimes evoked in therapists working with clients who have experienced trauma (Friedman 2015). Vicarious trauma can include the experience of being witness to the trauma, including the sight, sound, smell, touch, and body sensations of the survivor who may experience terror, guilt, shame, helpfulness, powerlessness, and sadness and may be searching for a way to heal. Vicarious trauma is manageable if the therapist recognizes it and takes early steps to address it. It may result in specific symptoms of psychological or emotional distress. It is important that the therapist takes time to process the experience by developing self-awareness inclusive of reflective practice. It can be important to work in supportive environments to debrief with a peer therapist or an expert therapist and to have regular supervision (Friedman 2015). Every individual's journey has its own pace and rhythm for healing and recovering from trauma. See Appendix C for a list of additional resources on vicarious trauma.

13 Reflective Questions

1. What strategies would you utilize to ensure your client is wanting to engage in collaborative and informed psychotherapeutic interventions for trauma?
2. How would you decide on your intervention or approach?
3. How would you engage in clinical supervision in managing vicarious trauma?

14 Case Vignette

14.1 Assessment

- The client is 37 years old, married with 2 children (ages 8 & 10) and works as a registered nurse in a private clinic.
- Trauma history: Nine months ago, their best friend was killed in an automobile accident and the client was the driver. The police investigated and it was found to be accidental.
- There is no past psychiatric history.

- No treatment has been attempted as the client has not engaged in psychotherapy previously.
- Normal early development.
- No significant medical history.
- No alcohol or substance use history.
- The client describes feeling irritable and has a lack of emotional connection with their family.
- The client feels guilty about the accident and states that "I should have been able to manage the situation... I should be over this by now... It feels like I am living it all over again." Stresses that otherwise wouldn't have caused feelings of being overwhelmed and less confident are currently doing so.
- The client reports frightening nightmares and their spouse notices they are screaming while sleeping, and reports irritability and argumentativeness with their spouse.
- The client's family has become frustrated with their family member's irritability and lack of emotional connection.

14.2 Plan/Intervention

- The nurse psychotherapist decides to begin one hour of manualized Cognitive Behavioural Therapy (CBT) once a week for 20 weeks to identify/address the thinking patterns and behaviours. They plan to guide the client to identify their own goals and interventions at the beginning of each session.
- Consider what the evidence-based recommended goals, journaling, and interventions might be regarding:
  - Problems list,
  - Reexperiencing memories and nightmares,
  - Feelings of numbness,
  - Ineffective coping & problem solving,
  - Irritability,
  - Impaired sleep (insomnia),
  - Conflict with spouse,
  - CBT manualized 20-session week treatment protocol, expectations, practice assignments, and rationale,
  - Monitor and teach sleep hygiene,
  - Progressive muscle relaxation, and
  - Grounding techniques.

14.3 Strengths/Resources

- Strengths and resources that are noted by the nurse psychotherapist
  - Client is motivated to deal with symptoms;
  - The partner is willing to engage in psychotherapy to support their spouse;
  - Client has family connections and support;
  - Mental health services are available and accessible to this person and their family.

14.4 Expected Outcomes

- Altered trauma-related beliefs and behaviours;
- Decreased anxiety;
- Feelings of safety and security through practicing stress reduction techniques;
- Improved coping through relaxation techniques and working with family;
- Normal sleep patterns by including positive sleep hygiene in their interventions.

14.5 Evaluation

- Regular review at individual sessions and at the end of therapy;
- Reduced hyperarousal;
- Feels rested, sleep improved;
- Decreased conflict with spouse;
- Provide client resources that support health teaching as needed;
- Continue the practice of skills learned;
- Identify goals for the future.

14.6 Case Vignette Reflective Questions

What trauma might the client be experiencing?
What might be triggering the client?
How could the CBT plan address thinking and behaviour?
Should the family be involved in the plan of care and if yes, how so?
How would you, as the clinician, engage in self-awareness and potentially protect yourself from vicarious trauma?
How can you help your client feel safe, self-empowered, and hopeful in the care and services you provide?

15 Summary

- Trauma can include:
  - Event(s) or circumstances (external threat) that are experienced by the individual that can overwhelm their coping resources and adversely affect their life.
  - Prevalence is high with approximately 76% of Canadian adults reporting a single or multiple trauma exposure(s) in their lifetime.
  - Trauma may be a single incident, complex or repetitive trauma, developmental trauma, intergenerational trauma, historical trauma, relational, and/or vicarious trauma.
  - Trauma activates the stress response and its neurobiological effects can be complex.
  - Trauma causes triggers that may feel and make the person act as though they are re-living the danger no matter whether or not the threat is a perceived threat or is real in the moment.
- Trauma-Informed Care (TIC) is a strength-based framework that:
  - Assumes that all clients have experienced some form of trauma.
  - Is grounded in an understanding of, and responsiveness to the impact of trauma.
  - Emphasizes physical, psychological, emotional, and spiritual safety for both providers and survivors.
  - Creates opportunities for survivors to rebuild a sense of control and empowerment.
  - Includes trauma awareness, safety, trustworthiness, collaboration, choice, connection, strengths-based approaches, and skill building.
- Trauma Specific Services (TSS)
  - Are clinical interventions, models of care, and treatments for addressing trauma and related symptoms.
  - Recognizes that individuals may be affected by trauma regardless of their exposure.
  - Offers clients safety and a chance to explore the impact of trauma, symptoms, strengths, creative adaptations in managing trauma histories, and resilience.
  - Recognizes that each individual's journey has its own pace and rhythm of healing and recovery.
  - Integrates screening and assessment tools (some may require formal training).
  - Requires the therapist to intentionally and regularly engage in self-awareness, self-reflection, and clinical supervision to better understand their response to clients with trauma, especially when experiencing vicarious trauma.

Appendix A Relevant Internet Links

Compassion Fatigue

Microsoft Word - ProQOL_v5_English.Docx (wsimg.com)

ProQOL Measure | ProQOL.

ACE and Resilience

Adverse Childhood Experiences (ACEs) (cdc.gov)

From-ACESTOOHIGH-ACES-and-Resilience-questions.Pdf (unc.edu).

Appendix B Screening and Assessment Tools

- Clinician-Administered PTSD Scale for DSM-5 (CAPS-5)—measures diagnosis, symptoms over the past week, 30 items, clinician-rated
- Evaluation of Lifetime Stressors (ELS)—measure trauma history, 56 items, clinician-rated
- Post Trauma Risky Behaviors Questionnaire—measures post trauma reckless & self-destructive behavior, 10 min., self-report
- Primary Care PTSD Screen for DSM-5 (PC-PTSD-5)—measures exposure to traumatic events, 5 min.
- PTSD Checklist 5 (PCL-5)—measures symptoms of PTSD, 20 items, self-report
- PTSD Symptom Scale Interview—identifies a single trauma that causes current distress, 17 items, clinician-rated
- PTSD Symptom Scale—interview for DSM-5 (PSS-1–5)—assess PTS symptoms, 24 items, self-report
- SPAN Self Report Screen—symptoms of PTSD, 4 items, self-report
- SPRINT Self Report Screen—PTSD symptom assessment, 8 items, self-report
- Structured Clinical Interview: PTSD Module—measures DSM-5 diagnosis & lifetime experience, 15 min., clinician-rated
- Structured Interview for PTSD (SI-PTSD)—assess PTSD symptoms, 17 items, clinician-rated
- Structured Trauma-Related Experience & Symptoms—measures lifetime exposure and symptoms, 25 items, self-report,
- Trauma History Questionnaire (THQ)—measures experience with potentially traumatic events, 24 items, self-report
- Trauma Screening Questionnaire—40 (TSC-40)—measures trauma symptoms, 40 items, self-report
- Trauma Symptom Inventory (TSI)—measures acute & chronic posttraumatic symptoms, 136 items, self-report
- Treatment-Outcome Posttraumatic Stress Disorder Scale—measures symptoms, 8 items, clinical-rated

Appendix C Internet Links on Vicarious Trauma, Trama-Informed Care, and Training

Organization	Web link
Aboriginal Peoples & Historic Trauma	www.ccnsa-nccah.ca/Publications/Lists/Publications/Attachments/142/2015-04-28-AguiarHalseth-RPT-IntergenTraumaHistory-EN-Web.pdf
Aboriginal Healing Foundation	www.ahf.ca
Academy of Cognitive Therapy	www.academyofcbt.org
ACE's Aware	www.acesaware.org/ace-fundamentals//principles-of-trauma-informed-care
Administration for Children and Families, Department of Health and Human Services	www.acf.hhs.gov/trauma-toolkit
Adverse Childhood Experiences (ACES)	www.cdc.gov/violenceprevention/aces/index.html
Adverse Childhood Experiences (ACEs): Impact on Brain, Body & Behavior. 6:02 min	www.youtube.com/watch?v=W-8jTTIsJ7Q
Alberta Health Services, Free eLearning Series	www.albertahealthservices.ca/info/page15526.aspx
American Academy of Experts in Traumatic Stress	www.aaets.org
Association for Behavioral & Cognitive Therapies	www.abct.org
Association for Psychological Therapies	www.aptcanada.com/trauma-focused-cbt-training.html
Acceptance and Commitment Therapy (with Dr. Ross Harris)	www.ImLearningACT.com
Canadian Mental Health Association	www.mha.ca/brochure/post-traumatic-stress-disorder-ptsd/
Canadian Psychological Association	www.cpa.ca/sections/traumaticstress/
CBT Training Centre of the North	https://rolespsychotherapy.com/cbt-training-of-the-north/
Center for Preparedness and Response, Center for Disease Control and Prevention	www.cdc.gov/cpr/infographics/6_principles_trauma_info.htm
Center on the Developing Child at Harvard University	www.developingchild.harvard.edu/science/key-concepts/toxic-str
Crisis and Trauma Resource Institute Inc. (CTRI)	www.ctrinstitute.com
Depression and Bipolar Support Alliance (DBSA)	www.dbsalliance.org
EMDR Institute	www.emdr.com/

(continued)

(continued)

Organization	Web link
Trauma and violence-informed approaches to policy and practice	https://www.canada.ca/en/public-health/services/publications/health-risks-safety/trauma-violence-informed-approaches-policy-practice.html
International Trauma Training Institute	www.traumaonline.net/certified-clinical-trauma-professional/cctp/
Klinic Community Health Center	www.klinic.mb.ca
Manitoba Training and Information and Education Center	www.trauma-informed.ca
Motivational Interviewing Network of Trainers. (MINT)	www.motivationalinterviewing.org www.motivationalinterview.org/trining/tnt2004.pdf
National Alliance for the Mentally Ill (NAMI)	www.nami.org
National Child Traumatic Stress Network	www.nctsn.org/trauma-informed-care
National Empowerment Center	www.power2u.org
National Mental Health Consumers' Self-Help Clearinghouse	www.mhselfhelp.org
National Technical Assistance Center (NATC)	www.nasmhpd.org/ntac
PILOTS database at Dartmouth	www.search.proquest.com/pilots/?accountid=28179
PTSD Association of Canada	www.ptsdassociation.com
Provincial Health Services Authority of BC 2013. Trauma-informed practice guide	www.bccewh/bc/ca/wp-content/upload/2012/05/2013_TIP-Guide/pdf
Recognize & Sustain Change Talk Round HD	www.youtube.com/watch?v=3iNl4tQuGNw
Roles & Associates Psychotherapy Services Inc	https://rolespsychotherapy.com/
SAMHSA's National Mental Health Information Center	www.mentalhealth.samhsa.gov
SAMHSA: Resources for Child Trauma-Informed Care	www.samhsa.gov/childrens-awareness-day/past-events/2018/child-traumatic-stress-resources
SAMHSA: TIP 57: Trauma-Informed Care in Behavioral Health Services	www.store.samhsa.gov/product/TIP-57-Trauma-informed-Care-in-Behavioural-Health-Services/SMA4816
SAMHSA: Trauma and Violence	www.samhsa.gov/trauma-violence
Sidran Foundation	www.sidran.org
Substance Abuse and Mental Health Services Administration: SAMHSA's Concept of Trauma and Guidance for a Trauma Informed Approach	www.samhsa.gov/resource/dbhis/samhsas-concept-trauma-guidance-trauma-informed-approach
The 7 Surprising Ways to Heal without Medication. Dr. Van Der Kolk. 1:45 min	https://www.youtube.com/watch?v=lrOBHyDRS-c

(continued)

(continued)

Organization	Web link
TF-CBT	www.tfcbt.org.training
Trauma-Informed Care Implementation Resources Center	www.traumainformedcare.chcs.org
Trauma Training Initiative	www.albertahealthservices.ca/info/page15526.aspx
Trauma and violence. (2019)	https://www.samhsa.gov/trauma-violence
Trauma Association of Canada	www.traumacanada.org/resources/links-and-resources/
Trauma- and Violence Informed Care (TVIC) Tool	www.equiphealthcare.ca/files/2021/05/G.TV-EQUIP-Tool-TVIC-Spring2021.pdf
Trauma-informed Practice Guidelines	www.cewh.ca/wp-content/uploads/2012/05/2013_TIP-Guide.pdf
Understanding the Effects of Trauma on Health	www.chcs.org/media/understanding-trauma-fact-sheet_071217.pdf
Understanding Trauma Later in Life	www.kmb.camh.ca/uploads/77b3ebd7-ec5c-412d-ac80-966fe52f9ddf.pdf

References

Arthur, E., Seymour, A., Dartnall, M., Beltgens, P., Poole, N., Smylie, D., North, N., & Schmidt, R. (2013). Trauma-Informed Practice Guide. BC Provincial Mental Health and Substance Use Planning Council. https://cewh.ca/wp-content/uploads/2012/05/2013_TIP-Guide.pdf

Bartoskova, L. (2015). Research into post-traumatic growth in the therapist: A critical literature. *Counseling Psychology Review, 30*(f3), 57-68.

Bellis, M. D. & Zisk, A. (2014). The biological effects of childhood trauma. *Child and Adolescent Psychiatric Clinics of North America, 23,* 185-222.

Bloom, S. (1999). *Final Action Plan: A Coordinated Community-Based Response to Family Violence.* Attorney General of Pennsylvania's Family Violence Task Force.

Bloom, S. (2006) *Human Service Systems and Organizational Stress: Thinking and Feeling Our Way out of Existing Organizational Dilemmas (Report for the Trauma Task Force).* Community Works.

Boyer, S. M., Caplan, J. E., & Edward, L. K. (2022). Trauma-related dissociation and the dissociative disorders: Neglected symptoms with severe public health consequences. *Del J Public Health, 8*(2), 78-84.

Canadian Centre on Substance Abuse and Addiction. (2014). *Essentials of Trauma-informed Care.* Author. www.ccsa.ca/trauma-informed-care-essentials-series

Cowling, T. & MacDougall, D. (2019, February 20). *Nabilone for the Treatment of Post-Traumatic Stress Disorder: A Review of Clinical Effectiveness and Guidelines.* Canadian Agency for Drugs and Technologies in Health. PMID: 31553551.

Earls, M. F. (2018). Trauma-informed primary care: Prevention, recognition, and promotion resilience. *NCMJ, 70*(2), 108-111.

Elliot, D., Bjelajac, P., Fallot, R., Markoff, L., & Glover Reed, B. (2005) Trauma-informed or trauma denied: Principles and implementation of trauma-informed services for women. *Journal of Community Psychology, 33*, 461-477.

Evans, A. & Coccoma, P. (2014). Trauma-informed care: How neuroscience influences practice. Routledge.

Felitti, V.J., Anda, R.F., Nordenberg, D., Williamson, D.F, Spitz, A.M., Edwards,V., Koss, M.P., & Marks, J.S. (1998). Relationship of childhood abuse and household dysfunctions to many of the leading causes of death in adults. The adverse childhood experiences study. *American Journal of Preventive Medicine, 14*(4), 245–258.

Fisher, J. (2017). *Healing the fragmented selves of trauma survivors: Overcoming internal self-alienation.* Routledge. Framo, J. (1981). The integration of marital therapy sessions with family of origins. In A. Gurman & D. Kniskern (Eds.) *Handbook of Family Therapy*, (pp. 133-158). Routledge

Freiven, P. & Lanius, R. (2015). *Healing the traumatized self: Consciousness, neuroscience, treatment.* W. W. Norton & Co.

Friedman, M. J. (2015). *Posttraumatic and acute stress disorder.* (6th Edition). Springer.

Gutierres, S. E. & Van Puymbroeck, C. (2006). Childhood and adult violence in the lives of women who misuse substances. *Aggression & Violent Behaviour, 11*(5), 497-513.

Harned, M. S. (2022). *Treating trauma in dialectical behaviour therapy.* The Guilford Press.

Harris, M. & Fallot, R. (2001). *Using trauma theory to design service systems. New Directions for Mental Health Services.* Jossey Bass.

Haskell, L. (2018, November 28). Understanding neurobiological consequences of trauma in the context of sexual and domestic violence. [Lecture].Woman Abuse Working Group meeting, Hamilton.

Heningberg, N., Kalember, P., Petrovic, Z. K., & Sicic, A. (2019). Neuroimagery research in post-traumatic stress disorder - focus on amygdala, hippocampus and prefrontal cortex. *Progress in Neuro-psychopharmacology and Biologic Psychiatry, 90*, 37-42.

Herman, J. (1992). *Trauma and recovery.* Harper Collins.

Howell, E. (2020). *Trauma and dissociation informed psychotherapy: Relational healing and the therapeutic connection.* W. W. Norton & Co.

Jean Tweed Centre. (2013).*Trauma Matters: Guidelines for Trauma-informed Practices in Women's Substance User Services.* Trauma-Matters-online-version-August-2013.pdf (jeantweed.com)

Kozlowska, K. Walker. P., McLean, H., & Carrive, P. (2015). Fear and defense a cascade: Clinical implications and management. *Harvard Review of Psychiatry, 22*(4), 263-287.

Lanius, R. A. (2015). Trauma-related dissociation and altered states of consciousness: A call for clinical treatment, neuroscience research. *Eur. J. Psycholol Traumatology, 6*, 1-9.

Malchiodi, C. A. (2020). *Trauma and expressive arts therapy.* The Guilford Press.

Mueser, K. T., Goodman, L. B., Trumbetta, S. L., Rosenberg, S. D., Osher, F. C., Vidaver, R., Auciello, P., & Foy, D. W. (1998). Trauma and posttraumatic stress disorder in severe mental illness. *Journal of Consulting and Clinical Psychology, 66*(3), 493–499. https://doi.org/10.1037/0022-006X.66.3.493

McHugh, L. & Egan, J. (2023). Psychological and somatic manifestations of dissociation: the role of childhood trauma, attachment and alexithymia. *Europea J of Trauma & Dissociation, 7*(1), 100316.

Middleton, J. S. & Potter, C. C. (2015). Relationship between vicarious traumatization and turnover among child welfare professionals. *Journal of Public Child Welfare, 9*(2), 195-216.

Nadew, S. (2012). Residential school related to increased female incarceration. *Windspeaker, 30*(4), 11-12.

Ponic, P. Varcoe, C., & Smutylo, T. (2016). *Trauma-(and violence-) informed approaches to supporting victims of violence: Policy and practice considerations.* Victims of Crime Research Digest, 9, 3–15. Government of Canada. https://www.justice.gc.ca/eng/rp-pr/cj-jp/victim/rd9-rr9/p2.html

Read, J. Fosse, R., Moskowitz, A., & Perry, B. (2014). The trauma genic neurodevelopmental model of psychosis revisited. *Neuropsychiatry, 4*(1), 65-79.

Schafer, I. (2009). Posttraumatic disorders in patients with substance use disorder: A German multi-center study. *European Psychiatry, 24*(1), S247.

Sotero, M.M. (2006). A conceptual model of historical trauma:Implications for public health practice and research. *Journal of Health Disparities Research and Practice, 1*(1), 93-108.

Substance Abuse and Mental Health Service Administration (2014). *SAMHSA's Concept of Trauma and Guidance for a Trauma Informed Approach* (HSS Publication No.(SMA) 14–4884). Author. https://ncsacw.acf.hhs.gov/userfiles/files/SAMHSA_Trauma.pdf

Sweeney, A., Felson, B, Kennedy, A., Collinson, L. & Gillard, S. (2018). A paradigm shift: Relationships in trauma-informed mental health services. *British J Psych Advances, 24,* 319-333.

Treleaven, D. A. (2018). *Trauma-sensitive mindfulness.* W. W. Norton & Company.

Van Der Kolk, B. (2014). *The body keeps the score.* Penguin Books.

Van Der Kolk, B. & Fisher, R. (1995). Dissociation and fragmentary nature of traumatic memories: Overview and exploratory study. *J of Traumatic Stress, 8,* 505-525.

Van Mol, M. M. C., Kompanje, E. J. O., Dominique, D. B., Bakker, J & Nijkamp, M. D. (2015). The prevalence of compassion fatigue and burnout among healthcare professionals in intensive care units: A systematic review. *PLoS ONE 10*(9), 1-22.

Walker, P. (2013). *Complex PTSD: From surviving to thriving.* CreateSpace Independent Publishing.

Wathen, C. N., & Varcoe, C. (2021). Trauma & violence-informed care (TVIC): A tool for health & Social Service Organizations & Providers. Gender, Trauma, and Violence Knowledge Indicator and Equip Health Care.

Part II
Current State of Nurse Psychotherapy—Being

Chapter 6
Delivery of Nurse Psychotherapy: Public Sector

Archna N. Patel and Siobhan Bell

Abstract Practicing psychotherapy as a nurse in public sectors may include government-funded facilities both in the community and in hospital. This chapter will give an overview of the dynamic role of the nurse psychotherapist in public-sector healthcare systems. The expectations, roles, and responsibilities of working within interdisciplinary teams will be outlined. The impact of government funding models will be introduced to better elucidate the extent of involvement for: (a) psychotherapeutic interventions, (b) individual and group sessions, (c) length of sessions and duration in care (d) additional responsibilities of coordinating care aspects within systems, (e) appropriate continuum of care and transitioning from one setting to another and (f) overall unique expectations and aspects in parameters of care. Components of care will be reviewed to better understand how to navigate care provisions in the public health system working in the role of the nurse psychotherapist including collaboration with family systems, legal aspects such as the Public Hospitals Act (1990), consent and capacity, Substitute Decision Maker, Power of Attorney, and the mental health act. Working within funding models will also be discussed.

Keywords Public practice · Hospital psychotherapy

Learning Objectives

After completing this chapter, the learner will:

1. Understand the different settings for public health care in Ontario.
2. Examine the models of care that exist within the public health setting for psychotherapy.
3. Articulate the scope of practice of nurse psychotherapists in the public sector.

A. N. Patel (✉)
Woodbridge, ON, Canada
e-mail: archnap@gmail.com

S. Bell
Mono, ON, Canada

S. Roles and K. Kalia (eds.), *The Nurses' Guide to Psychotherapy*,
https://doi.org/10.1007/978-981-97-4738-2_6

4. Examine the duration of care and different practices around psychotherapy sessions in the public setting.
5. Examine the roles and responsibilities involved in both individual and group sessions.
6. Examine the additional responsibilities of being a care coordinator within the public health system when working with mental health.
7. Articulate an understanding of the legal aspects of care.

1 Introduction

Nurse psychotherapists are found in many places across the world. Within Canada, nurse psychotherapists can be found in most provinces and territories, although potentially being called by a different name or being regulated by a non-nursing regulatory body. Specifically in Ontario, the role of the nurse psychotherapist has existed in hospitals for years, using the title mental health or addictions nurse.

The public health sector encompasses a vast and diverse landscape within our healthcare system including hospitals and community outreach and treatment programs. This chapter examines the intricate and dynamic role of nurse psychotherapists within these public sector domains. This chapter will explore the expectations, roles, and responsibilities that come with this multifaceted role, shedding light on the pivotal role of interdisciplinary collaboration in achieving holistic patient care. Nurse psychotherapists in the public sector operate in a constantly evolving environment, where government funding models play a pivotal role in shaping the extent and nature of psychotherapy access. Throughout this chapter, we will dissect the impact of these funding model changes, unraveling their implications for psychotherapy access. We will explore the importance of ensuring a seamless continuum of care and navigating transitions between different care settings, all while meeting the unique expectations and parameters of care set within the public sector framework.

2 Scope of Practice

The American Psychiatric Association (2023) defines psychotherapy as a type of treatment that can help individuals experiencing a wide array of mental health conditions and emotional challenges. Psychotherapy can help not only alleviate symptoms, but also, certain types of psychotherapies can help identify the psychological root causes of one's condition so a person can function better and have enhanced emotional well-being and healing. (para. 1).

This is a widely accepted definition of what the intervention of psychotherapy is. How that is applied or regulated differs from county to country and within Canada, from province to province. Each practitioner is responsible to seek out their own individual scope of practice understanding from the organizations that regulate psychotherapy in the place that they live and/or practice. Ontario is an exemplary province that regulates psychotherapy and that specifies how regulated health professionals like nurses are required to practice. In Ontario, psychotherapy is a controlled act and is defined as "...an intense client-therapist relationship which often involves the examination of deeply emotional experiences, destructive behaviour patterns and serious mental health issues" (Health Professions Regulatory Advisory Council, 2006). While registered nurses and registered practical nurses in Ontario do not require an order to perform the controlled act of psychotherapy in private practice, they may require one in public hospitals due to the interpretation of the Public Hospitals Act (1990). This regulation informs their ability to practice psychotherapy and leads to an understanding of the required scope of practice which is set out in the regulatory bodies' documents. It is important that nurses who are thinking of implementing a psychotherapeutic intervention, first ensure that they understand the regulatory requirements of their province and country.

3 Psychotherapeutic Sessions

Individual and group psychotherapeutic sessions are integral to the care plan for patients in public healthcare settings. Individual sessions can be as short as 20 min and as long as hours, depending on the need identified in the individual care plan. Group sessions are utilized routinely in in-patient and outpatient care settings. The benefits of group therapy are that groups can act as both peer support with psychotherapy and shorten waitlist times. Many clients are surprised by the benefits of group therapy and how much it can act as a grounding experience to be heard by people who are also likely to have experienced something similar. Speaking openly about your experiences can be cathartic and promote learning. Another benefit to group therapy is that within a group there is an array of personalities, backgrounds, beliefs, and experiences. This can provide many different lenses to the client's problem—beyond what a therapist can provide independently. Nurse psychotherapists in group sessions act as facilitators. They encourage engagement, honesty, assist in problem-solving, and hold all members accountable to the agreed-upon group norms, such as safety, privacy, and rules about socialization and relationships outside of the group. For more information on group psychotherapy, see Chap. 10.

4 Roles and Responsibilities in Individual and Group Sessions

Individual therapeutic sessions are founded on the therapeutic nurse-patient relationship. For more information on the nurse-client relationship, please see Chaps. 3 and 4. While the group therapeutic session also requires the nurse psychotherapist to have a therapeutic nurse-patient relationship with the group members, it does not usually have the same depth of therapeutic connection required in an individual session. In individual sessions, the nurse psychotherapist establishes a therapeutic alliance with their patient and guides the implementation of a therapeutic modality. For more on individual psychotherapy please see Chap. 9.

5 Coordinators of Care

Nursing regulatory bodies and associations across Canada put coordination of care as an important role that nurses play (College of Nurses of Ontario [CNO], 2023; British Columbia College of Nurses and Midwives [BCCNM], 2020; College of Registered Nurses of Alberta [CRNA], 2023; Saskatchewan Registered Nurses Association [SRNA], 2019). The College of Nurses of Ontario (CNO), British Columbia College of Nurses and Midwives (BCNM), College of Registered Nurses of Alberta (CRNA), and the Saskatchewan Registered Nurses Association (SRNA) all discuss that one of the unique roles of the nurse is as a coordinator of care (CNO, 2023; BCCNM, 2020; CRNA, 2023; SRNA, 2019). This is especially true in the work of the nurse psychotherapist. As nurses, we are acutely aware that a person's mental health and well-being are influenced by their world. Nurses are aware of the intersections of the social determinants of health and how they influence the client's journey. This unique awareness allows nurse psychotherapists to work as coordinators of care between the medical community, social supports, and clients in the community and within the public hospital system. As a coordinator of care, nurses ensure that services needed happen at "…the right time and in the correct sequence" (CNO 2019, p. 7). This includes ensuring that clients receive referrals and advocacy to appropriate service providers. Having a systems and population view of the healthcare system helps nurse psychotherapists provide this coordination of care in a way that supports patients and their needs.

6 Healthcare Settings

Canada's publicly funded healthcare framework is called Medicare. Rather than a unified national plan, Canada operates with 13 distinct provincial and territorial health insurance plans. Within this structure, all Canadian residents have access to essential healthcare services without paying out of pocket. The allocation of roles and responsibilities in healthcare services is a collaborative effort between provincial/territorial governments and the federal government. This allocation is contracted between the provincial and territorial governments in funding agreements and funding that comes to the provinces and territories through the Canada Health Transfer (Government of Canada 2023a). Provincial and territorial governments hold responsibility for managing, organizing, and delivering healthcare services to their respective residents.

In Canada, public health care is primarily governed by provincial healthcare funding arrangements which guarantee the right to access care. The provincial and territorial governments are: Ontario Health Insurance Plan (OHIP), Insured Benefits Branch of Manitoba, Alberta Health Insurance Plan, Government of Saskatchewan Fully Covered Health Services, Medical Services Plan for British Columbia, Health PEI (Prince Edward Island), Newfoundland and Labrador Medical Care Plan, Quebec Health Insurance Plan (RAMQ), New Brunswick Medicare, NWT (Northwest Territories) Health Care Plan, Nova Scotia Health, Nunavut Health Care Plan, Yukon Health Insurance Plan (YHCIP), Non-Insured Health Benefits for First Nations and Inuit (NIHB—federal health benefits for First Nations and Inuit peoples). Each provincial and territorial health plan decides what and how to provide funding. Not all provinces or territories provide funding for psychotherapy (Government of Canada 2023b). Within each of these provinces, there are three main settings in which psychotherapy is practiced: acute care, community/primary care, and residential/addiction care.

6.1 Community/Primary Care Settings

Primary care is often the first point of contact for individuals seeking health care. This includes family doctors, nurse practitioners, and community health centers. Individuals enrolled in their provincial and territorial healthcare plans including NIHB can visit these primary care settings for general health concerns, preventive care, and referrals to specialists such as psychiatry. Public health units and community health centers offer a variety of services, including immunizations, health education, and programs aimed at preventing and managing chronic diseases. These services are often community-focused and contribute to the overall well-being of the population. Mental health services are an integral part of public health care, with various programs and resources aimed at supporting individuals with mental health challenges. However, access specifically to psychotherapy is often limited or not accessible and differs by province and territory. Usually, healthcare plans only cover certain mental health services provided by psychiatrists and other mental health professionals employed within the healthcare system and programs funded by the province/territory (Government of Canada 2023a, 2023b).

6.2 Acute Care

Hospitals play a crucial role in providing acute care services, including emergency care, surgeries, and specialized treatments. Provincial, territorial, and the NIHB cover the costs associated with hospital stays, medical procedures, and necessary medications administered during a hospital visit. Psychotherapy is often provided within this setting by mental health nurses, nurse psychotherapists, social workers and social service workers, regulated psychotherapists, occupational therapists, psychologists, and physicians who are often psychiatrists (Government of Canada 2023a, 2023b).

Understanding these settings helps individuals navigate the public health care system ensuring access to essential health services and promoting overall well-being. Understanding these settings also means realizing the inequality that exists in accessing mental health services across Canada.

7 Legislation and Statutes

Each province and territory has their own legislation that governs nursing practice, healthcare and specifically, mental health and psychotherapy. In Ontario, for instance, this would include the *Nursing* Act 1991; Mental Health Act 1990; *Health Care Consent Act*, 1993; and the *Psychotherapy* Act 2007. Adherence to the standards set by the College of Nurses or the regulatory authority of the province/territory is paramount, and nurses are encouraged to engage in continuous professional development. Nurses must practice within their scope of practice and maintain the necessary competence in their role. This may include attending workshops, seminars, or webinars offered by legal experts and professional organizations in nursing. These events often cover current legal issues and updates related to practice.

8 Informed Consent and Capacity

Informed consent is a fundamental legal aspect of patient care, starting with the appropriate legislation for healthcare consent in that province. This includes examining in detail how to ensure nurse psychotherapists are obtaining valid consent. Prior to treatment, informed consent must be obtained from the patient, ensuring that they have the capacity to make decisions about their care. Capacity assessments may be required in certain cases.

9 Managing Conflicts of Interest

As a healthcare professional, nurses have a legal and ethical duty to identify and avoid conflicts of interest that may compromise the best interests of their patients. It is a critical aspect of practicing psychotherapy as a nurse. Some key aspects nurse psychotherapists need to examine related to conflicts of interest are:

- Any conflict of interest that may compromise the best interests of their clients.
- Always prioritizing the best interests of clients when making decisions or providing care.

- Avoiding any actions or decisions that could benefit the nurse financially or personally at the expense of clients or their well-being.
- Being transparent about any financial interests for themselves or that immediate family members may have in healthcare facilities, products, or services that are recommended to clients. Disclosure of these relationships to clients can help to maintain trust.
- Should a conflict of interest exist, ensuring that clients are fully informed about it and facilitate their transition of care to another provider as required.
- Continuously seeking guidance from regulatory bodies for specifics on ethical standards (code of conduct) and how to manage conflicts of interest within their province/territory.

10 Publicly Funded Mental Healthcare Programs

Nurses must understand the intricacies of publicly funded healthcare programs and how these programs affect patient's access to psychotherapy services. Publicly funded services may have limitations on the number of sessions or the duration of treatment, potentially affecting the depth of therapeutic work. Publicly funded services may have more standardized treatment protocols, and the range of available therapies and interventions may be more limited. Publicly funded services aim to provide access to care for a broad range of individuals, including those with financial constraints. However, there may be longer wait times due to higher demand, and clients might have less choice in selecting a specific therapist and may be assigned to one based on availability. Clients may have little to no direct cost for services, depending on their eligibility and the specific program.

11 Scope of Practice in Interdisciplinary Teams

Each healthcare professional in the interdisciplinary team must work within their defined scope of practice as outlined by their respective regulatory bodies. It's important to understand and respect these boundaries to avoid conflicts and to ensure effective teamwork with safe and effective client care. When healthcare professionals from different disciplines work together, it's often beneficial to establish formal collaboration agreements. These agreements should outline roles, responsibilities, and communication channels to ensure seamless client care. It is essential to understand the communication structure in order to ensure the maintenance of strict adherence to patient confidentiality and privacy laws, such as the Personal Health Information Protection Act (PHIPA), ensuring that information sharing within the team complies with PHIPA regulations and privacy laws. When multiple healthcare providers are involved in a client's care, nurses must ensure that informed consent is obtained for all aspects of treatment. Clients should be fully informed about their care plan and the roles of each team member. Proper documentation is crucial for record keeping and communication of care. All team members should maintain accurate and comprehensive client health records. This documentation can be legally significant in the event of disputes or legal actions. Disagreements or conflicts within the interdisciplinary team should be resolved through established protocols or policies, and in a manner that prioritizes client care. Failure to do so can lead to legal disputes or disciplinary actions. Being aware of the regulations and standards of practice specific to each profession within the team ensures that actions align with these standards to prevent legal issues. Effective and clear communication within the team is vital as miscommunication or misunderstandings can lead to subpar care, errors, or legal issues. Secure and approved channels for communication about patient care are important in maintaining confidentiality.

12 Reflective Questions

1. How does the definition of psychotherapy provided by the American Psychiatric Association resonate with your understanding of the scope of practice of nurse psychotherapists in your region of practice or one you have read about?
2. Have you personally witnessed instances within the public healthcare sector, where psychotherapy has not only alleviated symptoms but also identified root causes for improved functioning and emotional well-being? What were the key parts of this instance that made it useful?
3. Considering the variation in the application and regulation of psychotherapy across different provinces and territories, how do you think these differences may impact the quality and accessibility of mental health services?
4. Can you identify any potential challenges or advantages associated with diverse regulatory frameworks?
5. Using your understanding of national and provincial healthcare, how might the distinction between outpatient/community practice and acute settings impact the practice of nurses in mental healthcare?
6. What ethical considerations should healthcare practitioners consider when navigating these regulatory requirements, especially in terms of providing psychotherapeutic interventions?

13 Case Vignette

13.1 Navigating Public Health Settings as a New Nurse Psychotherapist

Salema, a nurse psychotherapist, begins their career in the public health sector in Ontario, Canada. Their role involves providing psychotherapeutic interventions to individuals with mental health challenges within an acute care hospital's acute care mental health unit. Salema is tasked with delivering psychotherapeutic interventions to acute inpatient mental health patients that support individuals experiencing acute psychiatric crises. Salema faces the unique challenges and opportunities presented in the acute care setting. The unit serves as a critical component of the broader public health system, offering specialized care to those in immediate need. Salema actively participates in individual and group psychotherapeutic sessions within the acute care unit. They also take on the role of a care coordinator, ensuring continuity of care for individuals transitioning between the acute care unit and community-based services.

13.1.1 Salema's Observations

- Salema witnesses the urgent nature of mental health challenges, where timely interventions are essential.
- Collaborative and interprofessional care are emphasized, with Salema working alongside psychiatrists, and other healthcare professionals.
- The acute care setting requires quick assessments and adaptable interventions to address the immediate needs of individuals in crisis.
- The duration of care varies, with some individuals requiring brief, intensive interventions, while others may benefit from ongoing support.
- Salema's responsibilities extend beyond direct psychotherapy to coordination with community resources, facilitating a seamless transition for individuals leaving the hospital.
- Salema ensures that individuals have the capacity to provide informed consent for psychotherapeutic interventions, considering the unique legal aspects related to mental health care.
- Confidentiality is maintained, with exceptions aligned with legal obligations, such as situations involving client harm to self or others.
- Salema navigates the legal framework of the Mental Health Act when engaging with individuals who may require involuntary psychiatric assessments.

13.2 *Reflective Questions for Case Vignette*

1. How does Salema's experience in the acute care mental health unit differ from other public health settings in Ontario, such as rehabilitative/addictions or outpatient clinics?
2. In the acute care setting, what psychotherapeutic models might be particularly effective in addressing the immediate needs of individuals in crisis? How do these models differ from those used in more preventive-focused settings?
3. What aspects of Salema's scope of practice are particularly relevant in the acute care hospital setting?
4. How does the acute nature of mental health challenges impact the autonomy and collaborative aspects of Salema's practice?
5. How does the acute nature of the mental health unit influence the duration and frequency of psychotherapeutic sessions?
6. Are there specific considerations in an acute care setting that affect the structure and content of sessions?
7. What unique roles and responsibilities would Salema encounter in individual psychotherapeutic sessions compared to group sessions within the acute care unit? How do these roles contribute to the overall care of individuals in crisis?
8. In what ways could Salema navigate the additional responsibilities of being a care coordinator in the acute care hospital setting?
9. How does this coordination contribute to the continuum of care for individuals transitioning from the hospital to the community? How can Salema ensure that this continuum is seamless?
10. How could Salema navigate legal considerations in obtaining informed consent for psychotherapeutic interventions in the acute care setting?
11. What steps could Salema take to ensure adherence to the Mental Health legislation in your province or a province or territory you've researched?

14 Summary

- Nurses may practice psychotherapy in the public sector, such as in hospitals or in the community.
- Funding models and practice settings influence the accessibility of psychotherapy and vary across Canada.
- Considerations for care provision such as consent and capacity, confidentiality, as well as managing conflicts of interest must be addressed in practice.

References

American Psychiatric Association. (2023). *What is psychotherapy?* Author. https://www.psychiatry.org/patients-families/psychotherapy

British Columbia College of Nurses and Midwives [BCCNM]. (2020). *Nurse practitioners and registered nurses standards of practice.* Author. https://www.bccnm.ca/Documents/standards_practice/rn/RN_NP_Professional_Standards.pdf

College of Registered Nurses of Alberta [CRNA]. (2023). *Practice standards for registrants.* Author. https://www.nurses.ab.ca/media/1mkkxvxi/practice-standards-for-registrants-2023.pdf College of Nurses of Ontario (2019). *Entry to practice competencies for Registered Nurses.*Author. https://www.cno.org/globalassets/docs/reg/41037-entry-to-practice-competencies-2020.pdf

Government of Canada (2023a). *Canada's healthcare system.* Author. https://www.canada.ca/en/health-canada/services/canada-health-care-system.html

Government of Canada (2023b). *Provincial and Territorial health care.* Author. https://www.canada.ca/en/health-canada/services/health-care-system/canada-health-care-system-medicare/provincial-territorial-health-care-resources.html

Health Care Consent Act, 1996, S.O. 1996, c. 2, Sched. A https://www.ontario.ca/laws/statute/96h02

Mental Health Act, R.S.O. 1990, c. M.7. https://www.ontario.ca/laws/statute/90m07

Nursing Act, 1991, S.O. 1991, c. 32. https://www.ontario.ca/laws/statute/91n32

Psychotherapy Act, 2007, S.O. 2007, c. 10, Sched. R. https://www.ontario.ca/laws/statute/07p10

Saskatchewan Registered Nurses Association [SRNA]. (2019). https://www.crns.ca/wp-content/uploads/2019/09/RN-Practice-Standards-2019.pdf

Chapter 7
Delivery of Nurse Psychotherapy: Private Sector

Siobhan Bell and Archna N. Patel

Abstract Psychotherapy is practiced by nurses in private and independent practice all over Canada. Nurses who practice psychotherapy are able to bring not only the practice of a psychotherapeutic modality but also their foundational nursing knowledge, their holistic and client-centred approach, and their knowledge of pharmacology. This chapter will explore the evolving world of private nursing psychotherapy, the supports available for independent practice, the practice requirements for nurses in independent practice, as well as the legalities and insurance considerations when operating as an independent practitioner.

Keywords Private practice · Independent practice · Nurse psychotherapy

Learning Objectives

After completing this chapter, the learner will be able to:

1. Examine the role of nurse psychotherapists in private or independent practice.
2. Identify challenges in private or independent practice with discrepancies in health insurance.
3. Identify the benefits and uniqueness that nurse psychotherapists bring to psychotherapy through their practice.

S. Bell (✉)
Mono, ON, Canada
e-mail: sbell@nursingatheart.ca

A. N. Patel
Woodbridge, ON, Canada

S. Roles and K. Kalia (eds.), *The Nurses' Guide to Psychotherapy*,
https://doi.org/10.1007/978-981-97-4738-2_7

1 The Nurse Psychotherapist in Private and Independent Practice

Nurse psychotherapists in private and independent practice play a multifaceted role in the mental healthcare landscape. They offer clients a unique blend of nursing expertise and psychotherapeutic interventions. One of the primary roles of the nurse psychotherapist is to offer a holistic approach to mental health and well-being. Drawing from their foundational nursing knowledge, they consider not only the psychological aspects of a client's condition but also their physical, emotional, and social well-being. This holistic perspective enables the nurse psychotherapist to offer comprehensive care to their clients that address the full spectrum of their needs.

Nurse psychotherapists in private practice are instrumental in delivering client-centred care. They prioritize their client's preferences and ensure that the goals of each client are tailored to their psychotherapeutic interventions. This client-centred approach fosters a therapeutic alliance built on trust, collaboration, and shared decision-making. It empowers clients to participate in their treatment journey actively and enhances the overall effectiveness of psychotherapy.

In private practice, nurse psychotherapists also navigate the complexities of legal and ethical considerations, ensuring they adhere to the regulatory framework set forth by their regulatory body. This involves maintaining a high standard of professional conduct, safeguarding client confidentiality, and adhering to ethical principles that underpin their practice. They ensure this by following any standards including their colleges' guidelines on scope of practice, code of conduct, independent practice, applicable ethical standards, and legislation governing private health information. By upholding these standards, nurse psychotherapists in private practice contribute to the integrity and credibility of the profession, fostering trust among clients and the broader healthcare community.

2 Determining Scope of Practice

When entering private psychotherapy practice, nurses must ensure that they know their individual scope of practice. Ontario is one of the only Canadian provinces to have psychotherapy clearly outlined in their nursing scope of practice and therefore will be used as an exemplar to learn from. In Ontario, the College of Nurses of Ontario (CNO) states that nurses must have the "...authority, context and competence" to practice psychotherapy (CNO, 2023, p. 2). For example, the CNO describes authority as knowing "...their legislated scope of practice, including controlled acts, and authorizing mechanisms" (CNO, 2023, p. 3). Nurses determine "... if their practice environment or setting supports the performance of an activity and has the available resources to support safe client care" and competence to practice as nurses ensuring that "...nurses have the individual knowledge, skill, and judgment to perform an activity (CNO, 2023, p. 3). Utilizing these three areas, nurses need to reflect on whether they meet these criteria to perform the controlled act of psychotherapy, or if they practice in regions without a controlled act, ensuring that they are following equivalent standards and guidelines. Nurses will need to seek out further education and training in psychotherapeutic modalities to complement their nursing education and practice experience in order to meet these criteria.

3 The Challenges of Private Practice

Private or independent practice is a place where practitioners can create unique client experiences. Challenges of private practice versus practicing in a public setting can include the loneliness and isolation that may arise from practicing in a solo environment. This means that nurse psychotherapists may need to seek out group practices or interactions with peers purposely, rather than as it typically occurs in a traditional nursing environment with other nurses in the public realm. Another potential challenge may be the fiscal responsibility of owning one's own practice (Barry, 2005). Like all entrepreneurs and small business owners, private practice overhead can be expensive. Specifically, some of the private practice expenses include things like business insurance, rent for office space, licensing for administrative and/or clinical tools, technology, and potentially additional staff. Nurses can take advantage of small business networks, discounts and participate in nursing associations for peer support to mitigate financial pressures (Barry, 2005). A third challenge in private nurse psychotherapy practice may also include the lack of recognition by insurance companies in billing for services. Unfortunately, many insurance companies have not updated their policies to reflect the changes in the ever-expanding scope of nurses and although nurses have been performing psychotherapy for decades, many insurance companies still do not cover nurses as a profession delivering these services to this day. Continued advocacy efforts are required to promote change. The practice of nursing "is the promotion of health and the assessment of, the provision of care for, and the treatment of health conditions by supportive, preventative, therapeutic, palliative and rehabilitative means in order to attain or maintain optimal function" (CNO, 2023, p. 3). This definition of nursing informs all nurses, including nurse psychotherapists in private and independent practice, demonstrating that their role in every client interaction needs to be nursing focused. Nurses have a uniquely holistic approach to well-being, with a licensing mandate to see a person and their reason for seeking support through that holistic lens. This lens can culminate in a client experience that incorporates many areas of their life and one that considers their mental health from all the areas that it intersects.

4 Reflective Questions

1. How does the incorporation of a holistic approach by nurse psychotherapists in private practice contribute to the overall well-being of their clients?
2. Give an example of how considering a client's physical, emotional, and social aspects of their life would improve the effectiveness of psychotherapeutic interventions?
3. Reflect on the significance of a client-centered approach in psychotherapy. How does prioritizing client preferences and involving them in shared decision-making contribute to a therapeutic alliance?
4. Can you think of a situation where client-centered care positively influenced the outcome of psychotherapeutic interventions?
5. Consider the complexities of legal and ethical considerations in private practice for nurse psychotherapists. How does adherence to regulatory frameworks, maintaining professional conduct, and safeguarding client confidentiality contribute to the integrity of the nursing profession in independent practice?
6. In your current practice or future aspirations, how would you approach determining your individual scope of practice as a nurse psychotherapist?
7. Reflect on the importance of having the authority, context, and competence as outlined by your regulatory body. Are there specific challenges you anticipate in meeting these criteria?
8. Consider the challenges outlined for nurse psychotherapists in private and independent practice, such as potential loneliness and fiscal responsibilities. How might you proactively address or mitigate these challenges in your own independent practice? Are there strategies, group practices, or support networks you envision utilizing to enhance your experience in a different environment?

5 Case Vignette

5.1 Providing Holistic Care for a Client with Depression in Independent Nurse Psychotherapy Practice

Sophia, a seasoned nurse psychotherapist, operates an independent private practice specializing in depression and anxiety. She begins her day with a new client, Alex, who is seeking support for depression. This case study explores Sophia's independent practice approach to providing holistic care and tailoring psychotherapeutic interventions to address Alex's unique needs.

5.1.1 Client Background

Alex is a 32-year-old professional experiencing persistent feelings of sadness, lethargy, and loss of interest in daily activities for the past 6 months. Alex identifies that these feelings have been getting worse over the past 3 weeks. Recognizing the impact of the depression on their work and personal life, Alex seeks assistance from Sophia to navigate and alleviate the symptoms of depression.

5.1.2 Holistic Nursing Assessment

Sophia begins with a thorough holistic assessment, taking into account not only the psychological aspects of Alex's depression but also their physical health, emotional well-being, and social connections. She explores potential triggers, coping mechanisms, and the impact of depression on the various facets of Alex's life.

5.1.3 Tailored Psychotherapeutic Interventions

Based on the assessment, Sophia tailors psychotherapeutic interventions to address Alex's specific needs. Cognitive Behavioural Therapy (CBT) and Compassion Focused Therapy (CFT) techniques are incorporated to explore and reframe the negative thought patterns that Alex is currently experiencing. Additionally, mindfulness and relaxation exercises are introduced to enhance emotional regulation.

5.1.4 Client-Centered Approach

Sophia ensures a client-centered approach by actively involving Alex in the treatment plan. They collaboratively set realistic goals and regularly review progress. This approach fosters a therapeutic alliance built on trust, openness, collaboration, and shared decision-making.

5.1.5 Legal and Ethical Considerations

Sophia adheres to legal and ethical standards in her practice. Confidentiality is maintained, and Alex is informed about the limits of privacy, particularly in situations involving harm to self or others. Sophia continuously monitors her practice to align with the ethical principles outlined by her regulatory body.

5.1.6 Case Vignette Reflective Questions

1. How does Sophia's holistic assessment contribute to a more comprehensive understanding of Alex's depression? In what ways might considering physical, emotional, and social aspects influence the development of a tailored treatment plan?
2. Reflect on the importance of tailoring psychotherapeutic interventions for clients with depression. How might a combination of cognitive behavioural therapy, compassion-focused therapy, and mindfulness techniques address both the cognitive and emotional aspects of Alex's condition?
3. Discuss the significance of a client-centered approach in treating depression. How does actively involving the client in goal-setting and treatment decisions contribute to the therapeutic alliance? Can you think of a situation where such an approach positively influenced the outcome of psychotherapeutic interventions?
4. Consider the legal and ethical considerations needed in Sophia's practice. How does maintaining confidentiality while ensuring necessary disclosures align with ethical principles? Can you identify specific legal aspects that Sophia needs to navigate while providing psychotherapeutic interventions?
5. What are some anticipated potential challenges Sophia might face in her independent private practice?
6. What strategies or support mechanisms can Sophia employ to address challenges such as maintaining professional boundaries, handling emergencies, and ensuring ongoing professional development in the evolving field of nurse psychotherapy?

6 Summary

- Nurse psychotherapists in private practice integrate nursing expertise with psychotherapeutic interventions, offering a unique and comprehensive approach to mental healthcare.
- In private and independent practice, nurse psychotherapists prioritize client preferences, tailoring goals to individual psychotherapeutic interventions. This approach fosters a therapeutic alliance built on trust, collaboration, and shared decision-making.
- Nurse psychotherapists navigate the complexities of legal and ethical considerations, adhering to regulatory frameworks. This includes maintaining professional conduct, safeguarding client confidentiality, and upholding ethical principles outlined by their regulatory body.
- Challenges in private practice include potential loneliness and isolation, fiscal responsibilities, and recognition of the role and stance taken by insurance companies.

- Nurse psychotherapists may need to proactively seek peer interaction, utilize business networks, and advocate for policy changes to address the current challenges.
- Owning a private or independent practice involves fiscal responsibility, including managing overhead costs. Nurse psychotherapists can benefit from small business networks, joining group practices, discounts, and peer support through nursing associations to navigate these challenges.

References

Barry, P. (2005). Questions and answers for the nurse psychotherapist in private practice. *Perspectives in Psychiatric Care*. 41(*1*), 42-44.

College of Nurses of Ontario [CNO]. (2023). Scope of practice. Author. https://www.cno.org/globalassets/docs/prac/49041-scope-of-practice.pdf

Chapter 8
Delivery of Nurse Psychotherapy: Digital Technologies and Psychotherapy

Kamini Kalia and Sheeba Narikuzhy

Abstract More than ever, technology is integrated into daily life inclusive of how health care is accessed, understood, and provided. Technology can serve as a foundational resource to increase the methods by which psychotherapy is delivered, as well as the accessibility of the service to a diverse range of populations. However, to maintain the safety of the client and nurse, it is imperative that these digital tools are utilized judiciously and competently. This chapter will outline different types of technologies that have been leveraged to support the delivery of virtual care psychotherapy, the opportunities, limitations, and risks presented through the use of digital technologies, as well as considerations for safe and ethical use as part of one's psychotherapy service.

Keywords Technology · Digital health · Virtual care

Learning Objectives

After completing this chapter, the learner will:

1. Distinguish between different digital technological modalities and how they may support the delivery of psychotherapy.
2. Understand the opportunities, limitations, and risks associated with the use of technology.
3. Determine the appropriateness of technology and additional considerations to support safe psychotherapy delivery.

K. Kalia (✉)
Trillium Health Partners, Mississauga, ON, Canada
e-mail: kaminikalia@gmail.com

S. Narikuzhy
Manipal Academy of Higher Education, Ajax, ON, Canada

S. Roles and K. Kalia (eds.), *The Nurses' Guide to Psychotherapy*,
https://doi.org/10.1007/978-981-97-4738-2_8

1 Introduction

The nurse psychotherapist will have opportunities to leverage technology to strengthen the care provided or augment how care is experienced by the client. The benefits of these tools may range from increased accessibility or engagement to improved client participation in care and increased self-efficacy. Despite the incredible opportunities that arise with these ubiquitous tools, there are pitfalls that have been known to bring about concerns that may impede the safe delivery of care and even lead to harmful impacts on the nurse-client relationship. There should be a thorough assessment of the appropriate use of these technologies prior to implementation into clinical practice. With the pace of technological advancement, it can be challenging to predict what may be a risk, however, guiding principles for judicious use of digital technologies can guide critical reflection prior to integration into practice. There are various terms used to describe digital health technology when considering psychotherapy. Terms used to describe technical modalities that may offer psychotherapeutic intervention(s) include but are not limited to: virtual care, video visits, ehealth, etherapy, telemedicine, telemental health, videoconferencing, telehealth, Internet-based therapy, and mhealth (mobile mental health). This chapter will highlight different types of technologies used in psychotherapy, explain the potential pitfalls of the use of various technologies, and describe considerations for safe and ethical use.

2 Digital Health Technologies

The nurse psychotherapist will have opportunities to leverage technology to strengthen the care provided or augment how care is experienced by the client. The benefits of these tools may range from increased accessibility or engagement to improved client participation in care and increased self-efficacy. Despite the incredible opportunities that arise with these ubiquitous tools, there are pitfalls that have been known to bring about concerns that may impede the safe delivery of care and even lead to harmful impacts on the nurse-client relationship. There should be a thorough assessment of the appropriate use of these technologies prior to implementation into clinical practice. With the pace of technological advancement, it can be challenging to predict what may be a risk, however, guiding principles for judicious use of digital technologies can guide critical reflection prior to integration into practice. There are various terms used to describe digital health technology when considering psychotherapy. Terms used to describe technical modalities that may offer psychotherapeutic intervention(s) include but are not limited to: virtual care, video visits, ehealth, etherapy, telemedicine, telemental health, videoconferencing, telehealth, Internet-based therapy, and mhealth (mobile mental health). This chapter will highlight different types of technologies used to support the provision of psychotherapy, explain the potential pitfalls of the use of various technologies, and describe considerations for safe and ethical use.

3 Digital Health Technologies Used in Psychotherapy Delivery

Telemedicine/Videoconferencing Telemedicine via videoconferencing has been identified as the most frequently used digital health technology (Strudwick et al. 2019). There are several studies examining the effectiveness of the delivery of cognitive behavioural therapy (CBT) with a real-time therapist via videoconferencing or over the Internet for health concerns (Carpenter et al. 2018; McGill et al. 2017; Tsuchiyagaito et al. 2017). Videoconferencing offers the potential for multiple service providers but also members of a client's family to participate in treatment, which may even strengthen the therapeutic relationship (Hummel et al. 2018).

Interactive Simulation Another novel telemedicine example is psychotherapy administered in an avatar virtual environment called "Second Life". In one case study, Quackenbush and Krasner (2012) describe a client who felt more comfortable with this medium rather than using videoconferencing, (i.e. Skype) as the option for psychotherapeutic service delivery. This three-dimensional computerized environment mimics the real world with physical simulations of both individuals and places and may utilize avatars, or characters, that are representations of the client and clinician. The therapist in this situation establishes a therapeutic relationship without common elements of psychotherapy, such as voice or visual cues (Quackenbush & Krasner 2012).

Internet-Based Therapy Internet-based psychotherapy modalities are identified as more effective than a waiting list for services and similar effectiveness when compared to face-to-face psychotherapy (de Bitencourt Machado et al. 2016). Research has repeatedly identified that Internet-based modalities are effective means for offering psychotherapy or psychotherapeutic interventions, particularly CBT, but additionally, dialectical behavioural therapy (DBT) and exposure and response prevention therapy (Netter et al. 2018), depending on the severity of the presentation or the individual needs of the client.

Blended or hybrid therapy models may also demonstrate to increase client adherence compared to face-to-face encounters (Mackie et al 2017). Blended therapy may include digital health technologies such as handheld devices or wearables in addition to videoconferencing or in-person visits (Bacchus et al. 2016; Shulver et al 2017). Remote care monitoring via these devices or applications (i.e. self-report questionnaires) may support ongoing real-time assessment, monitoring of progress or symptom severity aligned with psychotherapy, and be inclusive of reminders or alerts (Gual-Montolio et al. 2020).

4 Benefits of Digital Technologies and for Psychotherapy

Therapeutic Alliance and Client Satisfaction Jenkins-Guarnieri and colleagues (2015) completed a systematic review of measures of satisfaction and therapeutic alliance in studies that had comparisons of videoconferencing or telephone-based psychotherapeutic telemental health treatments. With respect to CBT, studies have reported satisfaction and preference with video-conference-delivered CBT in comparison to a face-to-face option (Jenkins-Guarnieri et al. 2015; Tsuchiyagaito et al. 2017). Authors suggest that perhaps online psychotherapy may be better offered as a compliment than a replacement for face-to-face psychotherapy (Cipolletta et al. 2018; Shulver et al. 2017). International studies on videoconferencing have consistently revealed that clients consistently rate the therapeutic alliance as high and that care providers rate lower levels (moderate to high) of therapeutic alliance in comparison to face-to-face or in-person psychotherapy (Simpson & Reid 2014). In comparison to videoconferencing and Internet-based interventions, text therapy treatment for various types of disorders using a mobile text platform identified that although there were improvements in symptoms, the rating of the therapeutic alliance was found to be low (Hull & Muhan 2017).

Although in the case of group therapy high therapeutic alliance has been rated by participants in some research, it should be noted that a few studies have also reported greater therapeutic alliance ratings in group therapy offered in-person than compared to video teleconferencing (Jenkins-Guarnieri et al., 2015; McGill et al., 2017). Videoconferencing platforms have demonstrated enhanced treatment, reduced symptoms, better time management, and planning problems from beginning to post-treatment (Sibley et al., 2017). Similar studies evaluating the feasibility, acceptability, and efficacy of real-time, in-home Internet-provided family-based CBT for child anxiety via videoconferencing show promise in terms of satisfaction, therapeutic alliance, and treatment retention (Carpenter et al. 2018).

Accessibility Digital technologies are increasingly versatile and enable remote connection for psychotherapy services to clients in rural settings that were perhaps limited or not traditionally available due to the cost or time of travel. Accessibility is furthered by technological infrastructures, such as secure and reliable Wi-Fi availability, helping to address waitlist challenges, and delays for general or specialty care. This type of offering is dependent upon the client having access to corresponding technology (i.e. mobile device) and required digital literacy as well. Patient portals, where available, also increase the participation of clients in their care with their therapist by potentially having access to therapist notes to increase transparency regarding stages of therapy, self-reporting (i.e. questionnaires), increased engagement in scheduling appointments, and secure messaging to the therapist for immediate support, when in need (O'Neill et al. 2019).

5 Pitfalls of Digital Health Technologies

Despite the abundance of opportunities that come with harnessing technology for psychotherapy, there are some pitfalls or cautions to raise. For example, in terms of access, health inequities may perpetuate or exclude specific individuals or populations, such as Indigenous persons, newcomers (immigrants and refugees), the 2SLGBTQIA+ community, the elderly, and the homeless (Canada Health Infoway & Healthcare Excellence Canada, 2022).

6 Common Challenges

Digital Literacy Digital literacy is "the skills needed to search, select, judge, transform, communicate, and use online health information" (Yu 2021, p. 3). Various factors of the individual such as gender identity, age, insurance coverage, education, and socio-economic status may influence their use or engagement of technology, and therefore, these persons may require support. Digital health literacy programs that are designed to target the needs of these clients can help to reduce health inequities (Yu 2021). Client education can include the basics of security measures such as username and password protection, to downloading of software and utilization. Online learning programs are available to support these needs to empower clients to be involved in their own care (Yu 2021).

Videoconferencing Technical Setup Challenges reported during videoconferencing include issues such as starting/setting up, interruptions or problems with technology, privacy, and the environment (Cipolletta et al. 2018). To proactively mediate these potential issues, client should be educated about the need for private environments with limited distractions, good lighting, and ensuring that technology is functional. Joining video visits early to test technology, such as microphone, video camera, and speakers, is recommended in advance of the appointment for both the nurse and client. Technical failures can lead to delays, such as Internet bandwidth interruptions as well. Identification of communication alternatives and emergency contacts, or mechanisms for easeful appointment rescheduling can mitigate these concerns or ensure a more seamless experience for both parties. Secure licensing of software and hardware ensures alignment with organizational policies and overall security of the client's care (Canadian Nurses Protective Society 2023).

Appropriateness Matching the right population to the right digital health modality is critical. An individual's symptom severity may dictate the choice to not employ technologies, for instance, a higher severity of symptoms would warrant face-to-face intervention whereas mild to moderate may be better addressed by leveraging these technical modalities (de Bitencourt Machado et al. 2016; Strudwick et al. 2019). For example, using an Internet-based therapy would not be appropriate for someone who has a primary issue related to an Internet use disorder, sexual or gaming addiction, avoidance, or social phobia. Development of eligibility requirements for the modes of therapy using technology can support appropriate identification for different client offerings, this can include additional clinical considerations, like stability, access to medical information and follow-up needs, and individual client factors such as insurance, availability of technology, language needs, or culture (Canada Health Infoway & Healthcare Excellence Canada 2022).

The first visit upon initiating psychotherapy might be in-person to support establishing trust and communication. The goals of therapy and the individual's needs may change the mode by which technology is used and when. For example, life-changing or emotionally charged discussions may be better suited in-person. Nurses practice using a bio-psycho-social model and thus may include physical examinations in-person to accompany nurse psychotherapy versus videoconferencing. Similarly, if there are new or worsening symptoms, the nurse may prefer to limit technology use to complete a comprehensive assessment. Applying clinical judgement in the appropriate mode of therapy is an ongoing assessment and consideration.

Considerations for Safe and Ethical Use of Technology for Psychotherapy. To ensure the safety of the client and nurse, there should be careful selection and responsible use of digital health tools for psychotherapy. In addition to employing an ethical framework to reduce the risk of harm, additional considerations must be well-thought-out when establishing psychotherapy practice.

Client Identification Positive client identification for either individual or group sessions is paramount like in any other mode of care delivery. Common requirements for the first encounter identification may include date of birth, valid health card, government-issued photo identification, and facial recognition after the initial in-person visit(s). Nurse psychotherapists can also leverage waiting rooms to mimic the in-person experience of being received and to ensure that the right person is attending the right session. Clients may also have approved proxy contacts that participate in care via technology. Ensuring there is required documentation of approvals for access in alignment with organizational policies and legislation is important to support the appropriate involvement of the client's circle of care. To maintain confidentiality in group contexts, limiting the client's first name to only be visible in video visits is also recommended.

Regulatory or Legal Considerations Review of regulatory standards, international practice standards, and, if present, organizational/agency policies may permit this extension of psychotherapy where healthcare is needed, however, healthcare roles or scopes of practices may differ enabling or hindering one's ability to provide care (Quackenbush & Krasner 2012). Strategies to promote collaboration and services to more than one nation or region should be addressed early and thoughtfully to safeguard clients and nurses. For example, governments and regulatory bodies must establish standards regarding which clinicians can safely provide clinical care remotely to other parts of the world and the criteria (such as type of technology, security, or privacy measures) to do so safely. Nurses have accountability to ensure they are licensed to provide psychotherapy in their own jurisdiction and in any other jurisdiction they wish to practice in (Canadian Nurses Protective Society 2023). Even if there are no laws or regulations preventing therapists from providing services in other provinces or countries, therapists should ensure adequate liability insurance coverage, consider the use of appropriate encrypted technology, challenges with technologies, and data storage (whether data will be stored in the home province/country or other countries) (Schell 2019).

Documentation and Consents Some digital technologies such as patient portals or video visit software can integrate with the secure organizational/agency electronic health record (EHR). This can support seamless clinical workflow, from ease of appointment scheduling to comprehensive review and documentation of the client's care. In some instances, self-reported questionnaires or remote care monitoring devices can also be integrated into the EHR to support monitoring of the client's progress. This limits fragmentation of care if an interdisciplinary team is engaged or the client is accessing additional services, such as emergency care or primary care. Some additional consent processes may be required in accordance with provincial or territorial legislative requirements to protect health information in terms of privacy and confidentiality, such as contacting the client via email or initiating video visits. Documentation of obtaining informed client consent after review of the limitations, benefits, risks, and alternatives is essential to maintain client rights and to abide by privacy laws.

7 Additional Considerations for Digital Technologies and Psychotherapy

Evaluation of Psychotherapy Leveraging Technology It is important for nurses to utilize validated tools to evaluate the quality of the therapeutic relationship when introducing new technology. Tools identified in the literature specifically regarding the evaluation of the digital 'therapeutic alliance' include the Penn (Penn Helping Alliance Scale), the Agnew Relationship Measure (ARM), the Videoconferencing Tele-Presence Scale, the Vanderbilt Psychotherapy Process Scale, Distance Communication Comfort Scale, Session Evaluation Questionnaire, and the Group Therapy Alliance Scale (Simpson & Reid 2014). A tool called the Internet-Specific Therapeutic Relationship Questionnaire (ITRQ) was created after a review of the literature specifically looking at characteristics of psychological treatments offered via the Internet, such as when utilizing CBT. This novel tool evaluates components such as the communication and attentiveness of the online therapist, sharing of information, the treatment environment, and client-reported outcomes, including treatment satisfaction, as well as improvements in coping and complaints.

Facilitation of Virtual Group Therapy It is recommended that virtual care psychotherapy groups are facilitated by two psychotherapists, especially if the information is presented by sharing the screen as facilitators may not be able to see participants while sharing screen. There can be designated roles for each facilitator, for example, one to lead the group and the other facilitator to monitor group process, team dynamics, and to monitor chat features. Determining the use of chat functions should also be taken into consideration in pre-planning and in some instances, a decision may be made to disable the chat function fully or restrict communications to facilitators only. Debriefing with co-facilitators after group sessions regarding any significant incidents can support follow-up, inclusive of management of urgent situations and documentation. In the event of being a single facilitator of a group psychotherapy session, it is imperative that a backup or on-call support is available in the event of an urgent situation. Private chat functions available in virtual platforms enable facilitators to check in with their clients, join one-to-one sessions, and address different learning styles. Group norms and safety plans with clients are as important, if not more essential, in the virtual session as they are in-person. Virtual waiting rooms can be used to establish group sessions to ensure the right people have joined for the right session and to prevent cybersecurity issues.

Training and Clinical Supervision Training and practice in the use of digital technology may be required to develop competencies for safe and effective use of various technology modalities such as virtual chats, telephone, video visits, and applications (Schell 2019). Clinical supervision regarding the use of these technologies is greatly encouraged both at the undergraduate level and post-licensure to exercise therapeutic relationship competencies such as empathy, non-verbal behaviours, assessment of the client and environment, and overall client engagement. There may be unconscious behaviours or patterns of interaction with the client that is perpetuated through technology that one would benefit from observation and feedback. Clients can still develop dependence on nurse-client relationships even over the Internet over time (transference), requesting more sessions or reassurance as the relationship develops (Quackenbush & Krasner 2012). A lack of confidence in the mode of therapy may impact authenticity in the therapeutic relationship and ultimately the ability to use a full range of psychotherapeutic techniques (Quackenbush & Krasner 2012). Although the technology offers and potentially extends psychotherapeutic interventions to other parts of the world that may not have access to traditional services, it poses the question about the culture competence of the care provider as well (Quackenbush & Krasner 2012).

User Design and Engagement End-user engagement in the design of a product used for psychotherapy will influence their engagement, whether for the nurse or the client (Baumel and Kane 2018). Baumel & Yom-Tov (2018) focused on understanding whether electronic health intervention design qualities predicted adherence to behavioural-based interventions and identified which qualities mattered most. Therapeutic persuasiveness design was the highest predictor of adherence. This data suggests that the design of digital technology should incorporate persuasive design and behaviour change techniques to enhance adherence (Baumel & Yom-Tov 2018). There is a great advantage for developers to work in collaboration with the healthcare industry, nurses themselves, as well as clients, to make more meaningful applications and connect or integrate them with existing or traditional ways clinicians understand or work with health information (Torous & Hsin 2018). Involving consumers, communities, and healthcare providers in the development of technology to improve the adoption and success of the technology as intended is encouraged. Collaborations with clients in the design process and implementation can enable feedback regarding what types of characteristics of a technology or its application may be needed to validate or create a humanistic, safe, and supportive interactive experience. Examples include ensuring the size of the video screen is adequate, speed at which responses are received or sent, and ways the virtual environment can be more conducive to supporting the therapeutic relationship (DeLucia et al. 2013).

8 Case Vignette 1

8.1 Virtual Group Psychotherapy (3rd Session of 10, Facilitated by 2 Therapists)

Janice is a 48-year-old female with a diagnosis of major depressive disorder and anxiety. Janice lives by herself with pets, and her extended family lives about 10 kms away from her house. Janice presented with blunted affect during initial check in; however, was able to participate in the icebreaker activity and provided updates regarding homework completion. Janice indicated that she practiced skills taught in group sessions; however, was unable to focus due to worried thoughts, and work-related stress. Janice turned the camera off informing the group via the chat function that she must take a washroom break. A few minutes later, Janice joined back. Janice expressed that she was in distress privately in the chat and asked if she could have a one-to-one conversation with the facilitator. The co-facilitator left the group and called Janice. Janice shared that she overdosed on her antidepressants while stepping away from the virtual group. She informed the facilitator that she was triggered when a fellow group member was talking about how she practiced coping skills to deal with anxiety while on vacation overseas. Janice noted that she was reminded of an early childhood traumatic incident when she heard about the vacation spot. The facilitator engaged the client on the phone while notifying a team member to call paramedics at her home. The paramedics arrived within 15 min and Janice was taken to hospital for urgent care.

8.1.1 Case Vignette 1 Reflective Questions

1. As a co-facilitator continuing to run the group session, how will you explain the situation that has just transpired to other clients?
2. Had you been the only psychotherapist facilitating this group session, how might you have handled the urgent situation?
3. What range of supports might you provide to a client in distress?
4. How might you document this situation?

9 Case Vignette 2

9.1 Individual Psychotherapy Video Session

Towards the end of a psychotherapy session, the therapist noted another individual entering the client's room and quickly leaving. Upon further exploring, the client shared that she was on vacation and did not have enough private space to do the virtual visit. The client had asked her family for private space for 1 h so she could attend her therapy session, however, was not clear why the family member entered the room during that time. The client also noted that she was out of the country and shared that it was great that she could still join the session while on vacation.

9.1.1 Case Vignette 2 Reflective Questions

1. What considerations might the therapist have in relation to: (i) privacy and confidentiality; (ii) regulatory requirements as they relate to the jurisdiction?
2. What might the therapist tell the client upon learning that they are not in the agreed-upon location established at the start of therapy? Note: the nurse is not registered to practice in the country the client was visiting.
3. What might you document in relation to this incident?
4. How might you have initiated this session with the client differently?

10 Summary

- The ongoing technical advancements in the provision of psychotherapy enable increased opportunities for clients to benefit from evidence-based practices.
- Despite advancements, not all clients, communities, or situations can effectively lend to virtual care.
- It is imperative that the nurse psychotherapist fully understands the technology, limitations, and ways to mitigate risks or potential pitfalls, such as technology failure or digital literacy.
- Access may be increased through user design and engagement in the development of new technologies, attention to social determinants of health, or cultural safety considerations during the delivery of psychotherapy.
- Clinical judgment can support the appropriate identification of clients who may benefit from this offering and ethical principles can ensure judicious use.

References

Bacchus, L., Bullock, L., Sharps, P., Burnett, C., Schminkey, D., Buller, A., & Campbell, J. (2016). Infusing technology into perinatal home visitation in the United States for women experiencing intimate partner violence: Exploring the interpretive flexibility of an mhealth intervention. *Journal of Medical Internet Research, 18*(11), 37–53.

Baumel, A., & Kane, J. (2018). Examining predictors of real-world user engagement with self-guided ehealth Interventions: Analysis of mobile apps and websites using a novel dataset. *Journal of Medical Internet Research, 20*(12), e11491.

Baumel, A. & Yom-Tov, E. (2018). Predicting user adherence to behavioral eHealth interventions in the real world: Examining which aspects of intervention design matter most. *Translational Behavioral Medicine, 8*(5) 793–98.

Canada Health Infoway & Health Care Excellence Canada. (2022). Providing safe and high-quality virtual care: A guide for new and experienced users: Clinician change virtual care toolkit. Version 1.0. Canada Health Infoway. https://www.infoway-inforoute.ca/en/component/edocman/6378-clinician-change-virtual-care-toolkit/view-document

Canadian Nurses Protective Society. (2023). *Twelve things to consider before joining a virtual care practice*. Author. https://cnps.ca/article/twelve-things-to-consider-before-joining-a-virtual-care-practice/.

Carpenter, A., Pincus, D., Furr, J., & Comer, J. (2018). Working from home: An initial pilot examination of videoconferencing-cased cognitive behavioral therapy for anxious youth delivered to the home setting. *Behavior Therapy,* 49(6), 917–30.

Cipolletta, S., Frassoni, E., & Faccio, E. (2018). Construing a therapeutic relationship online: An analysis of videoconference sessions. *Clinical Psychologist, 22*(2), 220–29.

de Bitencourt Machado, D., Braga Laskoski P., Trelles Severo, C., Bassols, A., Sfoggia, A., Kowacs, C., Valle Krieger, D., Benetti Torres, M., Bento Gastaud, M., & Wellausen, R. (2016). A psychodynamic perspective on a systematic review of online psychotherapy for adults. *British Journal of Psychotherapy, 32*(1), 79–108.

DeLucia, P., Harold, S., & Tang, Y. (2013). Innovation in technology-aided psychotherapy through human factors/ergonomics: Toward a collaborative approach. *Journal of Contemporary Psychotherapy, 43*(4), 253–60.

Gual-Montolio, P., Martínez-Borba, V., Bretón-López, J., Osma, J., & Suso-Ribera, C. (2020). How Are information and communication technologies supporting routine outcome monitoring and measurement-based care in psychotherapy? A systematic review. *International Journal of Environmental Research and Public Health, 17*(9). 3170. https://doi.org/10.3390/ijerph17093170

Hull, T. & Mahan, K. (2017). A study of asynchronous mobile-enabled SMS text psychotherapy. *Telemedicine and E-Health 23*(3), 240–47.

Hummel, S., van Lankveld, J., Oldenburg, H., Hahn, D., Broomans, E., & Aaronson, N. (2018). Internet-based cognitive behavioural therapy for DSM-IV sexual dysfunctions in breast cancer survivors: Predictors of treatment response. *International Journal of Sexual Health, 30*(3), 281–94.

Jenkins-Guarnieri, M., Pruitt, L., Luxton, D., & Johnson, K. (2015). Patient perceptions of telemental health: Systematic review of direct comparisons to in-person psychotherapeutic treatments. *Telemedicine and E-Health, 21*(8), 652–60.

Mackie, C., Dunn, N., MacLean, S., Testa, V., Heisel, M., & Hatcher, S. (2017). A qualitative study of a blended therapy using problem solving therapy with a customised smartphone app in men who present to hospital with intentional self-harm. *Evid Based Ment Health, 20*(4), 118–122. https://doi.org/10.1136/eb-2017-102764. Epub 2017 Oct 13. PMID: 29030503; PMCID: PMC10516399.

McGill, B., Sansom-Daly, U., Wakefield, C., Ellis, S., Robertson, E., & Cohn, R. (2017). Therapeutic alliance and group cohesion in an online support program for adolescent and young adult cancer survivors: Lessons from 'recapture life'. *Journal of Adolescent and Young Adult Oncology 6*(4), 568–72.

Netter, A., Hessler, J, Diedrich, A., Lehr, D., Berking, M., Pfeuffer, S., & Voderholzer, U. (2018). Usability and naturalness of videoconference-based exposure and response prevention for obsessive–compulsive disorder at the patients' homes: A pilot study. *Journal of Cognitive Psychotherapy, 32*(4), 303–14.

O'Neill, S., Chimowitz, H., Leveille, S., & Walker, J. (2019). Embracing the new age of transparency: mental health patients reading their psychotherapy notes online. *Journal of Mental Health, 28*(5), 527-535.

Quackenbush, D. & Krasner, A. (2012). Avatar therapy: Where technology, symbols, culture, and connection collide. *Journal of Psychiatric Practice, 18*(6), 451–59.

Schell, D. (2019). Guidelines for uses of technology in counselling and psychotherapy. Canadian Counselling and Psychotherapy Association. https://www.ccpa-accp.ca/wp-content/uploads/2019/04/TISCGuidelines_Mar2019_EN.pdf

Shulver, W., Killington, M., Morris, C., & Crotty, M. (2017). 'Well, if the kids can do it, I can do it': Older rehabilitation patients' experiences of telerehabilitation. *Health Expectations, 20*(1), 120–29.

Sibley, M., Comer, J., & Gonzalez, J. (2017). Delivering parent-teen therapy for ADHD through videoconferencing: A preliminary investigation. *Journal of Psychopathology and Behavioral Assessment, 39*(3), 467–85.

Simpson, S. & Reid, C. (2014). Therapeutic alliance in videoconferencing psychotherapy: A review." *Australian Journal of Rural Health, 22,* (6), 280–99.

Strudwick, G., Zhang, T. Inglis, F., Sockalingam, S., Munnery, M., Lo, B., Singh Takhar, S., Charow, R., & Wiljer, D. (2019). Delivery of compassionate mental health care in a digital technology-driven age: Protocol for a scoping review. *BMJ Open, 9,* (7), e027989.

Torous, J. & Hsin, H. (2018). Empowering the digital therapeutic relationship: Virtual clinics for digital health interventions. *NPJ Digital Medicine, 1*(1), 1–3.

Tsuchiyagaito, A., Hirano, Y., Asano, K., Oshima, F., Nagaoka, S., Takebayashi, Y., Matsumoto, K., Masuda, Y., Iyo, M., & Nakagawa, A. (2017). Cognitive-behavioral therapy for obsessive–compulsive disorder with and without autism spectrum disorder: Gray matter differences associated with poor outcome. *Frontiers in Psychiatry, 8,* 143. https://doi.org/10.3389/fpsyt.2017.00143.

Yu, E. (2021). Digital health literacy of Canadian adults: Evidence from the 2020 Canadian digital health survey. Canadian Association for Health Services and Policy Research. https://www.infoway-inforoute.ca/en/component/edocman/3882-digital-health-literacy-of-canadian-adults-evidence-from-the-2020-canadian-digital-health-survey/view-document?Itemid=103

Chapter 9
Population Needs: Individualized Nurse Psychotherapy in Public and Independent Sector

Alan Largo and Archna N. Patel

Abstract Nurses deliver individualized psychotherapy in various settings, from inpatient and outpatients to community clinics and private practice. Within these settings, there are similarities and differences in the professional and therapeutic responsibilities. This chapter examines the delivery of individualized nurse psychotherapy in hospital and community settings, comparing and contrasting the delivery of nurse psychotherapy.

Keywords Individual psychotherapy · Public sector · Hospital · Community

Learning Objectives

After completing this chapter, the learner will:

1. Understand similarities and differences in how nurses deliver individual psychotherapy in communities and hospitals.
2. Explain nurses' essential responsibilities when providing individual psychotherapy in communities and hospitals.
3. Demonstrate knowledge of the differences in hospital and community delivery of individual psychotherapy from referral, beginning treatment, measuring progress to discharge.

A. Largo (✉)
Roles and Associates Psychotherapy Services Inc., Toronto, ON, Canada
e-mail: largo.alan@gmail.com

A. N. Patel
Woodbridge, ON, Canada

S. Roles and K. Kalia (eds.), *The Nurses' Guide to Psychotherapy*,
https://doi.org/10.1007/978-981-97-4738-2_9

1 Introduction

Providing nurse psychotherapy to individuals requires similar qualifications and degree of competence in both community and hospital settings. Professional responsibilities in providing individualized nurse psychotherapy may include: referral processes, intake screening and treatment matching, crisis management, risk of harm assessments, identifying the duration of sessions and length of treatment, evaluating the effectiveness of care provided, discharging clients, advertising services, collaborating with allied health and most responsible clinicians, confidentiality, circle of care considerations, and diversity responsiveness. These responsibilities are critical in hospital and community settings to ensure the highest quality of care is established and maintained. There are also many differences in the responsibility of providing psychotherapy in both settings, including goals of care, collaborative case conceptualizations, the duty to warn, informed consent, the rights of the client, referring clients, the structure of therapy, and the maintenance and access of health records. This chapter will provide a comprehensive overview of the similarities and differences in delivering individualized nurse psychotherapy in hospitals and in the community.

2 Psychotherapy in Hospital and Community Settings

Nurse psychotherapists in hospitals and community settings must follow their regulatory body guidelines. These standards or guidelines for the provision of psychotherapy may differ from region to region. For example, in Ontario, nurses follow the College of Nurses of Ontario (CNO) requirements to practice. To competently practice psychotherapy, nurses need appropriate knowledge, skill, and judgment. Nurses are accountable for reflecting on their practice, determining their individual learning needs, and developing a learning plan for quality assurance purposes annually. Nurses continually reflect on their practice and choose what best helps them achieve their objectives, for example, enrolment in refresher courses or obtaining certifications. The CNO does not require nurses to obtain specific additional training or certification (e.g. courses, experience hours, supervision) for psychotherapy, nor does the CNO approve or endorse specific continuing education programs or certifications. It is up to the nurse and their employer, if not self-employed, to determine the appropriate training or requirements, such as certifications or degrees, necessary to perform psychotherapy safely (CNO 2023a). The criteria set by the CNO are non-specific to any particular training requirements. Thus, performing psychotherapy requires nurses to consider what training and qualifications would prepare them appropriately to practice safely, competently, and ethically.

3 Safe, Competent and Ethical Practice

Most regulatory bodies' entry-to-practice competencies address the required competencies of the generalist nursing roles and the CNO (2019) practice competencies are no different. In the case of a nurse psychotherapist, nurses must still be able to provide safe, competent, ethical, compassionate, and evidence-informed care. In Ontario's communities and hospitals, psychotherapy delivery is a controlled act established by the Regulated Health Profession Act (1991). If not applied appropriately, psychotherapy delivery has the potential to cause harm. Nurses are authorized to perform these acts and may initiate psychotherapy treatment if they possess the knowledge, skills, and judgment to provide psychotherapy to their clients. Part of this knowledge is a fundamental understanding of human rights to protect their client's dignity. While not an exhaustive list, a few essential legislative documents in the province of Ontario are the Mental Health Act (1990), Child, Youth and Family Services Act (2017), and Personal Health Information Protection Act (2004). Becoming aware of the legislative documents and requirements that may pertain to practicing psychotherapy in your jurisdiction of practice is crucial and required before establishing a practice.

4 Counselling/Therapy Responsibilities

The nurse psychotherapist also understands their area of psychotherapy expertise and limits, ensuring that the nurse has the training, experience, and education to treat, practice, and support clients. A nurse has the ability, knowledge, and skill to implement evidence-based psychotherapeutic modalities to treat various conditions and disorders but must also have the proper education and training to assess and evaluate the need to apply the psychotherapeutic modality to treat a mental health condition or disorder. When a clinical situation lies beyond their competence, the nurse must seek further support and education or refer the client to other, more appropriate services (CNO 2023b, 2023c).

4.1 Consent and Limits of Confidentiality

In both hospital and community settings, informed consent begins at admission or the beginning of treatment. The nurse therapist explains confidentiality and the limits of confidentiality to the client at the beginning of the initial session with the client. The nurse needs to ensure familiarity with the requirements and processes in their province or territory and place of work. An overview of the expectations of attending appointments, mode of therapy (i.e. in-person versus virtual), the code of conduct, goals, techniques and procedures, alternatives and risks are discussed with the client, and any questions are answered. This information may also be given to the client in writing, reviewed at the start of therapy, and can be signed by the client as consent (CNO 2022).

4.2 Duty to Warn

During a therapy session, the nurse therapist sometimes learns information that may represent imminent harm to the client, another person, or a minor. In the case of suicidal ideation or harm to self or others, the nurse therapist utilizes a risk assessment to determine the intent, plan, and lethality of the ideation. In the hospital, the duty to warn will include the circle of care, which may warrant escalating to the clinic psychiatrist. The nurse will conduct a thorough assessment, including screening tools to help inform the level of risk. Should the client be identified as a risk of harm to self or others, the client will likely be admitted to the hospital for supervision, assessment, and treatment in the inpatient psychiatric unit or the psychiatric intensive care unit of the hospital. In the community or private setting, the nurse would contact local authorities or crisis response teams to fulfill this duty to ensure the safety of the person in distress. In high-risk situations, the police may bring the client to the hospital for assessment, supervision, and possibly an inpatient stay in the psychiatric unit of a hospital (CNO 2022). The nurse should make themselves familiar with their reporting requirements and legislation as well as contact information for those to report to in the case of imminent risk of harm.

4.3 Diversity Responsiveness

Within hospital and community practice, nurse psychotherapists work with specific client populations and communities, such as child, youth, adult, geriatric, black, Indigenous, and/or people of colour. Programs are required to service the needs based on demographic and clinical data, thereby servicing the needs unique to the population and geographical area of the hospital or community clinic. The nurse bases their practice on principles of equality and equity. In private practice, nurse psychotherapists may choose specific populations of interest they would like to work with, having more choice in specializing in particular population characteristics or mental health conditions (CNO 2022).

4.4 Maintenance of Health Records

All nurses working in a hospital and community setting are required to follow the documentation standards of their regulatory college requirements and their place of work. Generally, it is expected to complete documentation after each visit and within 24 h of the visit. Some clinics and hospitals leverage an electronic health record with security and privacy provisions to ensure protection of the client's health data.

4.5 Third-Party Reporting

There may be times when a nurse needs to share psychotherapy information with other clinicians in the community. While in hospitals, this is often within the "circle of care." The assumed consent of the circle of care can extend to community settings and family members if formal consent has been obtained by having the client provide consent to release information. This would allow the nurse psychotherapist to share information such as client care plans, status updates and progress. These practices would be consistent with PHIPA (Information and Privacy Commissioner of Ontario [IPCO], 2015). The nurse would need to thoroughly understand what the privacy regulations for health care are in their jurisdiction as well as relevant workplace policies/procedures.

5 Delivery of Individualized Nurse Psychotherapy in Hospitals and the Community

Nurses must look to legislation and controlled acts within their regulatory bodies and regions to identify if they can independently practice psychotherapy in hospitals and community settings. In Ontario, Canada, nurses can independently perform the controlled act of psychotherapy without an order; however, if working within a hospital the nurse may be required to obtain an order to perform psychotherapy as per the interpretation of the Public Hospitals Act (1990) (CNO 2023a).

Different settings might present nurses with time limits and policy restrictions in how they practice. Typically, hospital settings host public service-funded therapy programs and often function in time-limited services targeted more at acuity and stabilization. After discharge, clients are generally referred back to mental health and addiction services in the community, either publicly funded or in private practice.

Hospital-based outpatient mental health and addiction services aim to establish acute stabilization of illness, strengths-based skills building, and safety for the client to cope with their symptoms of mental health outside of hospital care. The service is goals-based work with the client and the aim is to stabilize the client to return to their community and work towards decreasing the risk of re-hospitalization or deterioration of mental status.

In the community, nurses can find themselves with less structure and support than in hospital settings and can develop a strong independent practice. Community public therapy programs that employ nurse psychotherapists often function in time-limited episodic care formats due to limitations in funding. This allows public programs to provide access to many individuals in need despite limited resources. Usually, group psychotherapy or team approaches are used in these publicly funded settings. For more information on group psychotherapy see Chap. 10.

In private practice, nurses use their expertise to provide psychotherapy to clients who pay for psychotherapy using their private insurance, payment out of pocket, or are associated with different staff wellness or employee assistance programs. Usually, the client's finances or insurance benefits are the most common factors limiting service length. Still, outside of that, the client can receive psychotherapy for an undetermined length of time, depending on the needs the client presents with. Unfortunately, some insurance companies still do not recognize nurse psychotherapists and in these situations, clients may be required to pay out of pocket (Luczka 2022).

Nurse psychotherapists in both community and hospital can provide a variety of psychotherapeutic modalities such as cognitive behavioural therapy (CBT), dialectical behavioural therapy (DBT), motivational interviewing (MI), behavioural activation, addiction counselling, psychoanalysis, psychodynamic psychotherapy, and interpersonal psychotherapy. The type of modality the nurse psychotherapist chooses to work with can vary. Sometimes, in hospital settings and publicly funded community clinics, the clinic may be funded to treat a specific population and mental health diagnosis, for example, obsessive–compulsive disorder, or to provide a certain form of psychotherapy. In private practice, the nurse can specialize in a chosen modality and advertise to elicit referrals for their specialty. Nurses should strive to integrate evidence-based practices such as trauma-informed care practices (Chap. 5) and cultural sensitivity and therapeutic effects practices (Chap. 12) regardless of the modality they are practicing.

6 Treatment Process

Care is often grounded in frameworks such as the biopsychosocial model and trauma-informed care, see Chaps. 4 and 5. The treatment and care planning are a collaborative process. It can include the client, the therapist, members of the clinical team, family members as well as supportive people in the client's life depending on those the client wishes to include should they have the capacity to consent to their own treatment. For more on care planning, see Chap. 15.

6.1 Hospital Referrals

Hospital referrals typically go to the outpatient mental health services in the hospital setting. Referrals come to the outpatient mental health and addictions services from several sources—internally, referrals arrive through the emergency department or inpatient medicine, psychiatric, or surgery units. Clients typically can receive follow-ups in the mental health outpatient clinic after they are discharged from the inpatient unit. Other sources of referrals come from multiple outpatient programs within the hospital, such as cancer clinics, senior clinics, and mother/baby clinics.

External referrals to the hospital come from places such as primary care providers' clinics including family physicians, nurse practitioner-led clinics and community health clinics. Other hospitals may make hospital-to-hospital referrals if their hospital does not have the mental health or addiction services that the client may need. Not all hospital-based outpatient services are the same, nor do they have the same specialized clinics for specific conditions or presentations. Clients may also request follow-up at another hospital outpatient mental health and addictions clinic due to proximity to their residence, a preference for the services there, a shorter wait list, or if they have familiarity with the health care providers at another clinic. This ability to follow-up at a different location based on client preference changes based on the client's location such as in urban, rural, or remote areas.

6.2 Community Referrals

Receiving client referrals in the community happens in several ways. In most community settings, nurses may initiate psychotherapy independently without any order from a physician (Nursing Act 1991) and are not limited by requiring an order from a doctor or nurse practitioner as may be the case in hospital environments governed by the Public Hospitals Act (1990). Nurses in the community can accept psychotherapy clients through private practice or the public sector. In private practice, clients can self-refer and contact the nurse's private practice directly. Clients may be referred by primary care providers such as physicians, nurse practitioners, and other allied health sources. Also, community and government agencies and employee assistance programs can refer clients privately.

In the public sector, community referrals originate from primary care providers and health programs such as community nursing clinics, community health clinics, and case management teams and in some programs clients can also self-refer.

7 Beginning Individualized Therapy

In hospital and community settings, the nurse would receive a referral and then meet with the client for an intake screening appointment. This would often be a short phone call or meeting where the nurse and client meet each other, discuss the primary concerns and goals for treatment, and determine if the nurse psychotherapist's experience and knowledge match the client's needs.

Once treatment begins, a typical session length is 50 min. However, the length of treatment varies depending on the type of therapy, modality, and the type or severity of the condition being treated. See Chap. 16 for types of psychotherapy.

8 Course of Individualized Therapy

The length of therapy can vary based on symptom severity, therapeutic goals, resource limitations of public-based services, or in private practice, the finances and insurance coverage of the client. The therapy sessions can occur in-person or virtually. Measures and questionnaires can be used to monitor treatment progress and evaluate care effectiveness. These measurements can be completed at the start of therapy, at times during therapy, and near the end. Several common tools to measure symptoms related to psychotherapy interventions include the Patient Health Questionnaire (PHQ-9), General Anxiety Disorder-7 (GAD-7), Columbia Suicide Severity Rating Scale (CSSRS)–Screeners and assessments, The Clinical Institute Withdrawal Assessment Alcohol Scale (CIWA), the Quality Of Life (QOL) scale, the Life Events Checklist (LEC-5) and the Posttraumatic Stress Disorder Checklist for DSM-5 (PCL-5). An initial assessment is conducted when the nurse psychotherapist meets the client for the first time in session. Here, the nurse psychotherapist gets to know the client, their problems, and the therapeutic goals that the client would like to work on. The nurse explores the client's history and precipitating factors that led the client to seek treatment at this time. A mental status exam is typically conducted to achieve a baseline snapshot of the client's mental status and screen for specific symptoms and risk factors. The nurse may briefly conceptualize the client's problems and propose a method to explore. The nurse and client then work together through a psychotherapeutic modality to reach the client's therapeutic goals. This process varies and may take anywhere from a few sessions to years. Since every client's situation, risk factors, coping ability and problems are different, so is the length of time to recover, or resolve through psychotherapy. During each session, the nurse asks for feedback to determine if the client and nurse are still in alignment and on track to achieving the client's goals.

9 Discharge and Termination

Discharge planning and termination is a process that begins right from the start. The nurse psychotherapist discusses the estimated treatment time during the intake phase and revisits this throughout the treatment, adjusting as needed while monitoring symptoms. Termination of the nurse-client relationship can occur in multiple ways, but primarily occurs if the client chooses to end therapy, if the therapy goals have been achieved, and if the client feels that they have developed the skills to cope with their condition (Peplau 1992). After that, the frequency of visits is typically decreased to help the client transition from psychotherapy. In hospital and community settings, the nurse will work with the health care team involved in the client's care to support the client by ensuring a discharge plan incorporates support, which may include transitions to other local community centres and/or private clinics. Clients and therapists collaborate on an agreed-upon discharge time in a private practice setting. The paying clients can often continue therapy for as long as desired and financially feasible.

10 Case Vignette

Jonathan is a fully licensed RN who has just passed the RN licensing exam. He is interested in working as a nurse psychotherapist. Jonathan has learned about the psychotherapeutic modality of solution-focused therapy in his undergraduate mental health nursing course. He wants to provide this therapy to clients and decides to set up his private practice to provide solution-focused therapy. He creates a webpage advertising his services.

Jonathan later decides to work at a community pain clinic providing psychotherapy to treat individuals recovering from work-related injuries. The pain clinic is funded to provide clients with eight sessions of psychotherapy to help them with recovery, trauma, and adjusting to their lives post-injury.

The hospital that Johnathan's pain clinic is associated with asks Jonathan to work in their outpatient day hospital program part-time to provide cognitive behavioural therapy (CBT) to clients recently discharged from the hospital.

10.1 Reflective Case Vignette Questions

1. What considerations should Jonathan take to evaluate his readiness to provide safe and competent psychotherapy as he starts private practice? What suggestions would you make to help Jonathan become more prepared to work as a nurse psychotherapist in the community?
2. How could Jonathan evaluate his client's progress and response to therapy when he works in the outpatient pain clinic? At the end of the eight sessions, what elements would you include in a discharge plan for your clients to promote the best outcomes post-treatment?
3. When Johnathan is asked about providing CBT, what would he need to consider before he responds?

11 Summary

- Nurse psychotherapists must provide safe, competent, ethical, compassionate, and evidence-informed care.
- Nurse psychotherapists must be competent in relevant legislation about mental health issues, ethical principles, and practice standards such as boundaries of practice, duties, privacy, and consent.
- Delivering individual psychotherapy can be different in hospitals, outpatient community programs, clinics, and in private practice.
- Nurse psychotherapists ensure a comprehensive course of treatment starting with referrals, assessment, treatment, evaluation of progress, treatment goal attainment, discharge, and transition planning.

References

Child, Youth and Family Services Act, 2017, SO, 2017, c. 14, Sched. 1.

College of Nurses of Ontario (2019). *Entry to Practice Competencies for Registered Nurses.* Author. https://www.cno.org/globalassets/docs/reg/41042_entrypracrpn-2020.pdf.

College of Nurses of Ontario. (2022). *Confidentiality and Privacy—Personal Health Information.* Author. https://www.cno.org/globalassets/docs/prac/41069_privacy.pdf

College of Nurses of Ontario. (2023a). *Psychotherapy and the controlled act component of psychotherapy.* Author. https://www.cno.org/en/learn-about-standards-guidelines/educational-tools/ask-practice/answers-to-your-questions-about-psychotherapy/.

College of Nurses of Ontario. (2023b). *Scope of Practice.* Author. https://www.cno.org/globalassets/docs/prac/49041-scope-of-practice.pdf.

College of Nurses of Ontario. (2023c). *Code of Conduct.* Author. https://www.cno.org/en/learn-about-standards-guidelines/educational-tools/ask-practice/answers-to-your-questions-about-psychotherapy/.

Information and Privacy Commissioner of Ontario. (2015). *Circle of Care Sharing Personal Health Information for Health-Care Purposes.* Author. https://www.ipc.on.ca/wp-content/uploads/resources/circle-of-care.pdf.

Luczka, C. (2022, April 22). *RN psychotherapists push back on insurance providers not recognizing their practices.* Toronto Star. https://www.thestar.com/news/canada/rn-psychotherapists-push-back-on-insurance-providers-not-recognizing-their-practices/article_6acc55bc-dc8b-524b-9462-ee972e65c8f0.html.

Mental Health Act, RSO 1990, c. M.7.

Nursing Act, 1991 Reg. 275/94: GENERAL under Nursing Act, 1991, SO 1991, c. 32.

Peplau, H. E. (1992). Interpersonal relations: A theoretical framework for application in nursing practice. *Nursing Science Quarterly, 5*, 13–18.

Personal Health Information Protection Act, 2004, SO 2004, c. 3, Sched. A.

Public Hospitals Act, RSO (1990) c P.40.

Regulated Health Professions Act, 1991, SO 1991, c. 18.

Chapter 10
Population Needs: Group Psychotherapy

Emma Quinn, Archna N. Patel, and Alan Largo

Abstract Human beings are social beings. Group psychotherapy is regularly accessed in mental health care, not only because of the cost saving that occurs by reducing clinician-to-client ratios, but also because of the therapeutic benefit of interpersonal dynamics and learning that takes place within the group context. Yalom and Leszcz (The theory and practice of group psychotherapy. Basic Books, 2020) affirmed that the milieu of group psychotherapy processes can best accentuate mental health by using the dynamics of interpersonal connection. Furthermore, there is diversity in the types of groups that exist in mental health allowing for specific needs to be met, including some for psycho-educational purposes, mutual support groups and psychotherapeutic groups. Groups are often formed utilizing either specific or integrated models of psychotherapeutic practice (Corey in Theory & practice of group psychotherapy. Cengage, 2016). The intent of this chapter is to provide nurses with knowledge regarding the structures and processes of effective group psychotherapy interventions.

Keywords Group counselling · Group psychotherapy · Group psychoeducation

Learning Objectives

After completing this chapter, the learner will:

1. Understand how group work functions, how psychotherapy groups are created, designed, and delivered and how challenges in group work can be best remediated.

E. Quinn (✉)
Wasaga Beach, ON, Canada
e-mail: quinntheemma@gmail.com

A. N. Patel
Woodbridge, ON, Canada

A. Largo
Roles and Associates Psychotherapy Services Inc., Sunnybrook Health Science Center, Toronto, ON, Canada

S. Roles and K. Kalia (eds.), *The Nurses' Guide to Psychotherapy*,
https://doi.org/10.1007/978-981-97-4738-2_10

2. Have the knowledge to explain how group psychotherapy processes are relevant to mental health care delivery services and understand how they can integrate group psychotherapy processes into their clinical work.
3. Demonstrate a functional understanding of how group psychotherapy is formulated, structured, and delivered so that its efficacy is maximized, with knowledgeable reflection upon the established literature that describes what effective group work looks like.

1 Definitions

Counselling is identified as the provision of purposeful communication, intended to provide education and/or therapy, which is based upon both evidence-based practice; using evidenced-based theories, skills and interventions and practice-based evidence, such as the experiential learning gained through clinical practice. The Canadian Counselling and Psychotherapy Association (2023) affirms that

> [c]ounselling is a relational process based upon the ethical use of specific professional competencies to facilitate human change. Counselling addresses wellness, relationships, personal growth, career development, mental health and psychological illness or distress. The counselling process is characterized by the application of cognitive, affective, somatic, spiritual, developmental, behavioural, learning, and systemic principles. (para. 6)

Psychotherapy is a "type of treatment that can help individuals experiencing a wide array of mental health conditions and emotional challenges" (American Psychiatric Association 2023, para. 1). It is described as "an intense client-therapist relationship which often involves the examination of deeply emotional experiences, destructive behaviour patterns and serious mental health issues." (Health Professions Regulatory Advisory Council 2006). The College of Nurses of Ontario (2023) affirmed that psychotherapy: "includes a deep assessment of life processes that focus on behaviour modifications, thinking patterns, cognition, emotional response and social functioning" (para. 3).

2 Introduction

Group psychotherapy is a common intervention provided for clients in healthcare settings and has been noted to be an effective intervention for many individuals and presentations (Yalom and Leszcz 2020). Importantly, "people need people—for initial and continued survival, for socialization, and for the pursuit of satisfaction. No one—not the dying, not the outcast, not the mighty—transcends the need for human contact" (Yalom and Leszcz 2020, p. 40). Group psychotherapy takes many forms, with groups created to provide psychoeducation, groups formed as forums of peer support, and groups formed to provide specific psychotherapeutic modalities. Corey (2016) emphasized that group work is best provided when the group is well prepared, delivered with structure and purpose, and when the group is led effectively by facilitators who are skilled and competent in their group leadership skills.

Group psychotherapy must work towards goals agreed upon by the nurse psychotherapist and the clients, with trust and respect being present (Bordin 1979). Group work can involve utilizing the person-centered counseling tenets of Rogers (1957), which include the use of unconditional positive regard, genuineness, and empathy. Group work should recognize the common factors noted by Hubble et al. (2014), in that group psychotherapists believe in their work and clients have hope that the services that they are receiving will be helpful for them. While group psychotherapy is often seen as an expeditious way to provide psychoeducation or psychotherapy to a group of people, clinicians considering providing group psychotherapy must seek out experiences in training, supervision, and consulting with experienced clinicians. This could include shadowing a skilled clinician in delivering their group programming and receiving supervision from experienced clinicians when they begin delivering group work themselves.

3 Group Psychotherapy

Group interventions have been demonstrated to be an effective means of delivering psychotherapy (Yalom and Leszcz 2020). Much of the benefit of group psychotherapy is found to be that the members of the group provide each other with formative feedback, which adds to the interpersonal learning. As there are unique factors present when providing group psychotherapy compared to individual psychotherapy it requires appropriate training and appreciation of the unique factors that will present. Group psychotherapy is indeed an economical and effective means of providing psychotherapy, but must be delivered with planning, adequate training, and an appreciation for how the power of group psychotherapy can be best harnessed.

Corey (2016) affirmed that group facilitators must effectively utilize their presence when providing group work by being authentic, curious, and courageously interacting with groups, which can be demonstrated by not hiding "behind their special role as counselors" (p. 13). Corey (2016) illustrated as well that group psychotherapists must remember to use the essential counselling skills of listening actively while using effective questioning, reflecting thoughts and feelings, being empathetic, and providing feedback. It is important for group facilitators to know that "group members learn by observing the leader's behavior. If leaders value honesty, respect, openness, risk-taking and assertiveness, they can foster these in the members by demonstrating them in group" (p. 21). Corey (2016) also affirmed that clinicians must engage in self-care, that "self-care is not a luxury but an ethical mandate, and you need to commit to developing effective self-care strategies… you cannot provide nourishment to group members if you don't nourish yourself" (p. 14).

Preparation, Structure and Process

It is of crucial importance that group psychotherapy initiatives are well prepared before delivery (Corey 2016; Yalom and Leszcz 2020). When preparing for groups one must consider the goals, the membership, the structure and timing, the rules, and the leadership of the group. The primary task is to establish the goals of your group, identifying what the group is trying to accomplish. Next, the members of the planned group must be selected. Yalom and Leszcz (2020) suggest that selection is best focused on which potential group members should be ideally screened out of group membership. In this regard: "clients will fail in group therapy if they are unable to participate in the primary task of the group, be it for logistical, intellectual, psychological or interpersonal reasons" (Yalom and Leszcz 2020, p. 295). These might be called exclusionary criteria for group members, which can then lend to the development of inclusionary criteria for the group participants. Yalom and Leszcz (2020) affirmed that exclusion factors for groups can include circumstances that may overwhelm the work of the group, such as a person who is at risk for suicide or a person experiencing mental health concerns that will prevent the person from successfully being able to interact with the group or that can be damaging to other members of the group. Membership includes considering the group size. Yalom and Leszcz (2020) noted that: "the ideal size of a cohesive interactional therapy group is seven or eight members, with an acceptable range of five to nine members" (p. 344). The presence of two co-facilitators is ideal, since if one facilitator is away, the other co-facilitator can be present for the group and "when one leader's empathy and mentalization capacity falls short, the other can maintain the focus essential for the group" (Yalom and Leszcz 2020, p. 539). Group structures can be open, with new members welcome to join during the process of the group, or they can be closed, in that the membership of the group is set and does not change during the process of the group. Timing includes considering the length of time for each group session inclusive of breaks and how many times a week or a month the group meets as well as the total number of group sessions that will be offered. Timing also includes the time of the day for the members. For example, at times groups for clients with depression are strategically offered in the morning to assist with behavioural activation in getting the individual out of the house or bed earlier in the day, while some groups targeting individuals who are working may be planned in the evening to support the typical workday. It is important to establish rules for the group, such as the importance of confidentiality so that group members are aware of confidentiality obligations and limits to the confidentiality of the nurse psychotherapist, but also so that group members agree to not share information learned in the group outside the bounds of the group. Three ideal rules for group work are respect, participation, and feedback, along with others that can be brainstormed by the group members in the first group session.

Group facilitators assume the leadership of the group and this role must be taken very seriously. Planning and organizing the logistics of your group is of utmost importance. The location of the group must be selected and reserved and initial discussions prior to starting the group with each potential client and other group facilitators in planning and preparation need to be had. One way to accomplish a standardized plan can be to have group members review and sign a consent and group information sheet acknowledging that they agree with the terms established for the group. Consent documentation is essential. See Appendix A for a sample group consent form.

4 Reflective Considerations

1. Group work requires organization, structure, and purposeful leadership.
2. Group work is a very effective modality of delivering psychotherapy, especially due to the phenomena of interpersonal learning.
3. Group psychotherapists must learn from experienced clinicians and receive supervision in their work when they begin delivering group programming themselves.
4. It is recommended that psychotherapists wanting to engage in group facilitation seek out and utilize established group programming available.
   - Some examples include:
     i. The interpersonal, here-and-now focused group therapy described by Yalom and Leszcz (2020).
     ii. The cognitive-behavioural programming provided by Greenberger and Padesky (2016) in their book Mind over Mood (2nd Ed.). Purchasers of the Mind over Mood book are provided the electronic resources of Mind over Mood by Guildford Press via their website.
     iii. The Group Interpersonal Therapy (IPT) for depression as provided by the World Health Organization (WHO) (2016) in their publication *Group Interpersonal Therapy (IPT) for Depression*, which is available free on-line at: https://www.who.int/publications/i/item/WHO-MSD-MER-16.4.
     iv. The person-centered, humanist approach as described by Rogers (1957) in his article *The necessary and sufficient conditions of therapeutic personality change*, which is available for free online at: https://psycnet.apa.org/record/1959-00842-001.

5 Case Vignette 1

You are running a 6-week group psychotherapy program teaching coping skills and leveraging personal strengths to manage day-to-day stress. The attendees must meet the following criteria: stabilized mental health presentation, motivated to do the work required in the group, able to pay attention while attending group, have no active suicidality, and have a clear set of goals they are working towards.

During the sessions, you bring up a case scenario exemplifying a person struggling with a new life stressor which is then impacting various components of their pre-existing mental health condition. You then review together with the group members what might be the possible triggers for the person in the case example and then move on to review what possible coping strategies and skills might be able to support the person in their psychosocial functioning and working through the stressors in their life.

You ask attendees to draw upon the education they have earned in their group sessions and draw from personal experience. You notice that there is one member, Sally, who regularly shows signs of becoming triggered when case examples are reviewed and displays as visibly upset during the session. Sally then dominates the group discussion, talking about her struggles and how it has impacted her mental stability. When others try to share or when you try to redirect the discussion back to the whole group, she continues to take over the discussion with her own experiences thereby not allowing space for others to speak. Sally visibly shows feelings of anger and pain by vocalizing an angry tone and volume in her voice and by crying.

5.1 Reflective Question for Case Vignette 1

1. How would you, as a facilitator, manage this situation?

6 Case Vignette 2

As the nurse psychotherapist at a community clinic, you are developing a community program that services youth experiencing emotional distress. You design a Dialectical Behavioural Therapy (DBT) skills group to teach these valuable skills to youth. Taking time to research DBT skills, you develop a 12-week program that runs once a week on Monday mornings. The news of your new skills program is posted on the clinic's website. There is a significant response to the skills group, and you receive calls and emails from many individuals wanting to participate. The room you have for the skills group can hold 30 people, so you accept the first 25 people who have contacted the clinic. The first cohort meets on Monday morning, but only ten have shown up. You decide to start the group regardless. During a mindfulness meditation exercise, one of the members begins to cry. The other group members stop the practice and check on her, but the troubled member is inconsolable. When you attend to the troubled member, you notice scar marks on their wrist. You adjourn the group for the day and spend some time stabilizing and emotionally supporting the troubled member before she leaves. This member does not return to the skills group. Over the next few weeks, the attendance fluctuates. Some days, attendance increases to 15 members, and some days, it decreases to 2 members. Since there is room, you allow new members to join. On one particular day, you hear from another youth member that they visited the troubled member outside the skills group and discovered she was admitted to an inpatient hospital. The other youth members become concerned and start planning to visit the hospitalized member.

6.1 Reflective Questions for Case Vignette 2

1. What considerations, if any, to developing the structure of the skills group could the nurse psychotherapist have considered more carefully?
2. When selecting DBT skills group members, what factors likely contributed to low turnout and clients dropping out?
3. If you were to design a group such as this, would you make it a closed or open group? Explain your reasoning.
4. A member disclosed news of the other member's hospitalization in the group. Role play with another, how you might address that as the group leader. How would you balance the needs of the hospitalized member and the needs of the group?
5. Consider the local needs of your town/city/region. Is there a need for group psychotherapy where you live? Discuss what it is and how best it could be delivered in your area.

7 Summary

- To provide group psychoeducation or psychotherapy, clinicians *must* receive training and supervision from clinicians who are experienced in the delivery of such programming.
- Group work must build and maintain the working alliance so that psychotherapists and clients have mutually agreed upon goals and that there be trust and respect present.
- Group work should include the person-centered tenets of genuineness, unconditional positive regard, empathy, trust, and respect.
- Psychotherapists who provide group psychotherapy must believe in their work and provide group work processes that instill hope for clients.
- It is ideal to utilize established group programming to ensure that the group is constructed and facilitated with both evidence-based practice and practice-based evidence.
- Groups can be formed to provide psychoeducation regarding specific topics or can be formed to provide psychotherapy to assist the group members in providing attenuation of their symptoms of concern, such as symptoms of depression, anxiety or trauma-related symptoms.

Appendix A

Sample Group Consent Form

About This Group:

This (*add description of group*) group will be utilized to assist group members in (*describe focus of group*). This is a (*identify if a group is closed or open*) group, which means that the group (*does or doesn't*) add members throughout the course of the group and aims to begin and end with the (*same or different*) participants. The group is designed to operate for (*number of sessions*) sessions that occur weekly on (*note timing of group*) at (*location of group*). Participation is voluntary and group members can withdraw at any time; any person who withdraws from this group will be given a list of resources that are available to assist them, as needed.

Possible Risk and Benefits:

Engaging in group work can be challenging. The intent of this group is to teach and employ tools that provide the ability to (*add focus of the group*). The Centre for Addiction and Mental Health (CAMH) (2023) noted that group psychotherapy provides for the opportunity to learn from a community of other people and the opportunity to experience connectedness with others, which reduces the impact of stigma. CAMH (2023) also affirmed that group psychotherapy can be challenging because it involves exploring difficult areas in your life and therefore "therapy can sometimes be emotionally uncomfortable" (para. 6).

Group Exclusionary Factors:

Group membership will be deferred for factors including if we have serious concerns about a person possibly at risk of harm to themselves or others or when serious substance dependence is present, since these factors, when present, may interfere with ability to participate with the group. Further, when severe mental health concerns are present, such as symptoms of psychosis or mania, such persons would be directed to consult clinical resources that can assist with these concerns so that these concerns are best remediated so that a person can engage with the interpersonal processes of group work.

Roles and Responsibilities:

All group members, including facilitators, are expected to participate in group, provide feedback to others in the group, accept feedback in the group and to treat other people with respect. Facilitators are expected to provide their guidance and leadership to the group process. Group participants are expected to fully engage with the tools and resources provided, complete homework given, share work completed within their comfort level with their fellow group members, and provide feedback to their group peers.

Confidentiality and Record Keeping:

Clinical notes are made after every session and placed on each participant's individual clinical chart. Confidentiality will be ensured from the group facilitators, with the exception that information regarding possible harm to any individual will be immediately shared with the appropriate authorities so that the safety of all persons will be prioritized. The Canadian Nurses Protective Society (2023) affirmed that: "a nurse may be justified in divulging confidential patient information for the purpose of warning others of possible danger from a patient if there is credible, imminent risk or serious bodily harm or death to a known person or persons, perhaps to the police, out of a concern for others" (Are there exceptions to the duty to maintain confidentiality? section, para. 3). The College of Nurses of Ontario (CNO) (2022) noted that: "nurses have ethical and legal responsibilities to maintain the confidentiality and privacy of client health information obtained while providing care" (p. 3). The CNO (2022) also affirms that consent is not required for disclosure of information received from clients when there is any suspicion present regarding the safety and well-being of children and that such suspicions must be reported to your local child protective services, as directed by legal expectations regarding this matter. The Information and Privacy Commissioner of Ontario (2015) describes 16 different types of administrative and legal circumstances in which health information can be disclosed without consent, on pages 28 to 29 of their publication *Frequently Asked Questions: Personal Health Information Protection Act;* this document is found free, online, at: https://www.ipc.on.ca/wp-content/uploads/2015/11/phipa-faq.pdf.

Alternate Resources:

There are many resources present to assist you with your well-being. (*Describe the local relevant alternate and emergency mental health services in your area*).

Facilitator Information:

(*Provide information about the facilitators of the planned group, such as their professional certification, training and experience*).

In signing this form, I confirm that I have read this form, have had the ability to have any questions I may have answered, and consent with the information noted on the form.

Name (please print): ____________________

Signature (group member): __________________ Date: ________________

References

American Psychiatric Association. (2023). *What is psychotherapy?* Author. https://www.psychiatry.org/patients-families/psychotherapy

Bordin, E. S. (1979). The generalizability of the psychoanalytic concept of the working alliance. *Psychotherapy: Theory, Research & Practice, 16*(3), 252–260. https://doi.org/10.1037/h0085885

Canadian Nurses Protective Society. (2023). *InfoLAW: Confidentiality of health information.* Author. https://cnps.ca/article/confidentiality-of-health-information/

Centre for Addiction and Mental Health. (2023). *Group therapy.* Author. https://www.camh.ca/en/health-info/mental-illness-and-addiction-index/group-therapy

College of Nurses of Ontario. (2022). *Confidentiality and privacy—Personal health information.* Author. https://www.cno.org/globalassets/docs/prac/41069_privacy.pdf

College of Nurses of Ontario. (2023). *Psychotherapy and the controlled act component of psychotherapy.* https://www.cno.org/fr/exercice-de-la-profession/outils-educatifs/ask-practice/answers-to-your-questions-about-psychotherapy/

Corey, G. (2016). *Theory & practice of group psychotherapy* (10th ed.). Cengage.

Greenberger, D., & Padesky, C. (2016). *Mind over mood* (2nd ed.). Guilford.

Hubble, M., Duncan, B., Miller, S., & Wampold, B. (2014). Introduction. In B. Duncan, S. Millner, B. Wampold & M. Hubble (Eds.), *The heart & soul of change: Delivering what works in therapy* (2nd ed.) (pp. 23–46). American Psychological Association.

Information and Privacy Commissioner of Ontario (2015). *Frequently asked questions: Personal health information protection act.* https://www.ipc.on.ca/wp-content/uploads/2015/11/phipa-faq.pdf

Rogers, C. (1957). The necessary and sufficient conditions of therapeutic personality change. *Consulting Psychology, 21*(2), 95–103.

The Canadian Counselling and Psychotherapy Association. (2023). *The profession & regulation.* Author. https://www.ccpa-accp.ca/profession-and-regulation/

World Health Organization. (2016). Group interpersonal psychotherapy (IPT) for depression. Author. https://www.who.int/publications/i/item/WHO-MSD-MER-16.4

Yalom, I., & Leszcz, M. (2020). *The theory and practice of group psychotherapy* (6th Ed.). Basic Books.

Chapter 11
Population Needs: Vulnerable Populations

Siobhan Bell, Cheryl Forchuk, and Esther N. Monari

Abstract The intersectionality of sociocultural factors, both directly and indirectly, can impact situational health presentations, clinical decision-making for treatment, and outcomes. When treating vulnerable populations, nurses not only require an understanding of how these sociocultural factors impact the client but also require an awareness and understanding of concepts, such as the ways in which humility, oppression, and discrimination impact the person and family-centred approach, necessary to provide culturally safe care in the context of the client's situational need. Practitioners must continuously assess and reflect on their scope of knowledge when working with vulnerable populations. Acquiring the skills and experience necessary to provide culturally competent and trauma-informed care while taking a non-expert stance can increase the client's chances of positive outcomes from interventions by nurse psychotherapists. Several vulnerable populations that the nurse psychotherapist may encounter will be reviewed in this chapter, followed by the use of case vignettes to illustrate therapeutic application with some vulnerable populations.

Keywords Vulnerable populations · Intersectionality · Person-centered · Advanced practice · Sociocultural attunement

---

S. Bell (✉)
Nursing@Heart Inc., Mono, ON, Canada
e-mail: sbell@nursingatheart.ca

C. Forchuk
Nursing and Psychiatry, Lawson Research Institute, Western University, London, ON, Canada
e-mail: cforchuk@uwo.ca

E. N. Monari
Faculty of Nursing Health Sciences Centre, Memorial University of Newfoundland, St. John's, Newfoundland and Labrador, Canada
e-mail: enmonari@mun.ca

S. Roles and K. Kalia (eds.), *The Nurses' Guide to Psychotherapy*,
https://doi.org/10.1007/978-981-97-4738-2_11

Learning Objectives

After completing this chapter, the learner will be able to:

1. Analyze the concept of intersectionality within the context of vulnerable populations within nurse psychotherapy.
2. Examine the essential knowledge and skills needed to be able to apply concepts such as humility, oppression, and discrimination when providing person and family-centered care to vulnerable populations.
3. Assess the scope of one's own knowledge and recognize the importance of adopting a non-expert stance when working with vulnerable populations in nurse psychotherapy.
4. Examine the necessity of continuously acquiring skills and experiences to provide culturally safe and trauma-informed care.

1 Introduction

Providing psychotherapy for vulnerable populations means being morally and ethically aware of the intersecting needs that shape their world. Although as a practitioner, the nurse may be aware of these intersections, it is important to also remain as a learner, as an invitee into the client's world, allowing space to understand their lived reality. This learning will likely include creatively seeking ways to support their journey and attempting to gain an understanding of the ways in which they have been able to survive and thrive in their lives. The complexity of their worlds along with the potential for oppression, discrimination, and hostility that many face on a regular basis makes supporting them both a rewarding and trauma-laden experience. Vicarious trauma within this field of work is one of the most challenging aspects for the nurse psychotherapist. The continual need to practice from a space of humility while always utilizing a lens of trauma and violence-informed care can be challenging. This chapter is dedicated to all those patients who have shared their voices and pain with their nurse psychotherapist, trusting in them to hold space with a willingness to learn.

2 Intersectionality

Intersectionality is a critical concept in understanding and addressing the complex needs of vulnerable populations when providing psychotherapy. Coined by Kimberlé Crenshaw in 1989, intersectionality refers to the interconnected nature of social categorizations such as race, gender, class, and other identity markers, which can overlap and intersect, creating unique experiences of privilege and discrimination (Crenshaw 1989). In the realm of nursing psychotherapy, the concept of intersectionality underscores the importance of recognizing that individuals from vulnerable populations often face multiple layers of societal disadvantage and marginalization which in turn profoundly influence health presentations and behaviours, as well as therapeutic needs.

There is evidence that these intersecting factors, directly and indirectly, impact situational health presentations among vulnerable populations (Turan et al. 2019; Harari and Lee 2021). For example, a refugee who identifies as a transgender person may experience not only the trauma of forced migration but also discrimination and social exclusion based on their gender identity. This intersection of refugee status and gender identity significantly shapes their mental health needs and the therapeutic approach required. Nurse psychotherapists must be attuned to the intricate interplay of these sociocultural factors when assessing and addressing the mental health concerns of vulnerable populations (Crenshaw 1989). The concept of intersectionality emphasizes the need for culturally sensitive and safe person-centred care within nursing psychotherapy. Clients from vulnerable populations may carry experiences of systemic oppression, discrimination, and trauma related to their intersecting identities. This necessitates a deep awareness of humility, oppression, and discrimination, which are essential for nurse psychotherapists to provide effective and compassionate care. An awareness enables practitioners to create a therapeutic environment that respects the clients' unique experiences and situational needs, fostering trust and enhancing the therapeutic alliance (Crenshaw 1989). Nurse psychotherapists can tailor their approaches to meet the diverse and intersecting needs of their clients, promoting more equitable and effective mental health care.

3 Humility, Oppression, and Discrimination

Examination of essential knowledge and skills related to concepts including humility, oppression, and discrimination is paramount for healthcare professionals such as nurses, particularly when providing person- and family-centred care to vulnerable populations. These concepts are pivotal in fostering a therapeutic environment that respects the dignity and unique experiences of individuals from marginalized groups. Nurses need to continually examine and reflect on their ability to provide care that expresses humility, in addition to understanding, and whenever possible, to reduce systemic barriers that create oppression. Nurses must also be aware of how social inequities create discrimination and negatively impacts the outcome of basic survival needs and ultimately health (College of Nurses of Ontario [CNO] 2023, pp. 6–7).

Humility is a fundamental attribute that nurses must cultivate when working with vulnerable populations. It involves recognizing the limits of one's knowledge and expertise and approaching care with openness and receptivity. Nurse psychotherapists must acknowledge that they may not fully comprehend the lived experiences and challenges faced by individuals from diverse backgrounds. When nurses practice with humility they are encouraging learning and partnership, fostering collaboration with clients and tailoring care that aligns with the clients' values, preferences, and cultural contexts (Repo et al. 2017).

Oppression and discrimination are pervasive issues that impact the lives of many vulnerable individuals. Nurses must develop a deep understanding of these concepts to provide culturally competent and sensitive care. Oppression refers to the systemic and institutionalized mistreatment and discrimination that marginalized or racialized groups face (Mcleod 2021; Ontario Human Rights Commission n.d; National Museum of African American History & Culture 2014). It is essential for nurse psychotherapists to recognize how these structures affect the health and well-being of their patients. Discrimination, on the other hand, involves unjust treatment based on factors such as race, gender, sexual orientation, or socioeconomic status (Mcleod 2021; Ontario Human Rights Commission n.d; National Museum of African American History & Culture 2014). Nurses must be vigilant in identifying and addressing biases, prejudice, and discrimination within the healthcare system to ensure equitable care for all (Williams and Mohammed 2013). When applying these concepts to person- and family-centred care, nurse psychotherapists should strive to create a safe and inclusive environment that acknowledges the potential impacts of oppression and discrimination on their client's health. This includes actively listening to the patients' narratives, validating their experiences, and advocating for their rights within the healthcare system. By doing so, nurses can empower individuals and families to actively participate in their care decisions and promote more positive health outcomes (Repo et al. 2017).

Nurses must continually educate themselves on the unique needs and challenges vulnerable populations face. This involves ongoing professional development and a commitment to developing cultural competence and safety, knowledge of social determinants of health, and evidence-based practices (CNO 2023). By acquiring and applying this knowledge, nurse psychotherapists can offer more effective and tailored care that addresses the specific needs of the individuals and families they serve (Betancourt et al. 2005).

The examination of essential knowledge and skills related to concepts like humility, oppression, and discrimination is crucial for nurse psychotherapists when providing person- and family-centered care to vulnerable populations. These concepts inform a compassionate and culturally competent approach that respects the dignity and experiences of individuals and families, ultimately improving the quality of care and health outcomes for those who are most vulnerable (Betancourt et al. 2005; Repo et al. 2017; Williams and Mohammed 2013).

4 Specialized Populations

There are many populations of patients that fall into the category of vulnerable. Some may include persons who are: newcomers (refugees and immigrants), 2SLGBTQ+; military and veterans, those experiencing severe and persistent mental illness, teenagers and youth, those who may have experienced suicidal ideation or non-suicidal self-injury, those who have experienced eating disorders, perinatal and child grief and loss, or those who feel ostracized by choosing to live child-free, those with disabilities, survivors of sexual assault and interpersonal violence, the elderly, and racialized peoples. This chapter cannot possibly address all specialized vulnerable populations and is not attempting to do so. Rather, this chapter is bringing awareness to the nurse psychotherapist who may be working with a specialized population, some of which may not be listed in the sections ahead.

4.1 Severe and Persistent Mental Illness

Many healthcare practitioners often see those with severe and persistent mental illness frequently in the emergency departments, in crisis departments and accessing mental health and addictions services frequently. Oftentimes, these clients cannot maintain employment and frequently suffer from breaks in support from family or friends. When individuals are without work, housing becomes a challenge. Without housing, there is no fixed address and it is difficult if at all possible to access many social supports including healthcare and financial assistance from the government (Canadian Mental Health Association [CMHA] n.d). The inability to access support may continue until clients cannot function in any capacity within society, often left with no alternatives but to seek help or to involuntarily access support in emergency departments. Unfortunately, many emergency departments are not equipped to support this level of need or to coordinate community services. While many psychotherapists work with those with persistent mental illness, the nurse psychotherapist has a unique foundation in our holistic nursing practice to be coordinators of care. Being person-centred and aware of the intersections of health and the social determinants means that nurse psychotherapists can uniquely support this population. Nurses can accomplish this through liaising with social services (i.e. stable, affordable housing) to support clients with solution-focused steps as they transition through their journey to establish a balance in their lives.

4.2 Survivors of Sexual and Intimate Partner Violence

The World Health Organization (WHO) estimates that approximately 30% of women across the world have experienced physical and/or sexual violence (WHO 2024). Sexual and intimate partner violence is most often "...associated with the development of post-traumatic stress disorder (PTSD), drug and substance misuse, self-harm, increased risk of suicide, as well as relationship problems and long-term mental illness" (Stefanidou et al. 2020, p. 2). The high rates of post-assault mental health concerns make this population extremely vulnerable. The intersection of sexual and physical violence with multiple vulnerable groups such as the 2SLGBTQ+ community, sex workers and racialized community members make this a compounded psychological trauma. "Sexual minority Canadians [are] almost three times more likely to experience violence victimization in the previous 12 months than heterosexual Canadians" (Statistics Canada 2020, para 6). These many intersections mean that this vulnerable group can be complex to treat psycho-therapeutically. Current evidence suggests that present-focused psychotherapies (i.e. Dialectical Behavioural Therapy, Trauma-Focused Cognitive Behavioural Therapy, sensorimotor psychotherapy, or psychodynamic psychotherapy) are often better tolerated in this population, when complex, with the option to go into past-focused therapies after stabilization of current trauma symptoms (CAMH n.d; Cowan et al. 2020; Stefanidou et al. 2020; Najavits 2007). The exception to this is the utilization of a past-focused therapy solely on the current trauma such as the use of cognitive processing therapy (CPT), eye movement desensitization and reprocessing (EMDR) therapy, or prolonged exposure (PE) therapy (American Psychological Association [APA] 2017). For more information on the types of psychotherapies see Chap. 16. Nurse psychotherapists should present differing evidence-based treatments to these clients to empower psychotherapeutic choices and ensure constant reiteration of the safety of the client throughout the session. Nurses have a foundational understanding of the social and economic consequences for survivors of sexual and intimate partner trauma and the impact the stress response has on the clients' mental and physical health. These consequences can influence the client's ability to successfully heal psychologically. Whether working with a client alone or in conjunction with other providers, the nurse psychotherapist provides a holistic understanding necessary to navigate the complex challenges faced by survivors of sexual and intimate partner violence.

4.3 People Experiencing Homelessness

People experiencing homelessness are not a homogenous group. Experiences and needs can vary considerably, however, there are some common considerations.

Living on the streets, in shelters or in encampments tends to be very noisy and somewhat chaotic places that interfere with sleep. This can impact attention span and the ability to focus. Strategies for the nurse psychotherapist while working with these individuals can include careful observation of fatigue and offering breaks as needed (Billings et al. 2020). For some of these clients who are seeking psychotherapy, it may be necessary to have shorter sessions. The sleep issues can continue for the first period after being housed. People then often find being housed can be too quiet and may find they need several months to adjust to this new lifestyle.

People experiencing homelessness are often hungry, which can lead to symptoms appearing like or mimicking anxiety. The nurse psychotherapist should be mindful of this and consider having something like fruit juice, water or a biscuit handy which may be useful to increase the person's comfort. It is hard for a person to think and regulate their emotions when their body is in survival mode from malnutrition. The drive to find nourishment can be overwhelming. In order to provide a therapeutic space and interaction, you may need to first address the biological need to eat in order for the psychological need to be successfully considered.

Prior trauma issues are extremely common. The multiple losses that accompany losing one's home is in itself a traumatic experience These losses can include clothing, furniture, ability to safely store food, medication, kitchenware, pets, family mementos/photographs and any sense of privacy (Conalogueet et al. 2019). Multiple studies have found that the majority of people experiencing homelessness have also had multiple head injuries and these traumas should be taken into consideration (Cusimano et al. 2021; Hwang et al. 2008; Oddy et al. 2012; Stubbs et al. 2020; Topolovec-Vranic et al. 2014). Often the initial head injury precedes homelessness (Cusimano et al. 2021; Hwang et al. 2008; Oddy et al. 2012; Topolovec-Vranic et al. 2014) and people after becoming homeless frequently experience abuse and further head injuries (Cusimano et al. 2021). Head trauma issues may have rarely been treated and can interfere with cognitive functions (Synovec and Berry 2020). The social context of the various emotional, social, sexual, and physical traumas can add to the complexity of working through trauma and symptoms, therefore, trauma-informed practices need to be consistently employed.

Sexual exploitation is also common for those who have experienced sexual assault. Women and youth in particular may engage in survival sex in exchange for basics such as food and a place to stay (Li and Urada 2020). People from the 2SLGBTQ+ community are overrepresented in the homeless population (McCarthy and Parr 2022). Youth may have had a sexual identity as a source of family conflict prior to becoming homeless and or as a reason for becoming homeless. Sexual issues can be complex. For example, a young woman may have left home due to their family not accepting their attraction to other women. However, being homeless, they may be forced into situations involving sex with men. These issues overlap with trauma histories.

Substance use is very common while homeless. This can precede the experience of homelessness or happen after becoming homeless as a way to cope with their unhoused situation. Drug traffickers often target people experiencing homelessness and offer them work in high-risk drug sales situations. Harm reduction strategies can be a beneficial intervention as core approaches to treatment and support, as well as understanding that individuals may not be able to address substance use issues until stably housed. This does not mean that they cannot engage in deep meaningful discussions or planning phases in subsiding from substance use prior to being housed.

Vision and reading issues are also common in this population. Vision issues largely relate to not being able to keep glasses or contacts for those who require them (Jiang et al. 2020). Learning disabilities, including those related to fetal alcohol syndrome, can interfere with literacy (Gerber 2012; Kippin et al. 2021). Strategies for psychotherapy include considering the literacy level for any written material, considering reading material out loud and ensuring the font is plain and large (Evans and Randle-Phillips 2020).

Addressing homelessness is complex. However, there are many struggles that can benefit from psychotherapy. If providing psychotherapy to this vulnerable population, it would be helpful to also be aware of community resources and support for basic needs. Examples of these resources/supports include homelessness programs, housing programs, drop-in centers, food banks, harm reduction programs, and income supports.

4.4 *Racialized Peoples*

The role of nurse psychotherapy is crucial in the care of racialized people within vulnerable populations, contributing to increased diversity in health care. However, recognizing the heterogeneity of racialized peoples and understanding their unique cultural and supportive needs associated with substance use and related mental health are key factors for achieving successful treatment outcomes.

Racialized peoples are individuals from various ethnic, cultural, and racial backgrounds, including but not limited to Black, Indigenous, and people of color (Adames et al. 2023; Hagle et al. 2021). Many racialized people who suffer from substance use and mental health challenges encounter a range of difficulties associated with these issues, which include racial discrimination, stigma, shame, police arrest and harassment, which exacerbate the impact of substance and mental health problems and associated adverse effects such as psychosis and other mental health problems (Cénat et al. 2023; Godkhindi et al. 2022; Goldenberg et al. 2022; Perry et al. 2023). Additionally, racialized people may face barriers in accessing culturally and linguistically appropriate treatment interventions for mental health and substance use harm reduction (Kwok and Tam 2023; Matsuzaka and Knapp 2020; Monari and Taiwo 2023). Furthermore, a lack of awareness about available services compounds these challenges. Experiencing these challenges has been found to increase the risks of substance use and mental health complications, such as drug-related overdose, and death (Cénat et al. 2023; Banks et al. 2023). Addressing these barriers is essential to ensuring equitable access to comprehensive and culturally sensitive mental health and substance use support for racialized individuals (Joo and Liu 2021; Nguemo Djiometio et al. 2020).

4.4.1 Addressing Complex Challenges

Recognizing and eliminating racial discrimination, stigma, shame, police arrest, and harassment among racialized people is a complex and multifaceted challenge that demands a comprehensive approach (Goldenberg et al. 2022; Nguemo Djiometio et al. 2020). Nurse psychotherapists, in collaboration with the healthcare system and policymakers, are in a position to promote awareness and education, including cultural competency training that fosters an understanding of racialized population; addressing and implementing policies that address systemic racism and discrimination; establishing clear protocols for police interactions to ensure fair treatment and accountability; and creating safe spaces for racialized individuals to share their experiences and concerns without fear of reprisal.

4.4.2 Diversifying Nurse Psychotherapy Services

Racialized people often have unique needs that can be most effectively addressed by nurse psychotherapists with knowledge and expertise in racialized issues. Nurses providing psychotherapy services, equipped with an understanding of these specific needs, are well-placed to integrate culturally relevant programs facilitated by professionals from diverse racial backgrounds (Ilagan and Heatherington 2022). This may involve the inclusion of virtual and drop-in spaces, or the involvement of peer outreach psychotherapists conducting home visits and engaging in community outreach to enhance compliance and effectiveness in substance misuse and mental health treatment. The role of the nurse psychotherapist also extends to the development of culturally pertinent peer support group programs including initiatives such as youth-to-youth or peer group mentoring psychotherapy. These programs can foster a sense of belonging, facilitate the sharing of experiences related to substance misuse, and offer support for healing within racialized communities impacted by both substance use and mental health challenges (Banks et al. 2023; Monari and Taiwo 2023). Research indicates a distinct advantage in being cared for by someone from the same cultural background, as individuals tend to have a more positive perception towards therapists who share their race and ethnicity. This trust and relatability contribute to a more effective therapeutic relationship, emphasizing the importance of diversifying the healthcare workforce to better meet the cultural and contextual needs of racialized clients. Nurse psychotherapists who build an understanding of the factors contributing to these challenges will facilitate in providing a better approach that is culturally supportive of these populations (Ilagan and Heatherington 2022; Wilcox 2023).

5 Reflective Questions

1. Consider the losses that would accompany losing your home. How might this affect participation in psychotherapy?
2. As a nurse psychotherapist, how do you personally approach the cultivation of humility in your practice, especially when working with individuals from diverse backgrounds?
3. When has practicing humility positively influenced your collaboration with a client and the tailoring of care to align with their values and preferences?
4. Considering the pervasive issues of oppression and discrimination within healthcare, what steps can you take to identify and address discriminatory practices in your work as a nurse psychotherapist?
5. How will you create a safe and inclusive environment for vulnerable populations, actively listening to their narratives, validating their experiences, and advocating for their rights within the healthcare system?

6 Case Vignette

Alex, a 42-year-old individual experiencing homelessness in an urban setting, has been living on the streets for several months, facing the harsh realities of survival. Struggling with depression, anxiety, and substance abuse issues, Alex decides to seek psychotherapy to address the mental health challenges exacerbated by the circumstances of homelessness.

6.1 Psychotherapeutic Approach

Nurse psychotherapist Sarah takes on Alex's case, recognizing the unique challenges and vulnerabilities associated with homelessness. Sarah approaches the sessions with a person-centered focus, acknowledging the complex intersections of mental health, homelessness, and substance abuse.

6.2 Psychotherapy Nurse Assessment for Alex

Background Information:

- Demographics: Alex, 42 years old, currently experiencing homelessness in an urban setting.
- Living Situation: Alex has been living on the streets for several months, facing the harsh realities of survival. He has been robbed the 2 times he has previously tried to stay in the shelter system, the last time he was badly beaten and ended up in the hospital for 3 days with broken ribs. He will not return to the shelter system due to these experiences.
- Presenting Issues: Struggling with depression, anxiety, and substance abuse issues.
- Mental Health History: Alex has been previously diagnosed by a psychiatrist in hospital (5 years ago) with major depressive disorder, generalized anxiety disorder and PTSD.
- Family Mental Health History: Alex is aware that his parents likely had mental health concerns but they were both suffering from substance abuse disorder and so he is not sure what is mental health and what is substance abuse. He doesn't know the rest of his family.
- Substance Use Assessment: Alex routinely drinks alcohol, whenever he can get it and uses marijuana and methamphetamine.
- Impact on Daily Functioning: Drinking and using drugs consumes Alex's day, and trying to find money for drugs takes a lot of his day.
- Motivation for Change: Alex states that he wants help to stop using drugs and alcohol and if he could just get help to get into rehab, he wants to do it this time.

- Current Mental Health Status: Alex feels worthless and like life is not worth living. He wants to get better but doesn't think anyone will help him.
- Risk Assessment: Alex is at risk for self-harm as he does not know why he should still be alive; however, he is not at imminent risk as he does not have an active plan and states that he has no plans to die right now, he just doesn't know why he is alive.
- Coping Mechanisms: Currently he is using drugs and alcohol as his coping mechanisms.

6.2.1 Case Vignette Reflective Questions

1. Reflect on the complex intersections of homelessness, depression, anxiety, and substance abuse in Alex's case. How do these factors influence each other, and what potential challenges and opportunities do you anticipate in addressing this multifaceted presentation?
2. Consider the importance of building trust and rapport with a client experiencing homelessness. How might Sarah establish a therapeutic alliance with Alex, considering the potential barriers such as mistrust, fear, or previous negative experiences with healthcare providers?
3. Given the context of homelessness, how can Sarah tailor psychotherapeutic interventions to address Alex's mental health needs? What modalities or techniques might be particularly effective in addressing both the immediate challenges and the underlying issues contributing to depression, anxiety, and substance abuse?
4. Homelessness often involves struggles with meeting basic survival needs. How can Sarah incorporate strategies to address Alex's immediate needs, such as access to food, shelter, and health care, while also focusing on long-term mental health goals?
5. Reflect on the role of collaboration with other healthcare and social service providers in Alex's case. How can Sarah work collaboratively with shelters, addiction services, and other relevant agencies to ensure a holistic and coordinated approach to Alex's care?

7 Summary

- It is important to have moral and ethical awareness in providing psychotherapy for vulnerable populations.
- Social categorizations, such as race, gender, and class, create unique experiences of privilege and discrimination. Nurses must be attuned to the intricate interplay of sociocultural factors when assessing and addressing mental health concerns.
- Awareness of social inequity and its negative impact on survival needs and health outcomes is of importance. There are complex challenges faced by racialized people, including racial discrimination, stigma, and systemic issues. Nurse

psychotherapy focuses on caring for racialized peoples, recognizing diversity, and addressing barriers to mental health and substance use support.
- The examination of essential knowledge and skills related to concepts like humility, oppression, and discrimination is crucial for nurse psychotherapists. These concepts inform a compassionate and culturally competent approach, ultimately improving the quality of care and health outcomes for vulnerable populations.

References

Adames, H. Y., Chavez-Dueñas, N. Y., Lewis, J. A., Neville, H. A., French, B. H., Chen, G. A., & Mosley, D. V. (2023). Radical healing in psychotherapy: Addressing the wounds of racism-related stress and trauma. *Psychotherapy, 60*(1), 39. https://doi.org/10.1037/pst0000435

American Psychological Association. (APA, 2017). *Clinical practical guideline for the treatment of PTSD.* Author. https://www.apa.org/ptsd-guideline/ptsd.pdf

Banks, D. E., Duello, A., Paschke, M. E., Grigsby, S. R., & Winograd, R. P. (2023). Identifying drivers of increasing opioid overdose deaths among black individuals: A qualitative model drawing on experience of peers and community health workers. *Harm Reduction Journal, 20*(1), 1-9. https://doi.org/10.1186/s12954-023-00734-9

Betancourt, J. R., Green, A. R., Carrillo, J. E., & Park, E. R. (2005). Cultural competence and health care disparities: Key perspectives and trends. *Health affairs (Project Hope), 24*(2), 499–505. https://doi.org/10.1377/hlthaff.24.2.499

Billings, M., Hale, L., & Johnson, D. (2020). Physical and Social Environment Relationship With Sleep Health and Disorders. *Chest 157*(5), 1304–1312. https://doi.org/10.1016/j.chest.2019.12.002.

Canadian Mental Health Association. (n.d). Housing and mental health. Author. https://ontario.cmha.ca/documents/housing-and-mental-health/

Cénat, J. M., Dromer, É., Darius, W. P., Dalexis, R. D., Furyk, S. E., Poisson, H., Mansoub B. F., Diao, D. G., Gedeon, A. P., Shah, M.S., Labelle, P. R., Bernheim, E., & Kogan, C. S. (2023). Incidence, racial disparities and factors related to psychosis among black individuals in Canada: A scoping review. *The Canadian Journal of Psychiatry*, 68(10), 713–731. https://doi.org/10.1177/07067437231178957

Centre for Addiction and Mental Health. (n.d). Trauma. https://www.camh.ca/en/health-info/mental-illness-and-addiction-index/trauma

College of Nurses of Ontario. (2023). Code of conduct. https://www.cno.org/globalassets/docs/prac/49040_code-of-conduct.pdf

Conalogue, D., Maunder, N., Areington, A., Martin, K., Clarke, V., & Scott, S. (2019). Homeless people and health: a qualitative enquiry into their practices and perceptions. *Journal of Public Health 43*(2), 287–294. https://doi.org/10.1093/pubmed/fdz104

Cowan, A., Ashai, A., & Gentile, J. P. (2020). Psychotherapy with survivors of sexual abuse and assault. *Innovations in Clinical Neuroscience, 17*(1–3), 22–26

Crenshaw, K. (1989). Demarginalizing the intersection of race and sex: A black feminist critique of antidiscrimination doctrine, feminist theory and antiracist politics. *University of Chicago Legal Forum*, 1989(1), 139–167. https://chicagounbound.uchicago.edu/cgi/viewcontent.cgi?article=1052&context=uclf

Cusimano, M. D., Korman, M. B., Carpino, M., Feher, A., Puvirajasingam, J., Zhang, S., Hwang, S. W., & Tepperman, L. (2021). The temporal relations of traumatic brain injury, victimization,

aggression, and homelessness: A developmental trajectory. *Neurotrauma reports, 2*(1), 103–114. https://doi-org.proxy1.lib.uwo.ca/10.1089/neur.2020.0050
Evans, L. & Randle-Phillips, C. (2020). People with intellectual disabilities' experiences of psychological therapy: A systematic review and meta-ethnography. *Journal of Intellectual Disabilities, 24*(2), 233–252. https://doi.org/10.1177/1744629518784359
Gerber, P. J. (2012). The impact of learning disabilities on adulthood: A review of the evidenced-based literature for research and practice in adult education. *Journal of Learning Disabilities, 45*(1), 31–46. https://doi.org/10.1177/0022219411426858
Godkhindi, P., Nussey, L., & O'Shea, T. (2022). "They're causing more harm than good": A qualitative study exploring racism in harm reduction through the experiences of racialized people who use drugs. *Harm Reduction Journal, 19*(1), 96. https://doi.org/10.1186/s12954-022-00672-y
Goldenberg, S. M., Perry, C., Watt, S., Bingham, B., Braschel, M., & Shannon, K. (2022). Violence, policing, and systemic racism as structural barriers to substance use treatment amongst women sex workers who use drugs: Findings of a community-based cohort in Vancouver, Canada (2010–2019). *Drug and Alcohol Dependence, 237*, 109506. https://doi.org/10.1016/j.drugalcdep.2022.109506
Hagle, H. N., Martin, M., Winograd, R., Merlin, J., Finnell, D. S., Bratberg, J. P., Gordon, A.J., Johnson, C., Levy,S., MacLane-Baeder, D., Northup, R., Weinstein, Z., & Lum, P. J. (2021). Article commentary: Dismantling racism against Black, Indigenous, and People of Color across the substance use continuum: A position statement of the Association for Multidisciplinary Education and Research in Substance use and Addiction. *Substance abuse, 42*(1), 5–12. https://doi.org/10.1080/08897077.2020.1867288
Harari, L., & Lee, C. (2021). Intersectionality in quantitative health disparities research: A systematic review of challenges and limitations in empirical studies. *Social science & medicine,* 277, 113876. https://doi.org/10.1016/j.socscimed.2021.113876
Hwang, S. W., Colantonio, A., Chiu, S., Tolomiczenko, G., Kiss, A., Cowan, L., Redelmeier, D. A., & Levinson, W. (2008). The effect of traumatic brain injury on the health of homeless people. *CMAJ, 179*(8), 779–784. https://doi.org/10.1503/cmaj.080341
Ilagan, G. S., & Heatherington, L. (2022). Advancing the understanding of factors that influence client preferences for race and gender matching in psychotherapy. *Counselling Psychology Quarterly, 35*(3), 694–717.
Jiang, S., Mikhail, M., Slomovic, J., Pereira, A., Lebovic, G., Noel, C., & Lichter, M. (2020). Prevalence and impact of eye disease in an urban homeless and marginally housed population. *Canadian Journal of Ophthalmology 55*(1), 76–81. https://doi.org/10.1016/j.jcjo.2019.07.006
Joo, J. Y., & Liu, M. F. (2021). Culturally tailored interventions for ethnic minorities: A scoping review. *Nursing Open, 8*(5), 2078–2090. https://doi.org/10.1002/nop2.733
Kippin, N. R., Leitão, S., Watkins, R., & Finlay-Jones, A. (2021). Oral and written communication skills of adolescents with prenatal alcohol exposure (PAE) compared with those with no/low PAE: A systematic review. *International Journal of Language & Communication Disorders, 56*(4), 694–718. https://doi.org/10.1111/1460-6984.12644
Kwok, S. M., & Tam, D. M. (2023). The experiences of Chinese youth in drug treatment programs. In R. Csiernik, W. S. Rowe, & G. Novotna (Eds.). *Responding to the oppression of addiction* (4th ed.), (pp. 314–326). Canadian Scholars Press.
Li, J. & Urada, L. (2020). Cycle of perpetual vulnerability for women facing homelessness near an urban library in a major U.S. metropolitan area. *Environmental Research and Public Health 17*(5985), 1–16. https://doi.org/10.3390/ijerph17165985
Matsuzaka, S., & Knapp, M. (2020). Anti-racism and substance use treatment: Addiction does not discriminate, but do we? *Journal of ethnicity in substance abuse, 19*(4), 567–593. https://doi.org/10.1080/15332640.2018.1548323
McCarthy, L., & Parr, S. (2022). Is LGBT homelessness different? Reviewing the relationship between LGBT identity and homelessness. *Housing Studies, ahead-of-print* (ahead-of-print), 1–19. https://doi.org/10.1080/02673037.2022.210481

Mcleod, J. (2021). *Understanding racial terms and differences.* National Institute of Health. https://www.edi.nih.gov/blog/communities/understanding-racial-terms-and-differences

Monari, E. & Taiwo, A. (2023). The experience of addiction within the Black community: Treatments and Responses. In R. Csiernik, W. Rowe, & G. Novotna (Eds). *Responding to the oppression of addiction* (4th ed.), pp. 274–294. Canadian Scholars Press.

Najavits, L.M. (2007). Psychosocial treatments for posttraumatic stress disorder. In P.E. Nathan & J.M. Gorman (Eds.), *A Guide to Treatments That Work* (3rd ed.) (pp. 213–530). Oxford University Press.

National Museum of African American History & Culture. (2014). *Social identities and systems of oppression.* Author. https://nmaahc.si.edu/learn/talking-about-race/topics/social-identities-and-systems-oppression

Nguemo Djiometio, J. B., Buzuayew, A., Nelson, L. E., Maina, G., Njoroge, I., Kahan, M., & Wong, J. (2020). A scoping review of the prevalence of use of substance among African, Caribbean, and Black (ACB) people in Canada. *Journal of Substance Use, 25*(6), 575–590. https://doi.org/10.1080/14659891.2020.1760378

Oddy, M., Moir, J. F., Fortescue, D., & Chadwick, S. (2012). The prevalence of traumatic brain injury in the homeless community in a UK city. *Brain injury, 26*(9), 1058–1064. https://doi-org.proxy1.lib.uwo.ca/10.3109/02699052.2012.667595

Ontario Human Rights Commission. (n.d). Racism and racial discrimination: Systemic discrimination (fact sheet). Author. https://www.ohrc.on.ca/en/racism-and-racial-discrimination-systemic-discrimination-fact-sheet

Perry, C., Goldenberg, S., Deering, K., Patrick, L., Braschel, M., Shannon, K., & Bingham, B. (2023). Structural racism and violence: Routine healthcare access in a cohort of marginalized Indigenous women and Two-Spirit Peoples during the COVID-19 pandemic. [Manuscript submitted for publication]. https://doi.org/10.21203/rs.3.rs-3450143/v1

Repo, H., Vahlberg, T., Salminen, L., Papadopoulos, I., & Leino-Kilpi, H. (2017). The cultural competence of graduating nursing students. *Journal of Transcultural Nursing, 28*(1), 98–107. https://doi.org/10.1177/1043659616632046

Statistics Canada. (2020). Sexual minority people almost three times more likely to experience violent victimization than heterosexual people. Author, https://www150.statcan.gc.ca/n1/daily-quotidien/200909/dq200909a-eng.htm

Stefanidou, T., Hughes, E., Kester, K., Edmondson, A., Majeed-Ariss, R., Smith, C., Ariss, S., Brooker, C., Gilchrist, G., Kendal, S., Lucock, M., Maxted, F., Perot, C., Shallcross, R., Trevillion, K., Lloyd-Evans, B., & Edward, K.-L. (2020). The identification and treatment of mental health and substance misuse problems in sexual assault services: A systematic review. *PLoS ONE, 15*(4). https://journals.plos.org/plosone/article?id=10.1371/journal.pone.0231260

Stubbs, J., Thornton, A., Sevick, J., Silverberg, N., Barr, A., Honer, W., & Panenka, W. J. (2020). Traumatic brain injury in homeless and marginally housed individuals: a systematic review and meta-analysis. *The Lancet 5*(1), E19–E32. https://doi.org/10.1016/S2468-2667(19)30188-4

Synovec, C. E., & Berry, S. (2020). Addressing brain injury in health care for the homeless settings: A pilot model for provider training. *Work, 65*(2), 285–296. https://doi.org/10.3233/WOR-203080

Topolovec-Vranic, J., Ennis, N., Howatt, M., Ouchterlony, D., Michalak, A., Masanic, C., Colantonio, A., Hwang, S. W., Kontos, P., Stergiopoulos, V., & Cusimano, M. D. (2014). Traumatic brain injury among men in an urban homeless shelter: Observational study of rates and mechanisms of injury. *CMAJ Open, 2*(2), 69–76. https://doi.org/10.9778/cmajo.20130046

Turan, J.M., Elafros, M.A., Logie, C.H., Banik, S., Turan, B., Crockett, K.B., Pescosolido, B., Murray, S.M. (2019). Challenges and opportunities in examining and addressing intersectional stigma and health. *BMC Med 17*, 7. https://doi.org/10.1186/s12916-018-1246-9

Wilcox, M. M. (2023). Oppression is not "culture": The need to center systemic and structural determinants to address anti-Black racism and racial trauma in psychotherapy. *Psychotherapy, 60*(1), 76.https://doi.org/10.1037/pst0000446

Williams, D. R., & Mohammed, S. A. (2013). Racism and Health I: Pathways and Scientific Evidence. *The American behavioral scientist, 57*(8). https://doi.org/10.1177/0002764213487340

World Health Organization. (2024). Violence against women. https://www.who.int/news-room/fact-sheets/detail/violence-against-women

Chapter 12
Population Needs: Cross-Cultural Considerations

Hoodo A. Ibrahim, Myriam Innocent, and Archna N. Patel

Abstract Providing culturally competent and holistic nursing care is emphasized early in nursing school. However, what defines culturally sensitive holistic nursing care is an ever-evolving phenomenon given the varying insights that exist about what truly makes up culturally appropriate nursing interventions. Nurse psychotherapists need to understand how culture shapes people's beliefs and values, adding unique layers of health needs for Black, Indigenous, northern, and rural population groups among others. Nurse psychotherapists must respect clients' cultures, values, beliefs, and treatment preferences to achieve therapy goals. This chapter will provide some common client factors that nurse psychotherapists need to consider when conducting psychotherapy assessments and treatment interventions. Examples of cultural attributes include language, gender, the meaning of eye contact, age, experiences of illness, health and wellness, medicine/treatment, psychosocial care, historical trauma, and cultural safety. Cross-cultural considerations are complex and dynamic, and only a few models explain their basic components well. Helpful cross-cultural consideration strategies that nurses can use during their client interactions by applying the RESPECT model and case scenarios will be discussed.

Keywords Holistic · Cultural competency · Cross-cultural considerations

H. A. Ibrahim (✉)
St Joseph's Healthcare Hamilton/Hamilton Health Sciences, Hamilton, ON, Canada
e-mail: hoodo46@gmail.com

M. Innocent
Cobourg, ON, Canada
e-mail: info@manageyourlupus.com

A. N. Patel
Woodbridge, ON, Canada

S. Roles and K. Kalia (eds.), *The Nurses' Guide to Psychotherapy*,
https://doi.org/10.1007/978-981-97-4738-2_12

Learning Objectives

After completing this chapter the learner will:

1. Understand that being a culturally and ethnically sensitive nurse psychotherapist requires open-mindedness and a lifelong commitment to learning and unlearning.
   (a) This occurs by being intentional in the continuous scrutiny of one's own biases, beliefs, and perceptions about other cultures, ethnicities, religions, gender identities, and other cultural attributes.
2. Understand how to demonstrate cultural humility using therapeutic communication techniques to achieve optimal partnerships with one's own clients.
3. Demonstrate foundational competence to provide unbiased, non-judgmental, and inclusive nurse psychotherapy services for clients of various cultural and ethnic backgrounds.

1 Introduction

Nurses historically and presently continue to be the backbone of our healthcare system. It is no mystery that the nursing profession continues to evolve and gives title to work that nurses have always done, including psychotherapy. Nurses are at the forefront when a natural disaster strikes and are one of the first healthcare professionals to respond. Since nursing involves various specialized skills, it's difficult to find a nurse psychotherapist who would not also provide hands-on nursing during a crisis. When the 7.0 magnitude earthquake hit Haiti in 2010, thousands of nurses, including nursing psychotherapists, Ariane and Chanté, flew in to help (Pallardy, 2024). On the ground, what they saw was devastating. The earthquake tore families apart, left children orphaned, and made grief inescapable. They saw an already impoverished nation struggle to find its citizens and to make sense of what was happening as they continued to search in the rubble for families over one week later. The deadly impact of the earthquake was instant and catastrophic. It is estimated that anywhere between 100,000 to 200,000 people lost their lives that day (Pallardy, 2024). Human suffering cannot be quantified. The earthquake and the damage to the infrastructure of Haiti persist today. Earthquakes, floods, snowstorms, and other natural disasters could affect all regardless of nationality or ethnic affiliation. These calamities alter the course of peoples' lives, with immediate, acute, and long-term negative psychological effects. How can nurse psychotherapists help people cope with and overcome their emotional suffering most expeditiously? A variety of theoretical methods of psychological interventions are available for use. For years, psychological research lacked diversity. Research published in North America focused so closely on its citizens, both Canadians and Americans, who comprise less than five percent of the world's population; so much so that a detailed analysis of peer-reviewed publications in leading academic journals in psychology until the end of the first decade of this country showed that over 90 percent of research samples came from a small group of countries representing only 12 percent of the world's population (Henrich et al. 2010; Shiraev & Levy, 2021). The state of psychological research did not satisfactorily represent the global population (Arnett 2002). For over 100 years, white males, mostly of European descent, dominated psychological education and research (Lonner 2019).

Why is this relevant to note? The clients in both public and independent practice come from a variety of cultures and subcultures in Canada. In fact, 7 out of 10 Canadians indicate that multiculturalism is important to the Canadian identity (Berry 2013). Forty percent of Canadians identify either multiculturalism, the acceptance of immigrants and refugees, or the country's inclusiveness as part of the Canadian identity (Berry 2013). In 1971, Canada was the first country to pass a national multiculturalism law called the Canadian Multiculturalism Act (Berry 2013). Cross-cultural psychology advocates the idea that behaviour and experience are the products of interaction between culture and the individual (Shiraev & Levy, 2021). Discounting a person's culture can unintentionally cause harm even when the intention of it is to ease clients' suffering, not amplify it, or exploit it. The history of Canada and the provision of the Indian Residential School program where thousands of Indigenous children were taken from their families for the entire school year is an example of a tragic legacy that has manifested in intergenerational trauma for many generations in the Indigenous population.

The application of cultural psychology and cultural considerations is to not only help distinguish differences between groups but to identify and describe psychological phenomena that are common to all people and groups (Shiraev & Levy, 2021). The proper application of cross-cultural psychology and consideration is to avoid bias and to unite people worldwide through mutual understanding, curiosity, and appreciation (Shiraev & Levy, 2021).

2 Cultural Awareness and Responsiveness

Historically, healthcare professionals used a "one size fits all approach" (Hook et al. 2017, p. 4) to assess, diagnose, and treat patients based solely on their presenting symptoms and behaviors, without considering the individual's unique ethnicity, cultural background, values, or belief system. Although this approach might have benefited the dominant groups, it led to unintended harm for the ethnic minority and racialized groups i.e. high treatment dropout, poor engagement, and even negative treatment outcomes (American Psychiatric Association [APA], 2019, Hook et al. 2017; Hughes et al. 2020; Rogers-Sirin et al. 2015). People used to view culture as belonging to specific ethnic, racial, religious, or geographically bounded social groups in the past. However, it did not have a significant impact on considering cross-cultural factors in client encounters. Despite much work remaining, it's been a discovery that culture is a compelling force that is complex and ever-changing, and only those who have lived it can define it. The need for cross-cultural considerations in client care processes is periodically discussed in relation to how that culture influences how we feel, think, behave, and interact with one another (Hook et al. 2017; Osazuwa & Moodley 2023).

Similarly, it is being realized that achieving absolute multicultural competence is more complex than one might think and links clinicians who have a positive attitude toward lifelong learning about cultural diversity to favorable client health outcomes (Hook et al. 2017; Massaquoi 2023). In contrast, inaccurate assessment findings, misdiagnoses, and inappropriate treatment plans are some of the negative consequences associated with a clinician's cultural incompetence. Employing culturally responsive attitudes that foster cultural awareness (acknowledging that cultural differences exist), cultural sensitivity (recognizing cultural differences and similarities coexist without assigning values), cultural humility (embracing culture including your own and what you learn from each other), cultural competence (learning knowledge about varying cultures) and cultural safety (understanding, all humans carry social norms which influence how we view others) are important first step measures for nurse psychotherapists who wish to strive to provide holistic psychotherapy (APA, 2019; Rogers-Sirin et al., 2015; Substance Abuse and Mental Health Services Administration. [SAMHSA], 2014). For these reasons, it is vital that nurse psychotherapists are open-minded, flexible, and willing to learn from their own clients. Although cultural awareness is key in the development of a therapeutic relationship, it is even more important to be culturally responsive by getting to know one's clients. Cultural responsiveness is the ability to understand and consider the different cultural backgrounds of the clients you treat (APA 2019; Roche & Maxie, 2003). Clients possess unique knowledge about their own cultural background, ethnicity, values, belief system, socioeconomic status, and the presence of other influencing factors. It is equally important not to make generalized assumptions about how individuals from a specific culture or religion should or should not behave and/or conduct themselves (APA 2019; Rogers-Sirin et al., 2015; SAMSHA, 2014).

3 Themes in Provision of Culturally Sensitive Care

Culture touches all aspects of human life including language, customs, traditions, belief systems, spirituality, actions, values, behaviors, and knowledge. It shapes our social identity and impacts all the decisions we make, including how we choose to live our lives, our sense of belonging, the interpersonal relationships that we form, our worldview, and even how we seek treatment. This emphasizes how important it is for the nurse psychotherapist to work towards diversifying their own multicultural knowledge to have maximum impact on their client's treatment outcomes (Osazuwa & Moodley 2023). It is believed that not acknowledging the client's culturally shared norms, customs, beliefs, and values has a direct negative consequence on therapist-client therapeutic relationship building (Hook et al. 2017). The nurse psychotherapist's willingness to learn, explore, and honour the intersectionality of multicultural identities is vital for client engagement. Being a culturally considerate therapist facilitates respect and appropriate response to your client's unique cultural needs. Demonstrating the desire to accommodate a client's unique health and healing approaches, conveys an openness to engage in a collaborative partnership with the person being served (Aboriginal Nurses Association of Canada [ANAC], 2009; APA 2019; Hook et al. 2017).

Over the years, psychology researchers and theorists explored and adapted varying models and frameworks to identify how to best approach multiculturalism. Multicultural competence was the first model identified in the early 1980s by Derald Wing Sue and Colleagues to improve cultural competencies in counseling (Hook et al. 2017). The model emphasized three components (1) therapists' self-awareness, (2) therapist's knowledge development about various cultural groups, and (3) therapist-specific skill development. It encourages the therapist to be accountable by obtaining adequate knowledge about ethnicity, culture, and race, including one's own. It involves actively seeking knowledge about cross-cultures to appreciate the diverse human dynamics (U.S. Department of Health and Human Services [HHS], 2021). It accentuates that developing cultural competence is a lifelong process rather than an endpoint. Therapists are encouraged to engage in activities that promote skills acquisition (Rosario & Guzman, 2016). This concept is based on the premise that the therapist is motivated to explore various cultural identities of the people they serve. Nurse psychotherapists demonstrate cultural competence through ongoing self-awareness (reflective practice), cultural knowledge enhancement, and obtaining culturally specific psychotherapy skills. Being a culturally competent nurse psychotherapist promotes client empowerment while striving to provide unbiased, and non-judgmental trauma-informed client-centered care that values personhood (APA 2019, Hook. et al. 2017; St Catherine University, 2022).

The cultural humility concept stems from the criticisms of the multicultural competence model's limitations because of its difficulties in empirically verifying its validity (Benuto et al. 2018; Hook et al. 2017; Lekas et al. 2020). Cultural humility is a disposition to trust and learn from clients who are from various cultural backgrounds. It places emphasis on the therapist's attitude and engagement with the client. It requires flexibility, commitment to honest self-reflection (inward self-awareness, outward valuing of others, upward growth) as well as lifelong learning and unlearning. Cultural humility assumes that the therapist recognizes the power imbalance between oneself (provider nurse), and the person being served (client). It encourages the nurse to implement strategies to overcome the power imbalance while integrating culturally considerate therapy (First Nations Health Authority, 2024; Hughes et al. 2020; Lekas et al. 2020). Cultural humility is person-centered, and trauma-informed, and requires the use of therapeutic communication skills to develop a strong therapeutic alliance with the client. The nurse psychotherapist shows cultural humility by acknowledging any cultural knowledge gap, being open to learning from clients, and creating an environment that invites effective partnerships with culturally diverse individuals (Benuto et al., 2018; APA 2019: Hook et al., 2017). Cultural sensitivity is the awareness that everyone has cultural differences and similarities with one another. Part of this includes not assigning these differences a hierarchical value, nor labeling them positive or negative or right or wrong; but as differences that exist within humanity and society.

Components of having cultural sensitivity are:

- Remaining non-judgemental and non-reactive and intentionally practicing being open-minded and curious to understand the differences in each individual person's culture.
- Realizing that cultural differences impact each person differently. This may include their communication skills and styles, their understanding of health and wellness, their motivation to be well, and their willingness to learn and try different strategies to help them better cope with life events and stressors.
- Practicing self-reflections to understand our implicit biases and how they impact our cultural beliefs and how this can impact interpersonal effectiveness with our clients (Fig. 1).

The concept of cultural safety is a valuable concept as it influences how safe individuals being served feel about the nurse-client engagement. Cultural safety acknowledges the health adverse events encountered by members of cultural groups due to power imbalances and inequity between clients, healthcare providers, and

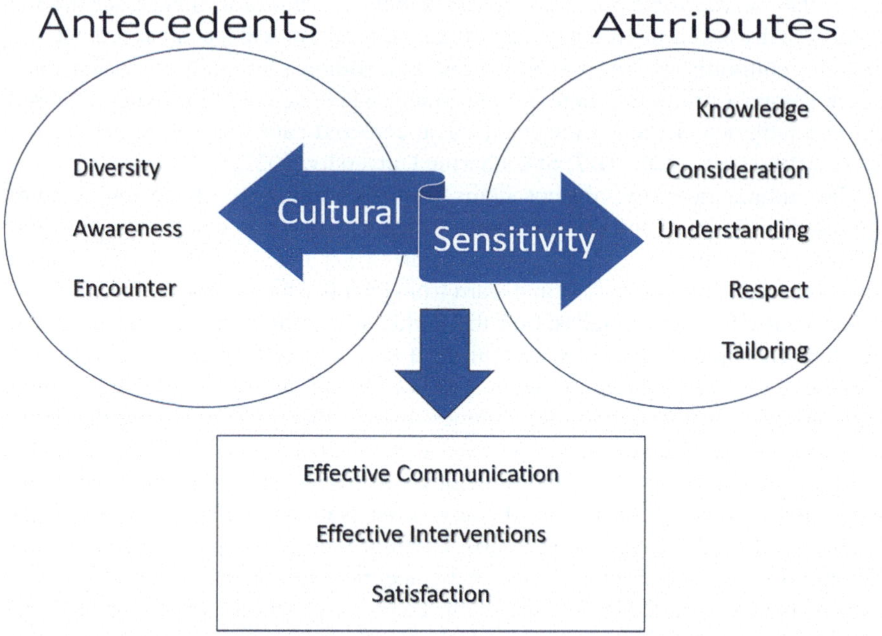

Fig. 1 Cultural Sensitivity. Adapted from Foronda, C. (2008). A concept analysis of cultural sensitivity: An improved understanding of the term as described within health care and in general would enhance nurses' understanding and communication with professionals and clients. *Journal of Transcultural Nursing, 19*(3), 207–12

healthcare organizations. Many minority and marginalized groups have encountered at least one traumatic experience within healthcare organizations (Benuto et al. 2018; Connecticut Women's Consortium 2023). While psychotherapy approaches are uniquely positioned as primary interventions by best practice guidelines, some cultures or individuals might not believe that talk therapy works (Cook et al. 2017; Koç & Kafa 2019). It is equally important to create an environment where the clients feel safe, and listened to, through the integration of their unique health and that healing approaches are respected. It is valuable before proceeding with any treatment interventions to always ask about the client's perception of psychotherapy and their experiences, ensuring to explore a client's current treatment expectations and what their priority goals are (ANAC 2009; Ball 2023; Chung et al. 2022). According to Ball (2023), engaging in mutual learning with clients, ensuring the focus is on client goals, and being aware of one's own cultural identity and biases, while respecting a client's cultural norms are the most effective facilitators of cultural safety. Poor self-esteem, poor or lack of commitment to the treatment plan, dismissal of suggested treatment options, and poor client–clinician therapeutic rapport are indicators of the client feeling culturally unsafe in the environment. It is vital that the clinician engage in racial/cultural humility practices to acknowledge their own cultural knowledge gaps and to minimize potential clinician–client power imbalance (Ball 2023; Bartholomew et al. 2023; Massaquol 2023).

To create a culturally safe environment, one must acknowledge, honor, and be open to discussing the experiences and traumas of historically marginalized populations such as Black, and Indigenous people. The client's cultural history and racial identity are important factors when assessing, diagnosing, and conceptualizing the presenting problems (Jones et al. 2018; Meyer, & Zane 2013; Nuttgens & Campbell 2010; Roche & Maxie 2003). The nurse psychotherapist must also be conscious about making generalized assumptions that every Black or Indigenous individual encountered similar traumas or practices cultural norms at the same degree as subculture or ethnic identities exist within the populations. Roche and Maxie (2003) state that maybe it is more appropriate to allow individuals to provide their own definitions of cultural identity and experiences instead of assigning broader definitions of culture.

Historically speaking, bear in mind that although African Americans and Whites have similar rates of mental health problems, African Americans are more likely to face unique health disparities compared to Whites (Jones et al. 2018; Meyer & Zane 2013). African Americans are more often underdiagnosed or misdiagnosed. They are unlikely to receive appropriate specialty mental health services. If they do receive any treatment, it is often inadequate resulting in higher rates of treatment dropout (Jones et al. 2018; Meyer & Zane 2013). These disparities are often linked to social exclusion stemming from slavery, racism, clinical biases in assessment tools, higher poverty rates, and incarceration. These issues lead to increased psychological distress, poor cognitive functioning, low self-esteem, and mistrust in the healthcare system which has a negative impact on client–clinician therapeutic rapport development (Jones et al. 2018; Meyer & Zane 2013).

Note, the term Indigenous is a global term that captures three subgroups (1) First Nation Aboriginal, (2) Inuit, and (3) Métis (Government of Canada, 2023).

This necessitates that the clinician asks the client to share their own self-identity in terms of which subgroup they self-identify with to avoid re-traumatization by utilizing the general term. Clinicians should take the time to explore the client's unique experiences in relation to colonization and residential schooling. As cited from the National Collaborating Centre for Indigenous Health (2020), colonization and its social structures such as the Indian Act (1876), residential schooling and Indian day schools resulted in a wide range of cultural traumas, loss of language, lack of social cohesion, high rates of family violence, disproportionate degree of mental health and addiction problems leading to lack of trust in the healthcare providers and the overall healthcare system (Canadian Nurses Association 2023; Nuttgens & Campbell 2010). Again, it is essential that the clinician explores the degree to which the client adheres to their own traditional cultural worldview. Nuttgens and Campbell (2010) assert that the following five acculturations apply to the First Nations People's degree of cultural adherence. *Traditional*—those who adhere to traditional cultural norms, values, and belief systems. These individuals only speak their native language. *Marginal*—these clients may or may not speak their mother language or English, and might not be compliant with the traditional norms or mainstream. *Bi-cultural*—clients amalgamate the traditional and mainstream cultures. *Assimilated*—the clients only practice mainstream cultural norms. *Pantraditional*—the client mainly practices mainstream culture but also tries to integrate traditional practices. These definitions highlight the importance of avoiding generalization based on someone's physical appearance or shared ethnic background.

Fragmented health services, poor living conditions, limited access to educational opportunities, lack of transportation, low socioeconomic status, and geographical social isolation may add to the challenges experienced by the northern rural and remote communities, particularly impacting the Indigenous population. Rural and remote communities self-report experiencing higher rates of mental health and addiction problems such as depression, anxiety, sleep disorders, substance use disorders, and higher suicide rates (Canadian Mental Health Association 2023). Although virtual health services have gained some popularity since the start of the COVID-19 pandemic, not everyone has access to technology to ensure the delivery of ethically responsive mental health services such as psychotherapy (Goodwin et al. 2023).

Regardless of the background of the client being served, researchers emphasize the need to adapt culturally tailored psychotherapy treatment approaches that are congruent with the client's cultural values, attitudes, practices, and beliefs.

Recommendations include that the clinician:

- Make an effort to communicate with honesty about their own cultural competence level.
- Be open to addressing traumatic experiences of racism, stereotypes, slavery, and colonization by allowing the client to unpack the historical traumas.
- Foster social cohesion to create a safe space that allows racial and ethnic identity growth.

- Integrate the client's holistic healing processes, spiritual values, and religious and other belief systems into the treatment plan to ensure the proposed treatment is relevant to the individual being served.
- Educate themselves regarding cultural awareness about marginalized populations' historical trauma as it serves a great purpose in providing culturally safe care and is an essential building block in creating a collaborative partnership with clients.
- Use clinician/client cultural differences as an asset instead of a barrier to foster therapeutic partnership.
- Be aware of difficulties associated with virtual care services in terms of providing a culturally safe environment given that the clinician is not in control of the client's immediate surroundings (Canadian Nurses Association 2023; Goodwin et al. 2023; Jones et al. 2018; Meyer & Zane 2013; Nuttgens & Campbell 2010; Roche & Maxie 2003).

Embracing the definitions of diversity and cultural competence as broader than simple terms can help to capture a range of characteristics. Committing to lifelong learning about these characteristics can enable the nurse psychotherapist to actively engage in activities that positively validate the strength of the nurse-client cultural differences and similarities (Registered Nurses Association of Ontario [RNAO], 2007). The U.S. Department of Health and Human Services [HHS] Office of Minority Health has put out a website called Think Cultural Health which has several helpful resources including two frameworks (ADDRESSING and RESPECT) that can be used as a starting point during client assessment (Hays 2016; HHS, 2021). The ADDRESSING framework can be useful in capturing some key social identities when exploring your client's cultural identity. The acronym stands for age/generational influences; disability status/developmental disability; disability status (acquired physical/cognitive/psychological disabilities); religion and spiritual orientation; ethnicity and race; socio-economic status; sexual orientation; Indigenous heritage; national origin, and gender identity. It is also noted that other influential social factors, such as educational level, food and security, housing, communication, and language must be considered to understand the complexity of the concept of culture (Hays, 2016; HHS, 2021).

The RESPECT model can assist nurse psychotherapists in remembering some important elements to consider during client assessment, diagnosis, and the treatment planning process. The RESPECT model includes Respect, Explanatory Model, Sociocultural Context, Power, Empathy, Concerns, and Fears, as well as Therapeutic Alliance and Trust. The following will illustrate how the components of the RESPECT Model can be applied during client assessment.

Respect The nurse psychotherapist must understand and or inquire about how respect is communicated within the client's unique culture or religion. It is important to remember even within the same culture or religion, generational differences exist. It is important not to assume that two individuals within the same cultural group would have the same expectations, values system, or set of social norms. Having cultural biases by expecting others to conform to popular societal norms can be a barrier to developing a nurse-client therapeutic relationship. For example, if you are a male serving a Muslim female or a female serving a Muslim male maintaining direct eye contact with the opposite gender or utilizing therapeutic touch would communicate signs of disrespect depending on how religious the client is. However, in North America, not maintaining good eye contact during clinical assessment is considered poor eye contact or avoidant eye contact which may communicate that the client might not be sharing the truth of his or her own health condition. It is crucial that the nurse psychotherapist communicates respect through verbal and nonverbal communication modes. The nurse psychotherapist must clarify the client's expectations and practices at the beginning of each session so there are no misunderstandings or implied disrespect (DuPraw & Axner 1997; HHS, 2021; College of Nurses of Ontario [CNO], 2006).

Explanatory Model The nurse psychotherapist allows clients to communicate their own understanding of their condition, the origin of their own illness, and its timeline then compares it with their own assessment findings. In acute psychiatry, this is rather difficult as some clients might have an altered sense of reality and it is often labeled as 'poor insight.' Furthermore, some cultures view mental illness as taboo. Therefore, admitting to being mentally ill is a difficult step for many. The nurse psychotherapist shows cultural sensitivity by asking the client his or her own cultural views about mental illness. What does having a mental illness diagnosis mean to the client? What impact would it have on the individual? How would clients' social support systems (life partner, children, parent, siblings, community members, etc.) view the client if they find out about their mental illness diagnosis? Asking these questions would assist the nurse psychotherapist in understanding the client's views about mental illness and would also assist the clinician in reaching less biased assessment findings. Always communicate with honesty and inform the client that the information shared with the clinician is protected by the law unless it imposes safety risk to the client or others, at which time you are bound by the law to intervene appropriately (Canadian Mental Health Association [CMHA], 2023; Hays, 2016).

Sociocultural Context The nurse psychotherapist must understand the varying factors that might influence client engagement. If the nurse psychotherapist has limited knowledge about the client's background, acknowledging this knowledge gap at the beginning of the assessment would be helpful. You want the client to openly share their unique cultural expectations and experiences. Gaining a basic understanding of how cultural influences shape an individual's interactions in society is crucial. Asking the client how important their cultural practices and perspectives on illness impact their health service encounters can provide clarity about client expectations. For example, culturally oriented individuals from Indigenous backgrounds might prefer to take holistic healing approaches including mind, body, and spirit before considering the other forms of treatment. Respecting their view of health and healing communicates the clinician's commitment to cultural safety practice (ANAC 2009; APA 2019; Ball 2023; Bartholomew et al. 2023; Hays 2016). When serving individuals from minority and marginalized subpopulations, one must remember significant cultural and historical traumas that might be a barrier to acquiring client trust and collaboration. Health service encounter-associated traumas often stem from mistrust, mistreatment, racist beliefs, prejudice discriminatory behaviors, and stereotyping. Racism may be subtle, systemic, embedded in assessment, and diagnostic tools, and even unintentional (ANAC 2009; Bartholomew et al. 2023; Massaquol 2023). Acknowledging and discussing openly historical systemic issues can reassure the client that you are committed to forming an unbiased and non-judgmental therapeutic alliance. Other factors that might impact positively or negatively on the client's level of engagement during the treatment process are their past experiences with health service encounters. It is good practice to explore any traumas associated with previous health service encounters to avoid similar missteps. This ensures a person-centered approach, promotes client's active involvement, and empowers them to have a voice in their care (ANAC 2009; APA 2019; Ball 2023; Osazuwa & Moodley 2023).

Power Keeping power dynamics between the therapist and the client in mind is always helpful. Individuals from certain cultures may view healthcare providers as authority figures and might never sagree with the treatment recommendations. Therefore, it is crucial that the nurse psychotherapist emphasizes the importance of a client's active participation in the process. Note, that culturally sensitive, client-centered care is one that supports the client to take the lead in identifying their own treatment goals and strategies to achieve them while the nurse psychotherapist is there to guide them and provide resources (CNO 2006, Curtis et al., 2019).

Empathy While the term 'empathy' can describe a wide range of experiences; in nursing, it refers to "the expression of understanding, validating and resonating with the meaning the health care experience holds for the client" (CNO, 2006, pp. 3–4). The nurse psychotherapist demonstrates empathy through verbal and nonverbal communication to emphasize the importance of each client's unique situation and/or service needs so the client feels heard.

Concerns and Fears Clarifying any pre-existing concerns and fears about health service engagement would allow the client to share any barriers that they might foresee. Actively listening to client's concerns, mainly what brought them to the clinic, what they understand about the psychotherapy treatment, and any fears, or apprehensions that they might have about the treatment modalities communicates the nurse psychotherapist's willingness to engage in the person-centered therapeutic alliance. Person-centered care promotes client trust in the nurse psychotherapist, allows clients to feel heard, and empowers them to share their most intimate health concerns. (CNO, 2006).

Therapeutic Alliance and Trust It is vital to recognize that the client's trust is not inherent but rather must be earned through nurse-client therapeutic engagement. Therapeutic alliance stems from mutual respect and honesty with appropriate self-disclosure. It is important to recognize that earning a client's trust might take some time therefore, the nurse psychotherapist would need to be patient and empathetic to the client's level of readiness. The use of effective communication and motivational interviewing skills would be vital during the early stages of the nurse-client therapeutic relationship in order to achieve the best possible client partnership (CNO, 2006).

4 Case Vignette 1

The nurse psychotherapist is from the same cultural and ethnic background as the client. The client comes from a family where premarital sex and dating are not permitted and against their religious beliefs. Her family believes she should have a marriage arrangement with someone of the same religious background. The nurse psychotherapist is from the same religious and cultural background as the client and has those same beliefs for herself and her children. The client is becoming increasingly depressed and seeking help. She has met a man through college who is of a different religion, and they have been dating for 15 months. She describes to the therapist the nature of their health and loving relationship. She feels guilty for having premarital sex and hiding the relationship from her family. She discloses that once they graduate from school next year, they hope to be formally engaged, plan their wedding, and be married. The client specifically wanted to see a therapist from her same religious and cultural background as she feels they will be able to relate to her circumstances, however, secretly the nurse agrees with her family's beliefs and plans for her. Therefore, the psychotherapist being of the same religious and cultural beliefs does not agree with her client's decision.

The therapist has seen the client for an initial intake appointment and for two follow-up appointments.

4.1 Case Vignette Reflective Questions *1*

1. What should the therapist do?
2. Can the therapist still objectively support this client?
3. What legal and ethical obligations does the psychotherapist have towards this client?
4. What cultural competencies, considerations, and frameworks should this nurse psychotherapist be examining?
5. What self-work does the nurse need to do if she continues to be this client's psychotherapist?

    (a) The therapist's challenge is that not everyone from their own cultural and ethnic background has similar views about their own culture or ethnic background.
    (b) The nurse psychotherapist is cautious about making assumptions about what similarities or differences the client and therapist might share.

5 Case Vignette 2

The psychotherapist is from different cultural and ethnic backgrounds than the client.

The therapist is uncomfortable treating this client due to not feeling culturally competent with this client's cultural and ethnic background. Note the client is from a minority subgroup.

Genevieve, a 20-year-old Canadian of Haitian descent, is taking a nursing undergraduate program at a local university. She is Black and identifies herself as female using she/her/sa/elle pronouns. Genevieve is coming to see you today because she is struggling with her program and hates it. She tells you that in her culture, education is very important, and she is afraid to tell her parents that she is not doing well and does not want to become a nurse. She has been having trouble sleeping, losing weight, having a poor appetite, and currently lives at home with her parents. Genevieve spends most of the day at the library but tells you she sleeps most of the time and has not been submitting her papers on time. She is having difficulty focusing and finishing her work. Genevieve would love to work part-time, but her parents want her to dedicate her time to her studies. When you ask her what she would prefer to be doing, Genevieve shrugs her shoulders and tells you she does not know. She considered no other options, but now regrets her high school decision and is unsure of what to do. Genevieve asks you what she should do. Upon further questioning, you discover she is a second-year nursing student, and she has started her clinical placements. Genevieve tells you she feels nauseous when she provides bedside care and sees bodily fluids. She describes that she cannot catch her breath and her palms sweat during these moments. She tells you that her heart races, and she feels like she is going to pass out. Her teacher took her aside and asked her what was wrong. She burst into tears and told her course instructor how she hates nursing, and she hates being here, but she feels like she has no choice; therefore, the instructor referred her to you, the nurse psychotherapist. When you ask about her parents, she tells you that both of her parents are "old school". They don't speak English very well. French is their first language. She informs you that she is the eldest of four and must set a good example for her siblings. Her father is a factory worker, and her mom works as a personal support worker. When you ask her if she told her parents how she feels and encourage her to speak to her parents- she becomes exasperated and says, "You don't get it! I can't tell my parents that I want to drop out and do something else after they have supported me for 2 years in school", she cries and says "why can't anyone help me". Frozen, you feel pressured to say the right thing.

The client is making herself vulnerable to you by opening up about her personal issues. You have a responsibility to set her at ease and that starts with a genuine interaction in wanting to know her story and to know who she is. Unconscious cultural bias manifests in the way we feel discomfort when interacting with someone who does not look the same way we do (Shiraev & Levy, 2021). This discomfort and or anxiety is felt by the client sitting across from us and most clients are oblivious to the way you feel but react emotionally with increased agitation in the session (Shiraev & Levy, 2021). That is not conducive to creating an effective therapeutic relationship (Shiraev & Levy, 2021). Paying no attention to physical characteristics would have made this conversation go smoother.

5.1 Case Vignette 2 Reflective Questions

1. What could have been done differently?
2. What kinds of questions might you have asked Genevieve to better understand her cultural background and personal experience?
3. Are there questions you could ask to learn more about the relationships in her life such as at home (i.e. her parents) and at school (i.e. friends)
4. What techniques could you apply to demonstrate cultural awareness and concern?

Note: asking the right questions at the start of the therapeutic relationship is an art. When the conversation begins organically, the person becomes more relaxed and more comfortable sharing more vulnerable pieces of information. She has already done the hardest part, which is showing up to see you. Genevieve is a first generation Canadian. It would be important to ask her why her parents immigrated to Canada. Most Caribbean parents put a large emphasis on education, particularly in Haitian culture. Knowing why Genevieve's parents came to Canada will help you understand the pressure she is feeling. Even without knowing a bit about the culture, you can ask questions that can give you a better sense of how her culture has shaped her life experience, such as:

- Was she allowed to go out with friends or to have a sleepover at a friend's house?
- How strict were her parents?
- Given, she is still living at home, is that common in her culture?

It is important to note typically, Haitian kids or adult children do not leave the home until they are married. Being aware of or asking about these types of information is important for the therapist to take the time to understand.

6 Case Vignette 3

The psychotherapist is from the same cultural, ethnic, and religious background as the client, however, the client doesn't feel comfortable sharing anything with the therapist as he doesn't trust the therapist.

Omar S. is a 24-year-old male who was brought to the clinic by his only male friend out of concern for his well-being. Omar initially hesitated to engage with you, as he noticed you are from the same background. However, his friend whom you provided psychotherapy before insisted that he give you a chance, given he desperately needs help. Omar agreed to sit down with you with great ambivalence. He was extremely guarded and withdrawn at the beginning of the session, but he became more relaxed and engaged mid-assessment after you answered all his confidentiality-related questions, including "Would other Somali community members know I saw you? Would you share my alcohol problem with other community members who might know my parents?".

Once his questions were answered satisfactorily, Omar tells you he uses too much alcohol and marijuana. He tells you that alcohol and marijuana use help him stay calm and not get ill to his stomach but feels that the alcohol use has destroyed his life. Omar tells you he did very well from kindergarten to middle school, as his siblings and parents were highly supportive of him. However, he started to moderately struggle with academics during high school. He completed high school and was accepted to college, in an electrical engineering program. Unfortunately, he dropped out of college in his first semester because of his substance use issues. Omar was told by his parents to either see a doctor for his mental health or leave the family home. Seeing a doctor about his mental health problems meant he was admitting to having a mental illness. He refused his family's advice, and he left home. Since leaving his family's home, he has been homeless, and unemployed, his substance use continues to worsen, and he is disconnected from his family, the Somali community, and his friends except for the one who just brought him in. Omar reports he receives food vouchers from the provincial financial assistance program, but he spends the money on substances to avoid withdrawal symptoms. He switches between shelters and attends wherever he can find food.

6.1 Case Analysis

Omar self-identifies as a Muslim young man; his parents migrated to Canada when he was two years of age. He acknowledges that he minimally adheres to his family's cultural background and Muslim religious boundaries. Omar expresses that his lifestyle is mainly influenced by his social peers. He carries massive amounts of guilt and shame due to not strictly following his family's culture, traditions, and Islamic values. Omar tells you that his hesitancy to engage with you was mainly driven by this guilt and shame as he worries that anyone with a similar background will judge him for not being a good Muslim. He informs you he spends most of his time avoiding engaging with anyone from a similar background for that same reason.

6.2 Application of Terms

In this scenario, the nurse psychotherapist shows cultural awareness and cultural competence by refraining from making statements that the client might perceive as judgemental, condescending, or belittling as those behaviors can hint that the client is a bad person by deviating from his religion and using substances. The nurse psychotherapist can demonstrate cultural safety by fostering a professional attitude that accepts the client's unique cultural identity and by integrating interventions that address the client's unique needs, considering Omar's visible apprehension to engage with someone from the same cultural background. The nurse psychotherapist can communicate cultural humility through building trust behaviors by remaining non-judgemental and displaying professional accountability to reassure the client that his personal health information will only be accessed by his circle of care team and anyone else outside of this organization would require his written consent to access his record. This may help to reduce Omar's apprehension to engage with the nurse. Regardless of the client's background, it's crucial to inform them that the nurse psychotherapist is legally obligated to keep their information confidential unless the limits of confidentiality apply. Clinicians should reflect on their biases and beliefs, regardless of a client's cultural background or identity. It is crucial that the clinician gains a therapeutic alliance with the client so they can feel comfortable sharing or disclosing their most intimate issues and struggles. The take-home message is that the nurse psychotherapist views and addresses the person being served as a unique individual who can decide their own destiny whether it aligns with their parents' background, religious expectations, values, and/or belief system. It is equally important to encourage your client to be in the driver's seat of their own treatment plan to ensure that the identified interventions serve their unique needs (First Nations Health Authority 2024; HHS 2021; Hughes et al. 2020).

6.3 Treatment Plan

It is essential that the nurse psychotherapist assist the client in identifying priority strategies and interventions to:

- Manage problematic alcohol and substance use.
- Reduce anxiety, guilt, and shame.
- Improve low mood, overall functioning, and social engagement/social isolation.
- Manage conflict and cultural/religious moral struggles.

Treatment Goals, Expected Success Indicators may include:
Omar shared that he:

- Values being accepted by his family and community as it is very important for him to reconnect.
- Feels getting back on his feet by engaging with acceptable social norms would be the only hope for him, but he doesn't know where to start.
- Hopes to stop drinking, find housing, and a job, go back to school to become an electrical engineer, rebuild his relationship with his family, and start his own family someday.

Treatment Facilitators:

- During this interaction, you noted that Omar's greatest treatment facilitator is his friend, and his strength is that he is motivated to change his life for the time being. Despite being hesitant to engage with you initially, he repeatedly requests your opinion about his treatment goals which is reassuring that he might be willing to continue working with you to achieve some of his goals.

Treatment Barriers/Maintaining Factors:

- Omar shared that he initially started substance use as symptom management but is currently driven by fear of alcohol withdrawal symptoms, social isolation, fear of criticism, shame, guilt, and poor self-esteem. He states that he is afraid of being judged by the Somali/Muslim community and worries about the lack of structure in his life, including being unemployed and not having permanent housing.

6.3.1 *Case Vignette Reflective Questions* 3

1. What other resources and support systems might Omar benefit from given his goal of quitting alcohol use?
2. What tools would you use to objectively assess the severity of this client's alcohol consumption:
   a. Alcohol use and marijuana use screeners and his level of readiness?
3. What would be your plan for the reported chronic mood and anxiety concerns?
4. How would you engage with or support a client who is from a similar background but does not trust you?
5. What is the most appropriate way of answering your client's mistrust, guilt, and fear-driven questions without taking it personally?
6. During the interaction, Omar asks you whether his dreams and aspirations are achievable given his current situation. How would you answer this question with optimism without giving an unrealistic outlook?
7. How would you determine which problem area to focus on?
8. Omar asks you how many sessions of psychotherapy would he require for his problems at hand, how would you answer his question conservatively?

7 Case Vignette 4

Leilani is a 25-year-old Cree woman who recently moved to town after leaving her home in a remote community in Northern Ontario. She tells you she is First Nation. She sees you today because she feels very sad since going through a 20-week miscarriage a week ago. She says that despite knowing what was happening and having advanced notice, she feels like she cannot shake off the dark blanket of depression. She is in town as a college student. Her partner works as a faculty member for a different school. Leilani states she misses her family and home. She cries profusely in your office. She recently moved in with her Caucasian partner and things are going well. She states that she is probably homesick and wishes her family were here to help support her. Leilani says that she has not been back home in over a year and used to be very submerged in her culture, going for sweat, and speaking to Elders. Leilani has been feeling out of touch and out of place. Upon further questioning, you ask her if she would like to be connected to a traditional Indigenous healer. She was surprised initially by this question but soon became excited to be making this connection. The nurse psychotherapist calls down to the Indigenous cultural center and requests a Traditional Healer that could help someone in her condition. You explain to her that there is no amount of grief that is considered 'normal' when one miscarries, but it sounds like she has multiple stressors that are compounding her grief, the missing of her home, culture, and a safe space to be herself. You ask if she had a service or ritual after her miscarriage; she shakes her head no. Leilani said she was told not to make a bigger deal of it than it is. The more she makes of it, the more it will hurt. You ask her what the practice back home would be like, and Leilani says that they would have a healing circle and she cries harder. You ask her if this is something that she would like to do, including planting a tree. Leilani is interested. With Leilani's agreement, you invite her partner to join the discussion. You provide condolences for the loss. The partner nods his head but remains non-verbal. Leilani's culture is a part of her identity and the lack of familiarity and not being back home amid her grief is augmenting her emotional pain. Her partner agrees to support her in returning home with family and hopes to learn more about her culture.

- What practice here was key to being able to connect with Leilani?
- What do you know about Indigenous teachings and cultural practices?
- Do you have enough knowledge to share and refer?
- Would you be willing to share what you know to empower someone else on their journey to wholeness?

Leilani, though away from home, has a good sense of who she is and what she needs for healing. She is away from her cultural safety net and does not feel as though she can grieve the way she needs to. Nurse psychotherapists can empower clients to make the decisions that they know they need to make. Every client is the expert in their own story and knows what they need to heal. The residential school system in Canada was a program focused on cultural genocide (Marsh et al. 2015). As a result, generations of Indigenous peoples have raised their own kids with no cultural context. This has created much harm and is the premise of intergenerational trauma (Marsh et al. 2015). Leaving the reserve meant leaving family, cultural roots, and identity. Truth and reconciliation in Canada begin with every single interaction one has with an Indigenous person (Marsh et al. 2015). While it is great that the referral to a Traditional Healer has been facilitated, there is more work to be done. The Indigenous peoples of Canada are a diverse population with many cultural practices unique to their heritage, band, and location in Canada (ANAC, 2009; Marsh et al. 2015).

7.1 *Case Vignette Reflective Questions 4*

1. What is your understanding of residential schooling in Canada?
2. What is your understanding of intergenerational trauma?
3. How might Leilani's partner support her in their grieving process?

8 Summary

- The concept of culture is complex and cannot be defined in simple terms.
- Intergenerational cultural differences exist within the same cultural groups.
- It is important not to make generalized assumptions or label a client's values and/or belief systems based on their cultural background.
- Achieving 100% cultural competency in every culture might not be possible but being a reflective practitioner is a choice that would help create spaces for strategies to engage in lifelong learning.
- The person being served is your greatest resource to understand their unique cultural identity, values, and belief system. Ensure to be unbiased, flexible, humble, and a good listener who is willing to learn from your own clients.
- Trauma-informed, culturally responsive practices are communicated through ongoing engagement in activities that enhance clinician's cultural awareness, cultural sensitivity, cultural competence, cultural safety, and cultural humility. These are not vocabulary terms to check off but rather skills and attitudes to gain your client's trust.
- Integrating practices that communicate your willingness to form effective and collaborative partnerships would augment the formation of therapeutic nurse-client relationships resulting in favorable client health outcomes.
- When clients are listened to and respected, they feel empowered, leading to better client engagement and treatment adherence.
- Tools like the ADDRESSING Framework and RESPECT model can support developing nurse psychotherapists to conduct organized culturally considerate client assessments.

9 Helpful Resources & Assessment Tools

- Essential Nurse Communication Skills: https://www.nursechoice.com/blog/profiles-and-features/essential-nurse-communication-skills-for-success/
- Developing Therapeutic relationships: https://rnao.ca/sites/rnao-ca/files/Establishing_Therapeutic_Relationships.pdf
- Nursing Assessment Process: https://www.ncbi.nlm.nih.gov/books/NBK499937/
- Nursing Diagnosis – NANDA: https://shop.thieme.com/nanda-international-nursing-diagnoses/9781684204540

- Nurse-client Therapeutic relationship: https://www.cno.org/en/learn-about-standards-guidelines/educational-tools/learning-modules/therapeutic-nurse-client-relationship/
- Stages of change Mode: https://www.therapistaid.com/worksheets/stages-of-change
- Understanding Alcohol Use Disorder:
  - https://www.niaaa.nih.gov/publications/brochures-and-fact-sheets/understanding-alcohol-use-disorder
  - https://www.verywellmind.com/dsm-5-criteria-for-substance-use-disorders-21926
- CAGE Questionnaire https://www.hopkinsmedicine.org/johns_hopkins_healthcare/downloads/all_plans/CAGE%20Substance%20Screening%20Tool.pdf
- CIWA: https://www.metaphi.ca/wp-content/uploads/WMS_6.1_CIWA-Ar.pdf
- DSM5 for alcohol use & Mood disorders—anxiety versus depressive symptoms: https://www.psychiatry.org/File%20Library/Psychiatrists/Practice/DSM/APA_DSM-5-Contents.pdf
- Trauma-Informed Approaches: https://bpgmobile.rnao.ca/sites/default/files/Key%20principles%20of%20a%20trauma%20informed%20approach.pdf
- Canadian Nurses Association (2017). Code of Ethics for Registered Nurses. https://www.nscn.ca/sites/default/files/documents/resources/code-of-ethics-for-registered-nurses.pdf
- Think Cultural Health Resources: https://minorityhealth.hhs.gov/omh/browse.aspx?lvl=2&lvlid=53
- Using Indigenous knowledge to address mental illness in Indigenous communities: https://www.canadian-nurse.com/blogs/cn-content/2023/01/23/indigenous-knowledge-address-mental-illness
- 10 Biggest Barriers to Black Mental Health Today: https://www.psycom.net/black-mental-health-barriers
- Manitoba Trauma Information Centre: https://trauma-informed.ca
- International Society for Traumatic Stress Studies: https://istss.org/public-resources/war-and-disaster-resources

References

Aboriginal Nurses Association of Canada (2009). *Cultural competency and cultural safety in nursing education: A framework for First Nations, Inuit and Metis Nursing*. Author. http://indigenousnurses.ca/resources/publications/cultural-competence-and-cultural-safety-nursing-education-framework-first

American Psychiatric Association. (2019). *Mental health disparities: Diverse populations*. www.psychiatry.org/psychiatrists/cultural-competency/education/mental-health-facts

Arnett, J.J. (2002). The psychology of globalization. *American Psychologist, 57*(10), 774-783.

Ball, J. (2023). *Cultural safety*. School of Child and Youth Care, University of Victoria, Canada. https//ecdip.org/cultural-safety/

Bartholomew, T., Pérez-Rojas, A. E., Bledman, R., Joy, E. E., & Robbins, K. (2023). "How could I not bring it up?": A multiple case study of therapists' comfort when Black clients discuss anti-Black racism in sessions. *Psychotherapy (Chic),60*(1), 63–75. https://doi.org/10.1037/pst0000404. Epub 2021 Nov 22

Berry, J.W. (2013). Research on multiculturalism in Canada. *International Journal of Intercultural Relations, 37*(6), 663-675.

Benuto, L. T., Singer, J., Casas, J., González, F., & Ruork, A. (2018). The evolving definition of cultural competency: A mixed methods study. *International journal of psychology and psychological therapy, 18*(3), 371-384.

Canadian Mental Health Association. (2023). *Cross Cultural Mental Health*. Author. https://cmha.bc.ca/documents/cross-cultural-mental-health-and-substance-use-2/#:~:text=Different%20perspectives%E2%80%94Culture%20plays%20a,use%20problems%20in%20different%20ways

Canadian Mental Health Association (2023). *Rural and Northern Community Issues in Mental Health*. https://ontario.cmha.ca/documents/rural-and-northern-community-issues-in-mental-health/

Canadian Nurses Association (2023). *Using Indigenous knowledge to address mental illness in Indigenous communities*. Author. https://www.canadian-nurse.com/blogs/cn-content/2023/01/23/indigenous-knowledge-address-mental-illness

Cook, S. C., Schwartz, A. C., Kaslow, N. J. (2017). Evidence-based psychotherapy: Advantages and challenges. *Neurotherapeutics, 14*, 537–545. https://doi.org/10.1007/s13311-017-0549-4

Chung, N., Barrett, K., & Matthews, T. G. (2022). Multicultural perspectives in co-occurring treatment. In *Co-occurring mental illness and substance use disorders* (pp. 143–155). Routledge.

College of Nurses of Ontario. (2006). Therapeutic Nurse-Client Relationship. https://www.cno.org/globalassets/docs/prac/41033_therapeutic.pdf

Connecticut Women's Consortium (2023). *A Guide to Building Trauma-Informed Practices and Organizations*. https://training.womensconsortium.org/building-trauma-informed-practices-and-organizations

Curtis, E., Jones, R., Tipene-Leach, D., Walker, C., Loring, B., Paine, S-J. & Reid, P. (2019). Why cultural safety rather than cultural competency is required to achieve health equity: A literature review and recommended definition. *International Journal for Equity in Health 18*(174) https://equityhealthj.biomedcentral.com/articles/https://doi.org/10.1186/s12939-019-1082-3

DuPraw, M.E., & Axner, M. (1997). Toward a more perfect union in an age of diversity: Working on common cross-cultural communication challenges. https://www.pbs.org/ampu/crosscult.html

First Nations Health Authority. (2024). *Cultural Safety and Humility*. Author. https://www.fnha.ca/what-we-do/cultural-safety-and-humility

Foronda, C. (2008). A concept analysis of cultural sensitivity: An improved understanding of the term as described within health care and in general would enhance nurses' understanding and communication with professionals and clients. *Journal of Transcultural Nursing, 19*(3), 207-12. https://doi.org/10.1177/1043659608317093.

Goodwin, S. L., Lints-Martindale, A., Carlson, A., Dean, M., Kinley, J., & Walker, S. (2023). A review of rural, remote, and northern competency in Canada: Cultural safety considerations for telepsychology and traditional psychological practice. *Journal of Rural Mental Health, 47*(4), 211–220. https://doi.org/10.1037/rmh0000239

Government of Canada (Dec, 2023). *Indigenous peoples and communities*. Author. https://www.rcaanc-cirnac.gc.ca/eng/1100100013785/1529102490303

Hays, P. (2016). *Addressing cultural complexities in practice: Assessment, diagnosis, and therapy* (3rd ed.). American Psychological Association

Henrich, J., Heine, S., & Norenzayan, A. (2010). The weirdest people in the world? *Behavioural and Brain Sciences, 33*(2/3), 123.

Hook, N., Davis, N., Owen, J. & Deblaere, C. (2017). *Introduction beginning the journey of cultural humility*. American Psychological Association.

Hughes, V., Delva, S. Nkimbeng, M., Spaulding, E., Turkson-Ocran, R-A., Cudjoe, J., Ford, A., Rushton, C., D'Aoust, R., Han, H-R. (2020). Not missing the opportunity: Strategies to promote cultural humility among future nursing faculty. *Journal of Professional Nursing*, 36, 24-33.

Jones, E., Huey jr, S. J. & Rubenson, M. (2018). *Cultural competence in therapy with African Americans*. Springer International Publishing.

Koç, V. & Kafa, G. (2019). Cross-cultural research on psychotherapy. *Journal of Cross-Cultural Psychology, 50*(1) 100–115, https://doi.org/10.1177/0022022118806577

Lekas, H-M., Pahl, K. & Lewis, C. F. (2020). Rethinking cultural competence: Shifting to cultural humility. *Health Serv Insights, 13*. https://doi.org/10.1177/1178632920970580

Lonner, W.J. (2019). A golden anniversary editorial. *Journal of Cross-Cultural Psychology, 50*(2), 151-163.

Marsh, T. N., Coholic, D., Cote-Meek, S. & Najavits, L. M. (2015). Blending Aboriginal and Western healing methods to treat intergenerational trauma with substance use disorder in Aboriginal peoples who live in Northeastern Ontario, Canada. *Harm Reduction Journal, 2*(14). https://doi.org/10.1186/S12954-015-0046-1

Massaquoi, N. (2023). Racial humility over competence: Addressing anti-Black racism and healthcare leadership responsibility. *Healthcare Management Forum, 36*(5), 280-284. https://doi.org/10.1177/08404704231186807

Meyer, O. L. & Zane, N. (2013). The influence of race and ethnicity in clients' experience of mental health treatment. *J community Psychol, 41*(7), 884-901.

National Collaborating Centre for Indigenous Health (2020). *Indigenous Experiences with Racism And Its Impacts*. Author. https://www.nccih.ca/docs/determinants/FS-Racism2-Racism-Impacts-EN.pdf

Nuttgens, S. A. & Campbell, A. J. (2010). Multicultural considerations for counselling First Nations clients. *Canadian Journal of Counselling, 44*(2), 115-129.

Osazuwa, S., & Moodley, R. (2023). "Will there be a willingness to actually engage with it?":Exploring attitudes toward culturally integrative psychotherapy among Canada's African community. *Journal of Psychotherapy Integration, 33*(1), 68-85. https://doi.org/10.1037/int0000289

Pallardy, R. (2023). 2010 Haiti earthquake. In T. Grant (Ed.), *Encyclopedia Britannica*. 9 Aug. 2023. https://www.britannica.com/event/2010-Haiti-earthquake. Accessed 1 September 2024.

Registered Nurse's Association of Ontario [RNAO], (2007). Healthy work environments best practice guidelines: Embracing cultural diversity in health care. Author. https://rnao.ca/sites/rnao-ca/files/Embracing_Cultural_Diversity_in_Health_Care_-_Developing_Cultural_Competence.pdf

Roche, M. J. L. & Maxie, A. (2003). Ten considerations in addressing cultural differences in psychotherapy. *Professional Psychology: Research and Practice, 34*(2). https://doi.org/10.1037/0735-7028.34.2.180

Rogers-Sirin, L., Melendez, F., Refano, C., & Zegarra, Y. (2015). Immigrant perception of therapists' cultural competence: A qualitative investigation. *Professional Psychology Research and Practice, 46*(4), 258–269. https://doi.org/10.1037/pro0000033

Rosario, M, T. & Guzman, D. (2016). Cultural competence an important skill set for the 21st century. https://extensionpublications.unl.edu/assets/html/g1375/build/g1375.htm

Shiraev, E. B., & Levy, D. A. (2021). *Cross-cultural psychology* (7th ed.). Taylor & Francis.

St Catherine University. (2022). How to practice cultural competence in nursing. Retrieved from https://www.stkate.edu/academics/healthcare-degrees/cultural-competence-in-nursing

Substance Abuse and Mental Health Services Administration. (2014). *Improving cultural competence. Treatment Improvement Protocol 59*. Author. https://store.samhsa.gov/system/files/sma14-4849.pdf

U.S. Department of Health and Human Services [HHS] office of Minority Health. (2021). *Think Cultural Health*. https://minorityhealth.hhs.gov/omh/browse.aspx?lvl=2&lvlid=53

Chapter 13
Population Needs: Ethics and Risk Management

Siobhan Bell and Stacey Roles

Abstract Delivering safe and competent psychotherapy in many different healthcare settings can present unique ethical and risk management implications. Nurse psychotherapists must consider these unique implications as they practice within the required standards of practice, legislation, and laws relevant to psychotherapy. To maintain the autonomy and dignity of all persons, the nurse psychotherapist practices from a lens that includes social justice, integrity, and collegial support. This type of ethical practice demonstrates excellence in professional psychotherapeutic practice. To uphold this standard, nurses must work to analyze ethical dilemmas and manage legal issues as they arise. To do this, nurses must actively participate in the process of ethical decision-making and receive supervisory or consultative support when needed. Nurses should safeguard the clients, practitioners, and the profession from both potential ethical and legal challenges by practicing within their scope of practice and by continuously attaining new clinical skills and knowledge. This chapter will cover ethical and legal concerns applicable to psychotherapy in nursing followed by case examples to illustrate ethical decision-making and legal implications.

Keywords Ethical practice · Risk management · Safe practice

Learning Objectives

After completing this chapter, the learner will:

1. Understand the ethical and risk management implications associated with delivering psychotherapy in various healthcare settings.
2. Demonstrate knowledge of the required standards of practice and legislation relevant to psychotherapy within the context of nursing.

S. Bell (✉)
Nursing@Heart Inc., Mono, ON, Canada
e-mail: sbell@nursingatheart.ca

S. Roles
Roles & Associates Psychotherapy Services Inc. & CBT Training Centre of the North, Sudbury, ON, Canada

S. Roles and K. Kalia (eds.), *The Nurses' Guide to Psychotherapy*,
https://doi.org/10.1007/978-981-97-4738-2_13

3. Apply principles of social justice, integrity, and collegial support in psychotherapeutic practice to ensure the autonomy and dignity of all individuals receiving care.

1 Introduction

Delivering psychotherapy within diverse healthcare settings places nurse psychotherapists at the intersection of ethical considerations and risk management practices. Risk management falls under the larger umbrella of patient safety and quality improvement. Nurse psychotherapists must consistently navigate a healthcare landscape defined by evolving standards of practice and changing legislations that are pertinent to psychotherapy and the treatment of individuals with mental health concerns. Nurse psychotherapists are called upon to uphold the principles of social justice, integrity, and collegial support while preserving the autonomy and dignity of every individual under their care. Ethical nursing practice is founded on proactive engagement with ethical decision-making processes and a readiness to manage legal issues as they emerge. By examining ethical dilemmas and legal challenges, nurse psychotherapists can develop a foundation for ethical decision-making. This chapter further underscores the importance of practicing within one's scope of practice, continually acquiring new clinical skills, and staying abreast of emerging knowledge. This is an approach crucial for safeguarding clients, practitioners, and the integrity of the profession.

2 Risk Management and Patient Safety

Delivering psychotherapy within diverse healthcare settings places nurse psychotherapists at the intersection of ethical considerations and risk management practices. Risk management, a problem-oriented approach within the broader realm of patient safety and quality improvement, is an ongoing and integral aspect of nursing practice (Healthcare Insurance Reciprocal of Canada 2017). While quality management focuses on prevention and experience, risk management involves daily screening, education, and intervention. As individual practitioners, nurse psychotherapists play a crucial role in applying risk management principles to their practice to identify potential risks and implement preventative measures.

The Canadian Patient Safety Institute Framework for Health Services (2020) serves as an example of an established framework that healthcare organizations may adopt to promote system-level risk management and patient safety. However, for nurse psychotherapists, the application of risk management principles extends beyond organizational frameworks. It involves a comprehensive risk assessment process, encompassing data collection, risk factor identification, prioritization, implementation of preventive measures, and continuous evaluation.

3 Ethical and Risk Management Implications

Understanding the ethical and risk management implications associated with delivering psychotherapy in diverse healthcare settings is paramount for nurse psychotherapists. Ethical considerations form the foundation of psychotherapeutic practice, requiring practitioners to navigate a complex landscape defined by evolving standards of care, a code of conduct, and legislation specific to mental health. At the heart of ethical practice lies the commitment to upholding principles such as nonmaleficence, beneficence, autonomy, and justice (Varkey 2021). Nurse psychotherapists, therefore, must be well-versed in the standards of practice and legislation relevant to psychotherapy, ensuring that their interventions align with the overarching goal of promoting the well-being and autonomy of individuals with mental health issues. Risk management is an ongoing daily program of screening, education, and intervention.

As individual practitioners, nurse psychotherapists can apply risk management principles to their practice to identify risks and implement preventative measures (Varkey 2021). These interventions are intended to prevent adverse events, promote patient safety, and improve health outcomes. Risk assessments can include multiple stages including collection of data, risk identification, prioritization, intervention and prevention, and evaluation. Gathering standardized information including past and current medical, physical, and mental health history, current condition(s), and psychosocial factors are critical components of a comprehensive assessment as discussed in Chap. 15.

Standardized tools to screen and assess risks including suicide and violence are used to identify behaviours of concern (Chap. 15). Following risk identification, the nurse psychotherapist can determine the likelihood and severity of each risk. Risk prioritization is used to develop an individualized plan of care. Evidence-based interventions address specific needs and minimize patient safety risks such as developing a personalized safety plan with coping strategies and resources alongside the client to reduce the risk of self-harm (Stevens et al. 2021). Lastly, continuous monitoring and regular assessments are essential in determining the effectiveness of clinical interventions and their impact on clients as they progress in their healthcare journey.

The delivery of psychotherapy introduces unique risk management challenges. The nature and extent of mental health issues require a nuanced approach to risk assessment and intervention. Practitioners must engage in continuous screening, education, and intervention to identify potential risks and prevent adverse events. The complexity of psychotherapeutic interactions requires the practitioner to have a solid understanding of risk factors, including but not limited to suicidal ideation, potential harm to self or others, or financial vulnerability. Nurse psychotherapists play a crucial role in developing and implementing preventive measures to promote patient safety and improve health outcomes. To ensure excellence, quality, and patient safety in a psychotherapeutic practice, nurse psychotherapists must strike a delicate balance between ethical considerations and risk management strategies. This involves not only adhering to established standards, professional values, organizational/agency policies and procedures, and legislation, but also actively participating in the ongoing process of ethical decision-making. By understanding the ethical and risk management implications associated with delivering psychotherapy in various healthcare settings, nurse psychotherapists can enhance the quality and safety of their practice, fostering an environment that prioritizes the well-being and autonomy of those under their care.

4 Required Standards of Practice and Legislation

Within nursing, particularly within the context of mental health care, it is important for practitioners to demonstrate an understanding of the requisite standards of practice and legislation governing psychotherapy. Adherence to these standards not only promotes the provision of high-quality care but also serves to protect the rights and well-being of individuals living with mental health challenges. The initial knowledge needed for nurse psychotherapists relates to each nursing regulatory body and varies from jurisdiction to jurisdiction as discussed in previous chapters. In regions where psychotherapy is not regulated by their nursing regulatory body, the nurse would need to determine if psychotherapy is regulated within the region of practice and by whom. Once this is understood, provincial and federal legislation and regulations can then be applied to practice if appropriate. It is also of importance to seek professional standards and policies established by organizations (i.e. regulatory bodies, hospitals/agencies), including those that support ethical practice, competency expectations, and principles guiding the conduct of psychotherapeutic interventions (Martin et al. 2013; Canadian Counselling and Psychotherapy Association [CCPA] 2024).

Nurses must possess knowledge of the legal frameworks governing their practice, particularly those addressing mental health issues. This includes familiarity with guidelines and legalities such as the Mental Health Act of 1990 (2015), for example, which delineates the rights and involuntary treatment procedures for individuals with mental illnesses (Mental Health Act of 1990 (2015)). Additionally, awareness of privacy laws, such as the Personal Information Protection and Electronic Documents Act (PIPEDA) and Personal Health Information Protection Act [2004] and other healthcare protection acts, which are essential for safeguarding vulnerable healthcare populations (Personal Health Information Protection Act 2004; Office of the Privacy Commissioner of Canada 2019). These acts and regulations are important in safeguarding the confidentiality and privacy of patient information, which is a foundational aspect of ethical mental health care.

The integration of evidence-based practices within psychotherapeutic interventions is another essential part of protecting clients, which includes staying up to date with the latest research findings and treatment modalities. Nurse psychotherapists who are providing psychotherapeutic interventions must ensure that they are providing care that is not only legally sound but also rooted in the most current understanding of effective interventions for mental health issues (Canadian Nurses

Association [CNA] 2018). Doing so aligns with the ongoing commitment of delivering client-centered care and continuously improving the quality of mental health services offered by the nursing profession.

5 Principles of Social Justice, Integrity, and Collegial Support

In psychotherapeutic practice, the application of principles grounded in social justice, integrity, and collegial support is important to ensuring the autonomy and dignity of all individuals receiving care (CCPA 2015; American Psychiatric Association [APA] 2021). Social justice principles emphasize the fair and equitable distribution of mental health resources, while acknowledging and addressing systemic barriers that may impact certain groups disproportionately. Practitioners must be attuned to the diverse needs of individuals and advocate for inclusivity and equal access to psychotherapeutic services (CCPA 2015; APA 2021; Elliott 2023).

Integrity, as a foundational principle, underscores the importance of honesty, transparency, and ethical conduct in psychotherapeutic practice (CCPA 2015; APA 2021). Maintaining the trust of individuals seeking care is essential for fostering a therapeutic relationship that respects autonomy and upholds dignity. Practitioners are obligated to uphold high ethical standards, ensuring that their actions align with the best interests of their clients and contribute to the overall well-being of individuals engaged in psychotherapeutic interventions (CCPA 2015). There are multiple areas where mental health and social justice intersect (Chap. 12) specifically as it pertains to the intersection of health and institutional racism and inherent practitioner bias.

Collegial support plays a crucial role in creating an environment conducive to the principles of social justice and integrity in psychotherapeutic practice. Collaborative relationships among practitioners in an interprofessional or intraprofessional team (Chap. 20) promotes ongoing professional development, ethical reflection, and the sharing of knowledge and insights (CCPA 2015; APA 2021, CNA 2017). Through collegial support, practitioners can collectively address challenges, enhance their competencies, and contribute to a culture of continuous improvement in the field of psychotherapy.

6 Case Vignette 1

Ian is a newly graduated nurse working at the intake department of a mental health and addictions program. Ian's role includes seeing many individuals who are new to the program, and he has therefore received extensive training in suicide assessment and risk management which included questions to pose to new clients presenting to his program. One day Ian recognizes a client who comes into intake that he has already completed an intake assessment with a few months ago. The client tells Ian that nothing has changed since his previous intake appointment, but that he had just decided it was not the right time for him to engage with mental health services, so he did not attend the programming. The client wants Ian to quickly go through the assessment as he said everything is the same as the last time. Ian is contemplating the client's request to "quickly go through the intake assessment" and is considering this option as he knows that clients can get frustrated retelling their story multiple times, but at the same time Ian wants to ensure that he is thorough in his current assessment.

6.1 Case Vignette 1 Reflective Questions

(1) What are the risks if Ian decides not to thoroughly go through the proper assessments as he would if it was a first-time client?
(2) What are the risks if he completes the intake with the client as though it is his first time meeting him?
(3) If Ian is going to modify the assessment, what areas must he address to reduce the safety risks to the client or to others?

7 Case Vignette 2

Suzy is a seasoned nurse psychotherapist who has worked on a busy inpatient psychiatric unit for 10 years. She knows, respects, and trusts the psychiatrists and other interdisciplinary team members and they respect her as well. One day a client's family member along with the client's psychiatrist approaches Suzy and states that they want Suzy, in her psychotherapy session with the client, to convince the client to move into a group home and to try to make it feel like it was the client's idea. Suzy feels ethically conflicted by this request and is contemplating how to handle it.

7.1 Case Vignette 2 Reflective Questions

(1) What, if anything, might be unethical if Suzy did as requested?
(2) Is there anyone Suzy can bring this ethical conflict to for further discussion?
(3) How can Suzy address this request with the psychiatrist and family members?
(4) If Suzy believes that the client moving into a group home is in the client's best interest, is there another way Suzy can broach this with the client?
(5) Are there other avenues that Suzy can take?

8 Summary

- It is imperative that nurse psychotherapists understand the ethical and risk management implications associated with delivering psychotherapy in diverse practice settings.
- Thorough risk assessments enable nurse psychotherapists to identify, prioritize and plan to mitigate or reduce risks for clients.
- Nurses must attend to high ethical standards and ensure that their actions align with the best interests of the client.
- The application of principles grounded in social justice, integrity, and collegial support are in place to ensure the autonomy and dignity of care recipients.

References

American Psychiatric Association. (2021). *APA commentary on ethics in practice.* Author. https://www.psychiatry.org/file%20library/psychiatrists/practice/ethics/apa-commentary-on-ethics-in-practice.pdf.

Canadian Counselling and Psychotherapy Association (2015). *Standards of Practice. 5th Edition.* https://www.ccpa-accp.ca/wp-content/uploads/2015/07/StandardsOfPractice_en_June2015.pdf.

Canadian Nurses Association. (2017). *Code of ethics.* Author. https://www.cna-aiic.ca/en/nursing/regulated-nursing-in-canada/nursing-ethics.

Canadian Nurses Association. (2018). *Evidence-informed decision-making and nursing practice.* Author. https://hl-prod-ca-oc-download.s3-ca-central-1.amazonaws.com/CNA/2f975e7e-4a40-45ca-863c-5ebf0a138d5e/UploadedImages/documents/Evidence_informed_Decision_making_and_Nursing_Practice_position_statement_Dec_2018.pdf.

Canadian Patient Safety Institute. (2020). *Canadian Patient Safety Institute Framework for Health Services.* Author. https://www.patientsafetyinstitute.ca/en/toolsResources/Canadian-Quality-and-Patient-Safety-Framework-for-Health-and-Social-Services/Documents/CPSI-10001-CQPS-Framework-English_FA_Online.pdf.

Canadian Counselling and Psychotherapy Association. (2024). *The profession & regulation.* Author. https://www.ccpa-accp.ca/profession-and-regulation/.

Elliott, T. H. (2023). Theory analysis and evaluation of emancipatory nursing praxis: A theory of social justice in nursing. *International Journal of Nursing Knowledge, 35,* (1), 32–39. https://doi.org/10.1111/2047-3095.12414.

Healthcare Insurance Reciprocal of Canada. (2017). *The link between risk management, patient safety, and quality improvement.* Author. https://www.hiroc.com/resources/risk-notes/link-between-risk-management-patient-safety-and-quality-improvement.

Martin, L., Turcotte, M., Matte, L., Shepard, B. (2013). The counselling and psychotherapy profession in Canada: Regulatory processes and current status. *British Journal of Guidance & Counselling, 41*(1), 46–57. https://doi.org/10.1080/03069885.2012.750271.org.

Mental Health Act, 1990, R.S.O. 2015, c. M.7.https://www.ontario.ca/laws/statute/90m07.

Office of the Privacy Commisioner of Canada. (2019). *The personal information protection and electronic documents act [PIPEDA].* Author. https://www.priv.gc.ca/en/privacy-topics/privacy-laws-in-canada/the-personal-information-protection-and-electronic-documents-act-pipeda/pipeda_brief.

Personal Health Information Protection Act, 2004, S.O. 2004, c. 3, Sched. A. https://www.ontario.ca/laws/statute/04p03.

Stevens, K., Thambinathan, V., Hollenberg, E., Inglis, F., Johnson, A., Levinson, A., Salman, S., Cardinale, L., Lo, B., Shi, J., Wiljer, D., Korczak, D., & Cleverley, K. (2021). Core components and strategies for suicide and risk management protocols in mental health research: a scoping review. *BMC Psychiatry* 21(13). https://doi.org/10.1186/s12888-020-03005-0.

Varkey, B. (2021). Principles of clinical ethics and their application to practice. *Medical Principles and Practice, 30*(1), 17–28.

Chapter 14
Nursing Competencies: Nursing Process

Mary-Lou Martin and Hoodo A. Ibrahim

Abstract This chapter describes selected considerations for mental health assessments, processes, and interventions that are essential components of psychotherapy. A bio/psycho/social/spiritual model and trauma- and violence-informed approach creates a safe structure for holistic comprehensive and focused assessments as well as treatment. Interpersonal skills are requirements for building and sustaining a trusting nurse-client therapeutic relationship. The nurse needs to understand the client's context, the connectedness of their problems, and their motivation for seeking care. Tools and scales to improve diagnostic reasoning set the foundation for further workup and tailored interventions. Screening for suicide, self-harm, and violence will be part of the assessment. Clients will respond to various interventions and the nurse's role is to empower them to find their own solutions. Pertinent health records and history may also be important. The nurse will guide the interventions so that a satisfactory outcome in the therapeutic relationship is achieved. The nurse recognizes their own personal and professional limitations. To be effective, the nurse requires supervised experience, and knowledge and skills in counselling theory and techniques. The nurse must familiarize themselves with the ethical standards developed by their jurisdictional professional association and regulatory body.

Keywords Assessment · Intervention · Nursing process

Learning Objectives

After completing this chapter, the learner will:

1. Describe therapeutic communication skills.
2. Understand nursing assessment and diagnosis.
3. Explain examples of specific tests and the rationale for these tests.

M.-L. Martin (✉)
St. Joseph's Healthcare Hamilton/McMaster University, Hamilton, ON, Canada
e-mail: martinm@stjosham.on.ca

H. A. Ibrahim
St Joseph's Healthcare Hamilton/Hamilton Health Sciences, Hamilton, ON, Canada

S. Roles and K. Kalia (eds.), *The Nurses' Guide to Psychotherapy*,
https://doi.org/10.1007/978-981-97-4738-2_14

4. Discuss the application of nursing interventions (goals, outcomes) for the bio/psycho/social/spiritual domains.

1 Introduction

Nursing assessment, diagnosis, planning, and intervention require critical inquiry, decision-making and evidence-based knowledge. A nurse-client relationship involves the phases of beginning, middle (working), and end. It is in the beginning phase that most assessments will occur although assessments will likely be ongoing. Therapeutic communication techniques build empathy, caring, and trusting relationships and help with effective communication. The factors affecting verbal communication such as the use of words both written and spoken, and nonverbal communication including kinesics, paralanguage and proxemics may produce anxiety, and change perception and communication style. The nurse's goal is to give the client the best support possible within a respectful, honest, fair, and equitable relationship using therapeutic communication techniques including listening, open-ended questions, reflecting, restating, clarifying, focusing, suggesting, providing feedback and including the use of silence. Person- and family-centered approaches provide examples of care that are based on current evidence and quality standards (Registered Nurses of Ontario [RNAO], 2015). Evidence-based theories, policies and practices need to be considered within all relationships and interactions. The nurse's goals in interacting with clients should include providing compassion, collaboration, and effective communication, thereby giving clients the best support possible. Throughout the nursing process, it is important to establish expectations and boundaries such as roles, techniques, costs, services, frequency of sessions (including time & length of meetings), responsibilities, confidentiality and limitations to confidentiality at the beginning of the interaction to clarify the context of the therapeutic relationship.

2 The Nursing Process

The nursing process is a systematic process of assessment, diagnoses, outcomes, planning, interventions, and evaluation over the lifespan. The bio/psycho/social/spiritual model (Abraham et al., 1992; Dent, 2021; Harrad et al., 2019; Saad et al., 2017) is a comprehensive and holistic approach to health and well-being that will inform the nursing process and can be used as an organizational framework. The domains of the model interact but can also be understood independently. It helps to understand the connectedness of a client's issues or problems. For example, comorbid physical health issues, such as chronic health diseases, can significantly affect the disease trajectory of mental health issues such as depression, while the reverse is also true. The therapist may need to address single or multiple issues in promoting the physical and mental health of clients. Medication assessment will include a review of past and current medications, herbal substances, the medication's therapeutic effects, and the client's adherence to the medication along with a review of the side effects. Medical history including acute health problems, chronic illness and other disease states, developmental function, family history and social history may be important to the overall assessment. An assessment will also include the social determinants of health with broad factors such as: housing, income, food security, social status, employment, working conditions, education, literacy, childhood experiences, physical environment, social and coping skills, health behaviours, access to health services, biology and genetic endowment, gender, culture and race and racism (Government of Canada, 2023). Exploring and asking questions about spiritual beliefs and how they impact the client's life and health may uncover spiritual needs. These domains will help the nurse to consider theories and interventions from the biological, psychological, social science, and spiritual lens (Harrad et al., 2019). The primary source of information is the client and additional collateral information can be collected from family and other sources as appropriate. An overall comprehensive assessment may be conducted first and then a more focused assessment can be helpful in the development of specific nursing diagnoses or case formulation.

3 Comprehensive and Focused Assessments

A collaborative, client-driven process designed to support and meet client goals is the main purpose of the assessment process. The nurse should determine what type of assessment is required in each client's situation. A comprehensive assessment can include a health history, a timeline of events, a physical examination, and a bio/psycho/social/spiritual, trauma and violence-informed approach to care. Comparatively, a focused assessment can be done in a brief timeframe, about a specific need or problem through the lens of the client's immediate needs. The practice setting where the nurse psychotherapist is interacting with the client might also determine if the assessment will be comprehensive or focused as in hospital settings the clients may be more acutely ill and might require a comprehensive assessment whereas in the community setting clients may be more stable, goal-oriented, and a focused assessment might be more appropriate. The opposite of this may also be true depending on the client's circumstances.

The mental status examination is an example of a focused assessment. It is used to systematically assess the client's appearance, motor, speech, affect, mood, thought content and process, perception, cognition, insight, judgment, and strengths. The goal of conducting a focused mental status assessment is often to collect the client's baseline mental status, to rule out or identify mental status alterations, to assess progress over time, or to assess elevated risk, and immediate thoughts and behaviours. Psychotherapy is best done with some focused assessment and planning, and this can be accomplished with trauma-informed (Chap. 5) and culturally sensitive care approaches in mind (Chap. 12). The nurse can employ therapeutic communication strategies to collect relevant and comprehensive data to determine the health patterns of the client.

The nursing diagnosis would then be based on assessment data including subjective data, objective data, and chart reviews if obtainable which can be accomplished through interview and observation. A nurse-client interview sheds light on the client's subjective view of the problem at hand. The nurse can then use the North American Nursing Diagnosis Association's (NANDA, 2023) compiled list of nursing diagnoses to integrate with the assessment of the clients' health patterns. Assessment tools such as the Patient Health Questionnaire (PHQ-9) used to screen for the severity of depression (Kroenke et al., 2001), the CAGE used to screen for alcohol or drug use (O'Brien, 2008), the Generalized Anxiety Disorder (GAD-7) used to screen for generalized anxiety (Spitzer et al., 2006), and the Hamilton Anxiety Rating Scale (Hamilton, 1959) may also be part of the overall assessment. The DSM-5 Diagnostic and Statistical Manual of Mental Disorders (DSM) may also be a point of reference to understand the client's presentation. Conceptual frameworks will influence all clinical judgements within the nursing process. Different clients with similar nursing diagnoses may respond to varying types of interventions in multiple ways. The nursing process is a series of steps, however, when there are signs that there is inherent risk to self or others, the nurse might need to intervene immediately. When the client is a danger to self or others, the use of critical thinking and clinical judgement to assess the type, for example, self-injury, suicide or violence, and the level of risk including other safety risks and hazards may require immediate effective interventions (Chap. 13). Strategies used to reduce risks may include crisis prevention, violence prevention, stress management, abstinence/harm reduction and cognitive restructuring. Additional support, such as emergency services or admission to the hospital, may be required if the client discloses a safety risk and plan.

Clinical reasoning and judgment involve logical reasoning and the assessment, analysis, interpretation, synthesis, and evaluation of information. Understanding the client's past and current behaviour, their story, and what is important to the client is necessary to develop an appropriate plan of treatment in partnership with the client. Nursing actions are goal-directed and best practice guidelines may be available for certain issues such as depression, anxiety, Post-Traumatic Stress Disorder (PTSD), and substance use disorders among others (American Psychological Association, 2023; Boeykens et al., 2022). The client is an active participant throughout the process and relationship. The nurse uses strength-based care and protective factors to promote resilience including flexibility, adaptability, perseverance, coping, connection, etc. (Reynolds, 2019). Only after discussion with the client will it be clear that these are issues the client wishes to work on with the nurse. Interventions may support health promotion, illness prevention, relapse management, risk mitigation, self-management, and client education. Based on the initial assessment, the nurse will help to determine which behaviours, thoughts or feelings require attention. The aim of the intervention(s) may be to reduce emotional distress, facilitate cognitive and behavioural change, and promote personal growth. It will be important to provide information and share about when and how to use therapeutic interventions. Short and long-term outcomes are identified by the client. Outcomes are identified, monitored, and evaluated throughout the care process. The therapist's techniques, strengths and quality of the therapeutic relationship can be associated with positive client outcomes in therapy (Noyce & Simpson, 2018).

Cultural norms, values and beliefs are important because we live within a cultural context, and this includes cultural identity, cultural competence, cultural humility, and cultural safety. Understanding the beliefs and behaviours of the client's culture of origin enables engagement and collaboration as well as the provision of culturally sensitive care (see Chap. 12).

Professional practice should be conducted in an ethical manner. Ethical standards as well as reflection of personal and professional limitations are safeguards for the client and nurse. Some considerations include competence of the nurse, documentation, confidentiality and client empowerment. Awareness regarding a lack of competence in a specific case may prompt a nurse to seek consultation with peers or a supervisor, in addition to seeking evidence-based resources to address the knowledge gap. It is important that the nurse ask permission to take notes and explain the purpose, including what they are doing with the notes and why. In accordance with regulatory requirements, documentation should be reflective of the nursing process such as to objectively and subjectively describe the assessment inclusive of the client's history, examinations, nursing diagnoses, interventions and the client's responses to treatment. A nurse psychotherapist must write accurate and informative case notes to meet legal requirements and to communicate relevant client information including health assessment findings, nursing diagnosis, imminent risks, client strengths and agreed-upon treatment plan. The foundation of trust in psychotherapy is client confidentiality. The nurse psychotherapist maintains privacy of the client's personal health information unless as aforementioned there is an immediate risk for harm to self or others. Lastly, person-centered care is established when the client is empowered, given choices, and engaged in an authentic partnership with the nurse. Only then can self-discovery and a fresh perspective be realized by both the client and the nurse. In the event of transference, countertransference, challenges of ethical standards or ethical dilemmas, clinical supervision with other psychotherapists would be recommended ensuring safety, objectivity and to seek additional expertise. Having the support of another colleague can enable deep self-reflection, sharing of the nurse-client experiences, addressing challenges and engaging in problem-solving.

The nurse is a therapeutic instrument, and purposely and thoughtfully uses the self. Self-awareness is a therapeutic tool for the nurse-client relationship where caring will be enhanced (Rasheed, 2015) and it is something that can be learned. The reflective nurse will be required to step back and reflect on the nurse-client interaction and develop self-awareness of their thoughts, feelings, and behaviors in their practice. In this way, the nurse will grow their capacity to practice psychotherapy and self-compassion.

Standardized Assessment Scales and Screening Tools

Standardized assessment scales and screening assessment tools are helpful aides during the assessment and evaluation phases of the nursing process, though clinical judgment must always be used for the collection and utilization of information and should not be replaced by these tools, rather nurses should strive to use actuarial tools and clinical judgement in tandem. Some tools may be more self-explanatory for use while others may require formal training. The following examples of standardized screening tools and assessments can be used to better understand the degree, severity, or specificity of a client's presentation:

- *Ask Suicide-Screening Questionnaire (ASQ)* measures suicide risk in youth and adults, five (5) items, clinician rated (National Institute of Mental Health, 2024).
- *Brief Psychiatric Rating Scale (BPRS)* measures psychotic & nonpsychotic symptoms in adult clients with major psychiatric illness. 18 or 24 items, clinician rated (Overall and Gorham, 1962).
- *Columbia-Suicide Severity Rating Scale (C-SSRS)* measures suicide risk, 18 items, clinician rated (Posner et al., 2011).
- *DSM-5-TR Substance Use Disorder Criteria* (American Psychiatric Association, 2022).
- *Generalized Anxiety Disorder (GAD) 7* A 7-item anxiety scale (Spitzer et al., 2006).
- *Geriatric Depression Scale (GDS)* measures depression in older adults, 15 items, patient rated (Yesavage, 1986).
- *Hamilton Rating Scale for Depression (HAM-D)* measures severity & change in depression, 17 items, clinician rated (Hamilton, 1959).
- *Montreal Cognitive Assessment (MoCA)* assesses cognition in Dementia & Alzheimer's, 30 items, clinician rated (MoCA Cognition, 2023).
- *Patient Health Questionnaire (PHQ-2) & PHQ-9* measures depression & functional health assessment, 9 items, patient rated (Kroenke et al., 2001).
- *Primary Care PTSD Screen for DSM-5 (PC-PTSD-5)* to identify individuals with PTSD, 5 items, patient rated (Prins et al., 2016).

4 Reflective Questions

1. What are some examples of open-ended questions to understand the client's chief complaint?
2. What strategies would you employ to prioritize nursing interventions if the client presents with multiple competing mental health issues? What would your focus be in therapy? Do your techniques include cognitive, affective, or behavioural interventions?
3. What strategies would you utilize to ensure the client is actively engaged with their own treatment goals and treatment plan?
4. How would you tackle motivating clients who might have poor insight into their illness or might not agree with the suggested treatment plan?

5 Case Vignette

5.1 Assessment

The client is a 62-year-old CEO, who recently retired after the company was bought out by their competitor. The client was planning on retiring at 65 years. Their spouse continues employment and has many social relationships. They own their own home and have no financial concerns. The spouse has noticed the client is withdrawn. They have three adult children who have children of their own. The family gets together four times a year and stays connected via telephone, video-conferencing, and email.

The client describes feeling depressed and having a sense of hopelessness. They voice sleep disturbances (insomnia) and describe not feeling rested upon awakening. They describe decreased energy, tiredness, and fatigue for over 3 months. They have lost 12 pounds and are not interested in food. The client describes a loss of interest and pleasure in hobbies as well as a decrease in libido.

Standardized Assessment Tool. Hamilton Rating Scale for Depression, Mental Status Examination, Columbia–Suicide Severity Rating Scale, etc.
Nursing Diagnosis. Ineffective coping for situation grief, disturbed sleep pattern, imbalanced nutrition, ineffective (reduced) activity planning.

5.2 Plan

Begin one-hour manualized cognitive behavioural therapy (CBT) once a week for 12 weeks to identify/address the current thinking patterns and behaviour that maintain the depression. Guide client to identify their own goals and priority interventions at the beginning of each session. Evidence-based recommended goals and interventions include:

- Develop satisfactory sleep hygiene.
- Establish satisfactory nutrition.
- Increase regular activity; starting with the current activity level and increasing it slowly.
- Assist the client in identifying home activities and strategies to achieve between sessions at the end of each session. Provide all necessary tools and resources to promote success.
- Review progress on mood, sleep, appetite, libido, social interactions, sense of meaning, interests in everyday activities and any other presenting areas and symptoms at each session.
- Always ask the client to report any noted improvements or barriers.
- Review last week's homework, barriers and facilitators of agreed-upon goals at each session.

- Allow the client to ask questions, clarify expectations and identify the next steps at the end of each session.

5.3 Expected Outcomes

- Decrease in depressive episodes or states.
- Normal sleep patterns (positive sleep hygiene).
- Normal health nutrition (well-balanced meals).
- Regular exercise and increase in activity.

5.4 Evaluation

- Provide feedback on response to treatment.
- Allow the client to express their own perception about their treatment progression, effectiveness and/or lack of effectiveness.
- If treatment was ineffective, present evidence-based alternative approaches and support the client to choose an alternative path.
- Self-reflection and awareness of own biases when suggesting alternative treatment options and staying true to evidence-based facts.
- Provide client resources that might support your health teaching as needed.

5.5 Case Vignette Reflective Questions

1. What loss is the client experiencing? What are the therapeutic benefits of the interventions listed above for the client?
2. How applicable is CBT to the problems the client presents with if at all?
3. What techniques may be used to engage the client in goal setting and care planning?

6 Summary

- Considerations for a bio/psycho/social/spiritual health assessment across the lifespan were discussed.
- Therapeutic communication is important to ensure the effectiveness of the therapeutic relationship.
- Assessment scales and screening tools are identified and may be self-explanatory or may require formal training to better understand a client's presentation.

- A collaborative nurse-client partnership and application of the nursing process (assessment, planning, intervention, and evaluation) are pertinent for the achievement of positive outcomes.
- Therapeutic interventions may support health promotion, illness prevention, relapse management, risk mitigation, self-management, and client education by reducing emotional distress, facilitating cognitive and behavioural change, and promoting personal capacity.
- Therapeutic use of self and self-awareness can be learned and can be helpful for professional growth.

Appendix 1: Organizations/Agencies

Organization	Internet links
American Group Psychotherapy Association (AGPA)	https://agpa.org
Canadian Alliance on Mental Illness and Mental Health (CAMIMH)	https://camimh.ca
Canadian Association of Schools of Nursing	https://casn.ca/education/5656-2
Canadian Collaborative Mental Health Initiative	https://ccmhi.ca
Canadian Federation of Mental Health Nurses	https://cfmhn.ca
Canadian Group Psychotherapy Association (CGPA)	https://cgpa.ca
Canadian Mental Health Association (CMHA)	https://cmha.ca
Canadian Psychiatric Association	https://cpa-apc.org
Centre for Addiction and Mental Health (CAMH)	https://www.camh.ca
Heretohelp	https://www.heretohelp.bc.ca
Mental Health Commission of Canada (MHCC)	https://mentalhealthcommission.ca/
Psychcentral	https://psychcentral.com
Substance Abuse and Mental Health Service Administration	https://samhsa.gov/nctic/trauma-interventions
Manitoba Trauma Information Centre	https://trauma-informed.ca
Registered Nurse of Ontario	https://rnao.ca/bpg/guidelines
World Federation for Mental Health	https://wfmh.com
The World Health Organization (WHO)	https://www.who.int

References

Abraham, I.L., Fox, J. C., & Cohen, B. T. (1992). Integrating the bio into the biopsychosocial: Understanding and treating biological phenomena in psychiatric-mental health nursing. *Archives of Psychiatric Nursing, 6*(5), 296–305.

American Psychiatric Association. (2022). Diagnostic and statistical manual of mental disorders (5th ed., text rev.). https://doi.org/10.1176/appi.books.9780890425787

American Psychological Association (2023). Clinical practice guideline for the treatment of depression across three age cohorts. Author. https://www.apa.org/depression-guideline

Boeykens, D., Boeckxstaens, P., De Sutter, A., Lahousse, L., Pype, P., De Vriendt, P., & Van de Velde, D. (2022). Goal-oriented care for patients with chronic conditions or multimorbidity in primary care: A scoping review and concept analysis. *PLoS One 17*(2):e0262843. https://doi.org/10.1371/journal.pone.0262843

Dent, A. (2021). Heart led psychotherapy. A biopsychosocial spiritual model for clinical practice. *Transpersonal Psychology Review, 23*(1), 20–31. https://doi.org/10.53841/bpstran.2021

Government of Canada. (2023, June 1). *Social determinant of health and health inequalities.* https://www.canada.ca/en/public-health/services/health-promotion/population-health/what-determines-health.html

Hamilton, M. (1959). The assessment of anxiety states by rating. *Br J Med Psychol 32,* 50–55.

Harrad, R., Cosentino, C., Keasley, R., Sulla, F. (2019). Spiritual care in nursing: an overview of the measures used to assess spiritual care provision and related factors amongst nurses. *Acta Biomed for Health Professions 90*(4): 44–55 https://doi.org/10.23750/abm.v90i4-S.8300

Kroenke, K., Spitzer, R. L., & Williams, J. B. (2001). The PHQ-9: Validity of a brief depression severity measure. *J Gen Intern Med, 16*(9), 606–613.

MoCA Cognition. (2023). *MoCA test.* Author. https://mocacognition.com/paper/

North American Nursing Diagnosis Association (NANDA), 2023. https://nanda.org/

National Institute of Mental Health (2024). *Ask Suicide-Screening Questionnaire (ASQ).* Author. https://www.samhsa.gov/resource-search/dbhis?rc%5B0%5D=issues_conditions_disorders%3A20579

Noyce, R., & Simpson, J. (2018).The experience of forming a therapeutic relationship from the client's perspective: A metasynthesis. *Psychotherapy Research, 28*(2), 281–296. https://eprints.lancs.ac.uk/id/eprint/80056/1/RNlitrevjune2016anon.pdf

O'Brien, C. (2008). The CAGE questionnaire for detection of alcoholism. JAMA 300(17), 2054–2056.

Overall. J. & Gorham, D. (1962). The brief psychiatric rating scale. *Psychological Reports, 10,* 799–812.

Posner, K., Brown, G, K., Stanley, B., Brent, D. A., Yershova, K. V., Ouendo, M. A. ... Mann, J. J. (2011). The Columbia severity rating scales; initial validity and internal consistency from three multisite studies with adolescents and adults. *American J of Psychiatry, 168*(12), 1266–1277.

Prins, A., Bovin, M., Smolenski, D., Marx, B., Kimerling, R., Jenkins-Guarnieri, M., Kaloupek, D., Schnurr, P., Pless Kaiser, A., Leyva, Y., & Tiet, Q. (2016). The primary care PTSD screen for DSM-5 (PC-PTSD-5): Development and evaluation within a primary care sample. *Gen Intern Med 31*(10), 1206–1211.

Rasheed, S. P. (2015). Self-awareness as a therapeutic tool for nurse/client relationship. *International Journal of Caring Sciences, 8*(1), 211–216.

Registered Nurses Association of Ontario (RNAO). (2015). *Person-and family-centered care.* Author. www.rnao.ca

Reynolds, C. (2019). Building resilience through psychotherapy. *World Psychiatry, 18*(3), 289–291.

Saad, M., De Medeiros, R., & Mosini, A. C. (2017). Are we ready for a true biopsychosocial spiritual model? The true meanings of "spiritual". *Medicines, 4,* 79. https://doi.org/10.3390/medicines4040079.

Spitzer, R., Kroenke, K., Williams, J., & Lowe, B. (2006). A brief measure for assessing generalized anxiety disorder: The GAD-7. *Arch Intern Med, 166*(10), 1092–1097. https://doi.org/10.1001/archinte.166.10.1092

Yesavage, J. A. (1986). The use of self-rating depression scales in the elderly. In L. W. Poon, T. Crook, K. L. Davis, C. Eisdorfer, B. J. Gurland, A. W. Kaszniak, & L. W. Thompson (Eds.), *Handbook for clinical memory assessment of older adults* (pp. 213–217). American Psychological Association.

Chapter 15
Nursing Competencies: Assessment and Case Formulation

Mary-Lou Martin, Natalie Castonguay, and Stacey Roles

Abstract This chapter presents and explores concepts foundational to assessment with case formulation, treatment planning, and evaluation. The concepts of trauma and violence-informed care along with cultural identity, cultural competence, and cultural safety will be highlighted. Collecting, processing, and organising information and formulating an approach will be reviewed. Clinical judgement skills and actuarial screening tools to determine the level of strengths, vulnerabilities, risks, and resources will be discussed. Critical pathways and case formulation will be highlighted. Clinical knowledge, theory, judgement, and collaboration with clients will be discussed including how it helps to determine the selection of the intervention. Utilising evidence-based information to provide confidential, ethical, culturally competent, safe, effective, and efficient care consistent with mental, physical, spiritual, emotional, social, and cultural needs of the individual are paramount. These will be discussed using the bio/psycho/social/spiritual model as a conceptual framework for understanding and responding to health problems in partnership with clients, to promote health and foster recovery and resilience.

Keywords Assessment · Formulation · Intervention · Evaluation · Risks · Reflection

M.-L. Martin (✉)
St. Joseph's Healthcare Hamilton/McMaster University, Hamilton, ON, Canada
e-mail: martinm@stjosham.on.ca

N. Castonguay · S. Roles
Roles & Associates Psychotherapy Services Inc. & CBT Training Centre of the North, Sudbury, ON, Canada
e-mail: stacey@rolespsychotherapy.com

S. Roles and K. Kalia (eds.), *The Nurses' Guide to Psychotherapy*,
https://doi.org/10.1007/978-981-97-4738-2_15

Learning Objectives

After completing this chapter, the learner will:

1. Describe assessment. Case formulation, treatment planning, and evaluation.
2. Describe the important issues in selecting an approach.
3. Identify examples of specific screening and assessment tools.
4. Discuss self-awareness and reflection.

1 Introduction

The value of therapeutic work relies on the ongoing assessment, planning, implementation, and evaluation of the therapeutic alliance and its effectiveness over the course of the nurse-client relationship. Therapeutic work uses a collaborative trauma and violence-informed approach in the assessment and plan of care, and recognizes the positive and negative effects of the social determinants of health on the client.

Multicultural processes and outcomes are also important factors to consider (Chap. 12). The multicultural orientation (cultural humility and cultural comfort) of therapists has been shown to positively associate with therapeutic outcomes, whereas cultural missed opportunities have been demonstrated to negatively relate to the working alliance and therapy improvements (Davis et al., 2018). Recent research indicates that there are improvements in therapy outcomes when clients have a high cultural identity and therapists have high cultural humility (Anders & Kivlighan, 2023).

Collaboration in the treatment process is also important to the therapeutic rapport and outcomes. Clients seek psychotherapy for a variety of reasons including past or current physical stress (injury, insomnia, pain, physical illness, trauma/abuse, violence), psychological stress (colonization, discrimination, finances, housing, loss or altered relationships, mental health issues, racism, self-harm, trauma, unemployment, work), spiritual stress (existential crisis, loss of hope or purpose), developmental stress (becoming a parent, retiring), and/or situational stress (sexual assault, limited social support, unexpected injury or illness). The client who identifies as part of the 2SLGBTQIA+ community may experience health inequities due to stigma and discrimination (Comeau, Johnson, & Bouhamdani, 2023), and this can also contribute to multiple areas of the stressors listed above. Collaboration throughout the assessment and in treatment planning allows the nurse psychotherapist an opportunity to explore the clients' stressors from their own perspective and enables an opportunity for the client to set goals for treatment.

The therapeutic relationship (Chap. 3) and the value it lends to psychotherapy inclusive of the assessment and case formulation process has resulted in the development of Best Practice Guidelines in Canada (Forchuk et al., 2006; Gallop et al., 2002). These standards identify that honest, reciprocal, and intentional communication is key to developing a respectful and trusting relationship with clients (Forchuk et al., 2006). Curiosity and empathic listening are necessary for identifying, expressing, and exploring silence, emotions, thoughts, and behaviours in the assessment process. Nurse psychotherapists use these skills in the assessment phase, which helps to determine the use of case formulation and/or clinical pathways, and throughout the therapy process. While critical pathways may be useful for clients who have typical symptoms and who have an expected course of treatment, case formulation may be more appropriate for more individualistic care and to identify past life experiences that have brought today's goals to the forefront.

2 Assessment, Clinical Formulation, and Treatment Planning

Assessment in relation to psychotherapy is defined as a complex, systematic, and co-created process of collecting and evaluating information from a variety of sources (observing, case history, interviewing, instruments) of the clients' emotions, thoughts, and behaviours that may contribute to the client's problems/issues (biological, psychological, social, cultural, environmental) to inform treatment planning and the course of treatment (Guilli & Nasser, 2019; Pathak, 2016; Peterson et al., 2015). Assessment is ongoing and is required throughout the therapeutic process. Assessment provides the first opportunity to begin building rapport and helps the therapist to develop an overall understanding of the client through their past experiences, present problems, strengths, and future goals (Friedman & Markey, 2023).

A thorough holistic assessment will allow the nurse psychotherapist to complete a comprehensive clinical case formulation, which includes the presenting issue(s), global history, the primary concern, and the proposed plan (Baird et al., 2017). An in-depth assessment via a healthy therapeutic relationship can help to uncover a clear purpose and expectations. Clinical case formulation is defined as a process of developing hypotheses and organising information about the origins, predisposing, precipitating, protective, psychological, interpersonal, and behavioural factors as a guide for treatment that gives directions on how the goal(s) may be benchmarked and reached, from session to session and throughout the course of therapy (Eells, 2022). The goal(s) or problem(s) to be worked on are established and the therapeutic approach can then be determined through the client's active involvement in decision-making.

Clients are multidimensional, each with their own individual goals, abilities, and preferences. Clients may contemplate several issues when initiating psychotherapy including the psychotherapist they choose and this is important to discuss in the assessment process. When choosing a psychotherapist client may consider their own and the psychotherapist's personal characteristics, such as gender, socioeconomic status, religious beliefs, race, ethnicity, cultural background, sensitivity, and overall life experiences as well as the therapeutic approaches they are interested in exploring (Noyce & Simpson 2018). To disclose personal information, clients identify the need for openness, honesty, and receptivity to needs and for the psychotherapist to use some form of self-disclosure to help the therapeutic process grow (Noyce & Simpson, 2018). Attunement is the process of relating to another at the moment and is important to the therapeutic process as the client and psychotherapist tend to connect on a deeper level when the client feels truly listened to and understood by their psychotherapist (Noyce & Simpson, 2018). The psychotherapist then listens for communication patterns and themes for example, identifying patterns in communication that cause frustration, anger, and conflict which can aid in the assessment process. Clients will vary about the need for adequate time and space to build a trusting therapeutic relationship (Noyce & Simpson, 2018). Clients' patterns of attachment are formed by their childhood experiences and how they negotiate relationships in their life. The impact of transference and countertransference in a therapeutic relationship can be positive or negative for both the client and therapist and must be observed and reflected upon within the course of treatment. A person-centred approach, using flexibility, safety, and promoting a collaborative relationship while allowing the client to pace the work can enhance the case formulation and treatment outcomes (Noyce & Simpson, 2018).

The clinical formulation and treatment plan encompasses a holistic approach to the client's problems which best fits the individual and the therapeutic modality being used as intervention. One example of assessment, formulation and treatment planning is based on Dr. Aaron T. Beck's cognitive behavioural model (2021) and can be found in Table 1, Case History, Formulation and Treatment Plan. Cognitive behavioural therapy uses a range of techniques to make connections between maladaptive assumptions, conditions and behaviour whereby the goal is to engage in cognitive restructuring leading to new ways of thinking, behaviour change, and emotional shifts. For more on different types of psychotherapy see Chap. 16.

Screening tools can also be an important part of the assessment, case formulation, diagnosis, monitoring, and evaluation process. There are a variety of screening tools that exist, for a multitude of presentations, some requiring training to use in clinical practice. For a non-inclusive list of screening tools see Appendix A.

Treatment planning in relation to psychotherapy is an organised conceptual effort to develop a plan in advance of and throughout therapy. This type of planning seeks to provide the most effective strategies and methods to reach the identified goals and to assist clients with measurable outcomes within a reasonable time in duration and frequency (Makeover, 2016). The choice of psychotherapy is dependent on the psychotherapist's expertise and the client's problems and preferences and is never begun without informed consent from the client. See Appendix B for Internet links to resources on assessment, case formulation, and mental health resources.

Table 1 Case history, formulation & treatment plan. Adapted from Academy of Cognitive Therapy (2014). Academy of Cognitive Therapy Handbook, pp. 67–69. https://www.academyofcbt.org

Case history
Identifying information Include age, gender, ethnicity, marital status, living situation, and occupation
Chief complaint Consider using the client's own words
History of presenting symptoms Describe emotional, cognitive, behavioural, and physiological symptoms. Consider environmental stressors. Briefly review treatments (if any) that have been attempted
Past psychiatric history Summarise past psychiatric history including substance abuse
Personal and social history Summarise most salient features. Include observations on formative experiences, traumas (if any), supports and interests
Medical history Note any medical problems (e.g., endocrine disturbances, heart disease, cancer, chronic medical illnesses, chronic pain) that may influence psychological functioning or the treatment process
Mental status observations List a few salient features of the mental status exam during the evaluation phase. Include observations on general appearance and mood
DSM V diagnoses (if applicable)
Case formulation
Precipitants Large-scale events that may play a significant role in precipitating current symptoms. If no psychosocial precipitants can be identified, note any other features of the client's history that may help explain the onset of symptoms
Cross-sectional view of current cognitions and behaviours The cross-sectional view should conceptualise how the cognitive model applies to the client early in treatment. Observations of the predominant cognitions, emotions, behaviours (and physiological reactions if relevant) that the client demonstrates in the "here and now"
Longitudinal view of cognitions and behaviours The longitudinal view is developed fully as therapy proceeds and the therapist uncovers underlying schemas (core beliefs, rules, assumptions) and enduring patterns of behaviour (compensatory strategies). It includes key schemas (core beliefs, rules, or assumptions) and compensatory behavioural strategies. For those without premorbid history, consider major belief(s) and dysfunctional behaviour patterns present only during the evaluation period
Strengths and assets Describe strengths and assets (e.g., physical health, intelligence, social skills, support network, work history, etc.)
Working hypothesis (summary of conceptualization) Summarise the principal features of the working hypothesis that directs treatment interventions. Link the hypothesis with the cognitive model for the client's disorder(s)
Treatment plan
Problem list
Treatment goals

(continued)

Table 1 (continued)

Plan for treatment
Course of treatment
Therapeutic relationship Nature and quality of the therapeutic relationship and any problems encountered
Interventions/procedures Describe cognitive interventions being considered and rationale
Obstacles
Outcome Describe outcomes and/or barriers

3 Evaluation

Evaluation in psychotherapy includes considering the quality, efficiency, and effectiveness of the treatment effects (or the lack thereof), and the evaluation and health-related outcomes important to individualised person-centred care (Fairburn & Cooper, 2011; Gerger et al., 2020). Summarization, evaluation and ensuring understanding of the client's meaning is not only important to case formulation, but also to the therapeutic relationship and its resolution. Measurement outcomes are important quality indicators and are valued by the therapist and client to measure progress in therapy. The psychotherapist and client should monitor progress and evaluate therapeutic outcomes as established at the beginning of the relationship. The therapist and client can take this opportunity to evaluate and share their mutual understanding of perspectives, priorities, growth, and achievement of goals (Forchuk et al., 2006; Gallop et al., 2002). The nurse psychotherapist may want to inquire as to if the psychotherapy made a significant positive difference in the situation of the individual client and what changes the client and therapist noticed in relation to symptoms, problems, perceptions, emotions, thoughts, behaviours, function, and relationships? In the final evaluation, alongside the resolution of the relationship, there may be feelings of loss or ambivalence, but can be redirected to focus on the evaluation of the benefit of the therapeutic process, the goals achieved and future goal planning for the client. For more on the evaluation of psychotherapy, see Chap. 17.

4 Case Vignette

4.1 Assessment

- A 35-year-old graphic designer is living through the unexpected rupture of a primary relationship with a significant other.

- The client has been in the relationship for 4.5 years. They share a home together and many of the same friends. The client is labile, emotionally dysregulated, and thinking of taking a drug overdose. There is a recent increase in the use of alcohol and drugs. The client reports difficulties related to sleep, feelings of isolation, and abandonment.
- No treatments attempted. Has not engaged in psychotherapy previously.
- No past psychiatric history.
- Normal early development.
- No history of trauma.
- Family is supportive however the immediate family lives 1,000 km away. Enjoys work. Interests such as working, are at the same gym as partner. Friends are shared with partner.
- No significant medical history.
- Partner says that they have wanted to end the relationship for some time. Does not see any chance for reconciliation.
- Patient appears distressed and somewhat dishevelled.
- "My partner is leaving me; they are sleeping on the couch at night and only come back when they have to. We don't talk… and when we do it's about selling our house. I don't know what to do. I can't sleep. I don't have anyone. My friends have abandoned me. The only thing that helps is using a little something to help me get through the pain. At times I think it might be easier to end it."

4.2 Standardized Assessment Tools

- Columbia Suicide Rating Scale,
- CAGE Alcohol Questionnaire,
- CAGE Drug Abuse Questionnaire.

4.3 Treatment

Discuss main responsibilities and function, clarifying therapy goals, targets for therapy

Problem List

- Potential for self-harm,
- Abuse of substances,
- Impaired coping and problem solving,
- Feels abandoned,
- Impaired sleep.

Strength/Resources

- Has fairness, honesty, kindness, creativity,

- Has generally good health,
- Has family connections/support,
- Has high value in helping others,
- Enjoys photography, gardening.

Interventions (collaborate on the plan)

- Safety planning—coping skills and problem-solving skills,
- Cognitive therapy—manualized 12–20 week treatment protocol with cognitive restructuring, connections between events, thoughts, feelings, and behaviour,
- Grounding techniques, progressive muscle relaxation, mindfulness,
- Sleep hygiene,
- Maintaining some previous relationships and developing new relationships for support.

Expected Outcomes

- No self-harm,
- Reduced use of substances,
- Improved coping,
- Feels secure,
- Improved sleep,
- Does homework,
- Reassess symptoms.

4.4 Evaluation

Regularly review at individual sessions and at the end of therapy to determine if they are improving with:

- Feeling emotions rather than using avoidance (no self-harm, reduced use of substances);
- Developing a balanced & realistic beliefs about the event, self and others;
- Developing and maintaining meaningful relationships;
- Using self-soothing and coping;
- Decreasing the use of alcohol and drugs;
- Feeling rested with improved sleep;
- Reflecting on work, progress, and changes made;
- Continuing practice of skills learned;
- Identifying goals for the future.

5 Case Vignette Reflective Questions

1. What loss is the client experiencing?
2. What is your primary role as a therapist?
3. What might be the clients' goals?
4. What are the client's preferences regarding intervention?
5. What tools might you use in your assessment to develop a case formulation and treatment plan?
6. What resources might you pull from to assist the client?
7. How have you personally dealt with the loss of a relationship and how did you cope with it?
8. Reflect on your personal values, beliefs, privileges, and social position—how does it influence your nurse-client relationship?
9. How would you navigate the therapeutic relationship if your values and beliefs are not in line with the client?
10. What is the difference between a crisis intervention session and a psychotherapy session?
11. How would you evaluate the client's overall experience?

6 Chapter Summary

- Clinical assessment, formulation, treatment planning, and evaluation are important psychotherapy interventions.
  - An example of assessment, formulation, and treatment plan for cognitive behaviour therapy was provided.
- Therapy and approaches to care involve a variety of factors.
  - A review of some tools that can be used for screening, diagnosis, monitoring, and evaluation of psychotherapy were listed.
- Strengths, vulnerabilities, and risks are important to highlight and address.
- Therapeutic relationship, alliance, and the change process are important for positive psychotherapy outcomes.

Appendix 1: Screening and Assessment Tools

There are many screening tests, assessment guides and tools that can be used to screen, monitor or to complete ongoing assessments. When selecting these tools, it is important to consider their type, utility, reliability, and sensitivity. Some are completed by the clinician, some require specific training to use while others do not and others are completed by the client. Below in a non-inclusive list, many can be found online.

- Adult Attitude to Grief Scale—Measures changes to reactions and responses to grief, 9 items, self-rated
- Anticipatory Grief Scale—Measures aspects of multidimensional grief, 27 items, self-rated
- Beck Depression Inventory (BDI)—Assesses intensity of depression, 21 items, self-report
- Brief Psychiatric Rating Scale (BPRS)—Measures psychopathology, 16 items, self-report
- CAGE Alcohol Questions—Indicates potential problems with alcohol use, 4 items, clinician rated
- CAGE Drug Abuse Questions—Indicates potential problems with substances, 4 items, clinician rated
- Columbia-Suicide Severity Rating Scale (C-SSRS)—Assesses the severity and immediacy of suicide risk, 3 versions
- Composite Abuse Scale (Revise) Short Form (CASR+SF)—Measure physical, sexual, and psychological abuse, 15 items, self-rated
- Diagnostic and Statistical Manual of Mental Disorders (DSM_5-TR)—Classification of mental disorders
- Dissociative Experiences Scale-II (DES-II)—Measures the percentage of time they experience a dissociative symptom, 28 item, self-report
- Eating Attitude Test (EAT-26)—Screens for eating disorder, 26 items, self-report
- Edinburgh Postnatal Depression Scale (EPDS)—Assesses woman with perinatal depression, 10 items, self-report
- Generalized Anxiety Disorder (GAD-7)—Screening tool for generalized anxiety disorder, 7 items, self-report
- Geriatric Depression Scales (GDS)—Assesses depression in older adults, 15 items, self-report
- Geriatric Suicide Ideation Scale (GSIS)—Factors associated with suicide ideation in older adults, 31 items
- Hamilton Depression Rating Scale (HAM-D)—Measures depression, 21 items, self-report
- International Classification of Diseases, Tenth Revision, Clinician Modification (IC-CM)
- Mini Mental Status Exam-screening for cognitive function, 11 items, self-report
- Montreal Cognitive Assessment (MoCA)—Measures cognitive function, 30 item, self-report
- Mood Disorder Questionnaire (MDQ)—Screening for bipolar symptoms, 17 items, self-report
- Opioid Risk Tool (ORT)—Screening tool to predict opioid use disorder among individuals prescribe opioids for treatment of chronic pain, 11 items
- Patient Health Questionnaire (PHQ-9)—To screen, diagnose, monitor and measure severity of depression, 9 items, self-report

- Post Traumatic Stress Disorder Checklist (PCL-5)—Measures DSM-5 Symptoms of PTSD, 17 items, self-report
- Post Traumatic Stress D Checklist for DSM-5 (PCL-5)—Global assessment of PTSD severity at the time of diagnosis and over the course of treatment, 20 items, self-report
- Primary Care PTSD Screen for DSM5 (PC-PTSD-5) – screening tool to identify probable PTSD, 5 items
- Rapid Mood Screener—To differentiate bipolar I disorder from major depressive disorder, 6 items, self-report
- Rosenberg Self-esteem Scale—Measuring both positive and negative feelings related self-esteem, 10 items, self-report
- Screening, Brief Intervention and Referral to Treatment (SBIRT)—Universal screening for individuals who use alcohol and substances at risky levels; early intervention and treatment
- Short Form Health Survey (SF-36)—Measures quality of life, 36 items, self-report
- Short Term Assessment of Risk and Treatability (START)—Assesses vulnerabilities, strengths and risks, 20+ items, clinician-rated
- Social Functions Questionnaire—Measures social functioning, 8 items, self-report
- Trauma Screening Questionnaire (TSQ)—Screens for all types of traumatic stress; experienced at least twice in the past week, 10 items, self-report
- Zung Self-Rating Depression Scale—Measures severity of depression, 20 items, self-report.

Appendix 2: Internet Links for Assessment, Case Formulation, and Mental Health Resources

Organization	Web link
Alcoholics Anonymous	www.aa.org
Al-Anon	www.al-anon.org
BPD Central	www.bpdcentral.com
BPD World	www.bpdworld.org
Bulimia Anorexia Nervosa Association	www.bana.ca
Canadian Alliance on Mental Illness and Mental Health	www.camimh.ca
Canadian Association for Suicide Prevention	www.suicideprevention.ca
Canadian Centre of Substance Use and Addiction	www.ccsa.ca
Canadian Mental Health Association	www.cmha.ca

(continued)

(continued)

Organization	Web link
Canadian Network for Mood and Anxiety Treatment	www.canmat.org
Canadian Network for the Prevention of Elder Abuse	www.cnpea.ca/en
Canadian Nurses Association	www.cna-aiic.ca/en/home
Canadian Psychological Association	www.cpa.ca
Canadian Red Cross	www.redcross.ca/how-we-help/violence-bullying-and-abuse-prevention/youth/bullying
Centre for Addiction and Mental Health	www.camh.ca
Centre for Addiction and Mental Health	www.camh.ca/en/education/continuing-education-programs-and-courses
Canadian Research Initiative on Substance Misuse	www.crism.ca
Centre for Suicide Prevention	www.suicideinfo.ca
Cleveland Clinic: Communicating with patient in a new world of virtual visits	https://my.clevelandclinic.org/departments/patient-experience/depts/experience-partners/licensed-programs/rede-to-communicate
College of Nurses of Ontario	www.cno.org
Eating Disorders Association of Canada	www.edac-atac.ca
Danger Assessment	www.dangerassessment.org
First Nations Youth Suicide Prevention Program Curriculum	www.canada.ca/en/department-national-defense-services-benefits-military/military-mental health.html
FUTURES Without Violence	www.futureswithoutviolence.org
Health Canada	www.canada.ca/en/health-canada
International Bipolar Foundation	www.internationalbipolarfoundation.org
International Initiative for Mental Health	www.iimhl.com
International Society of Bipolar Disorder	www.isbd.org
Lifeline Canada Foundation	www.thelifelinecanada.ca
Manitoba Trauma Information Centre	www.trauma-informed.ca
Mental Health Commission	www.mentalhealthcommission.ca/English
Mental Health First Aid	www.mentalhealthcommission.ca/training/mhfa
Mental Health First Aid	www.mhfa.ca
Mind	www.mind.org.uk
myPlan Canada	www.myplanapp.ca/en
National Collaborating Centre for Aboriginal Health	www.nccih.ca
National Eating Disorders Information Centre	www.nedic.ca
National Initiative for Eating Disorders	www.nied.ca

(continued)

(continued)

Organization	Web link
National Institute of Drug Abuse	www.drugabuse.gov
Preventative Online Mental Health Program for Youth	www.OurYouthWellbeing.com
Registered Nurses of Ontario Best Practice Guidelines	www.rnao.ca/bpg/guidelines
Substance Abuse and Mental Health Services	www.samhsa.gov
US National Institute of Mental Health	www.nimh.nih.gov/health
World Federation for Mental Health	www.wfmh.global
World Health Organization: Mental Health	www.who.int/iris/handle/10665/329602
World Health Organization Recovery practices for mental health & wellbeing: Training. Course Guide	www.who.int/health-topics/mental-health#tab=tab_1

References

Academy of Cognitive Therapy. (2014). *Academy of Cognitive Therapy Handbook,* Author. https://www.academyofcbt.org

Anders, C., & Kivlighan, M. (2023). Identity salience: An intersectional approach to understanding multicultural processes and outcomes in psychotherapy. *Journal of Counseling Psychology, 70*(5), 477–485.

Baird, J., Hyslop, A., Macfie, M., Stocks, R., & Van der Kleij, T. (2017). Clinical formulation: Where it came from, what it is and why it matters. *BJPsych Advances, 23*(2), 95–103. https://doi.org/10.1192/apt.bp.115.014670

Beck, J. (2021). Cognitive Behavior Therapy: Basics and Beyond (3rd ed.). Guilford Press.

Comeau, D., Johnson, C. & Bouhamdani (2023). Review of current 2SLGBTQIA+ inequities in the Canadian health system. Frontiers in Public Health, July 18, 11.

Davis, D. E., DeBlaere, C., Owen, J., Hook, J. N., Rivera, D. P. Choe, E.,Van Tongeren, D. R., Worthington, E. L., Jr., & Placeseres, V. (2018). The multicultural orientation framework: a narrative review. *Psychotherapy: Theory, Research & Practice, 55*(1), 89–100.

Eells, T. D. (Ed.) (2022). Handbook of psychotherapy case formulation, 3rd ed. The Guilford Press.

Fairburn, C. G. & Cooper, Z. (2011). Therapist competence, therapy quality, and therapist training. *Behaviour Research and Therapy, 49*(6–7), 373–378.

Forchuk, C., Carmichael, C., Golea, G., Johnson, N. Martin, M-L., Patterson, R., Ray, K., Robinson, T., Sogbein, S. A., Srivastava, R. & Shov, T. (2006). Nursing best practice guideline: Establishing therapeutic relationships (rev. supp) Registered Nurses of Ontario. https://rnao.ca/bpg/guideline/establishin-therapeutic-relationship

Friedman, H. S., & Markey, C. H. (editors) (2023). Encyclopedia of Mental Health (3rd ed.). Elsevier Inc. ISBSN: 978-0-323-91498-7

Gallop, R., Choiniere, T. Forchuk, C., Golea, G., Johnsons, N., Levac, A., Martin, M-L., Robinson, T., Sogbeing, S., Sutcliffe, H., Wynn, F. (2002). *NBPG: Establishing Therapeutic relationships.* Registered Nurses Association of Ontario. https://rnao.ca/sites/rnaofiles

Gerger, H. Nascimento, A. F., Locher, C., Gaab, J., & Tachset, M. (2020). What are the key characteristics of a 'good' psychotherapy? Calling for ethical patient involvement. Front Psychiatry, June 2, 11, 406.

Guilli, L. F. & Nasser, B. (2019). Assessment and diagnosis. Retrieved on Jan. 11 2024. https://www.encyclopedia.com

Makeover, R. B. (2016). Treatment Planning for Psychotherapy. A Practical Guide to Better Outcomes (3rd ed.). American Psychiatric Association Publishing.

Noyce, R, & Simpson, J. (2018). The Experience of forming a therapeutic relationship from the client's perspective: A metasynthesis. *Psychotherapy Research, 28*(2), 281–296

Pathak, P. C. (2016). Assessment in Counselling: A Perspective. *Indian Journal of Community Psychology, 12(*2), 293–306.

Peterson, R. L., Peterson, D. R., Abrams, J. C., Stricker, S., & Ducheny, K. (2015). Training in clinical psychology in the United States: Practitioner model. In James D. Wright (Ed.), *International Encyclopedia of the Social & Behavioural Sciences* (2nd ed.) (pp. 517–523). Elsevier.

Chapter 16
Nursing Competencies: Types of Psychotherapy

Stacey Roles, Madison Moxam, Natalie Castonguay, and Carly Valiente

Abstract Psychotherapy covers a broad range of multi-modal treatment approaches, some adhering to theoretical foundations and structured protocols while others are considered more fluid, utilising an integrated approach built on an assortment of theoretical foundations. Case formulation and treatment planning methods are developed and adjusted throughout the treatment trajectory, in alignment with the theoretical underpinnings from which they emerge. This chapter will discuss psychotherapies from a multi-generational and multi-modal lens, considering both structured and unstructured psychotherapy perspectives. This chapter is not meant to be exhaustive but will discuss a range of therapies including cognitive behavioural therapy, dialectical behavioural therapy, eye movement desensitization and reprocessing therapy, compassion-focused therapy, internal family systems, polyvagal-informed therapy, acceptance and commitment therapy, cognitive processing theory, psychoanalysis, psychodynamic, and brainspotting therapy. This chapter will help readers understand some of the history of psychotherapy, how some modern psychotherapy approaches were construed, and the types of evidence-based psychotherapies available to explore and learn in more depth.

Keywords Psychotherapy · Structured psychotherapies · Unstructured psychotherapies · Interventions

---

S. Roles (✉) · N. Castonguay · C. Valiente
Roles & Associates Psychotherapy Services Inc. & CBT Training Centre of the North, Sudbury, ON, Canada
e-mail: stacey@rolespsychotherapy.com

M. Moxam
Laurentian University, Sudbury, ON, Canada

S. Roles and K. Kalia (eds.), *The Nurses' Guide to Psychotherapy*,
https://doi.org/10.1007/978-981-97-4738-2_16

Learning Objectives

After completing this chapter, the learner will:

1. Understand some of the history of psychotherapy, which includes evidence-based psychotherapies from a historical and modern-day lens.
2. Explain the theoretical foundations of multiple psychotherapy approaches and their applicability to individual clients.
3. Demonstrate the types of client presentations that would warrant the use of certain psychotherapeutic approaches.

1 Overview of Psychotherapy

Psychotherapy is a therapeutic treatment approach which includes a range of interventions targeting thoughts, feelings, and behaviours, both conscious and unconscious, that can be used with clients facing a range of mental health adversities (Lambert et al., 1994). Clinicians adjust the therapeutic approaches in alignment with the intentions of the treatment plan, ultimately supporting the clients' self-awareness and decisions with the goal of improved quality of life and overall wellness of the client (Lambert et al., 1994). Psychotherapy intends to support individuals through transformative shifts in multiple aspects of life including behaviours, beliefs, attitudes, lifestyle, relationships, and overall well-being (Psychotherapy and Counselling Federation of Australia, 2020). The transformations that may occur are dependent on the values and goals of the psychotherapist and client (Psychotherapy and Counselling Federation of Australia, 2020). Within the scope of psychotherapy, there are many specialised skill sets and practices that can be considered and integrated within the treatment plan (Lambert et al., 1994).

The American Psychiatric Association (APA) Committee on Psychotherapy developed the Y model to meet accreditation board standards in structuring the teaching of residents about supportive, cognitive behavioural, and psychodynamic psychotherapy (Goldberg & Plakun, 2013). The Y model and an adaptation of it will be discussed in this chapter to help outline the different types of psychotherapy one can learn. At the base of the Y model (Fig. 16.1 Y-Model) are the core skills and foundational principles for psychotherapists-in-training which they often begin developing during undergraduate studies when learning counselling skills (Binder & Betan, 2013).

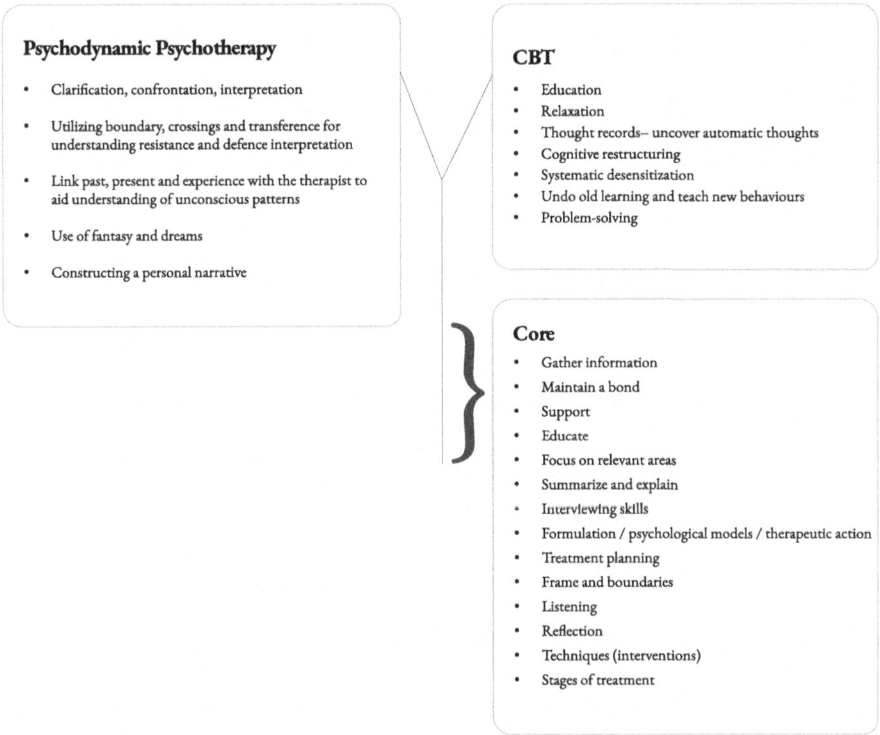

Fig. 16.1 Y-Model Interventions Techniques. Adapted from Goldberg, D. & Plakun, E. (2013). Teaching Psychodynamic Psychotherapy with the Y Model. *Psychodynamic Psychiatry, 31*(1), 111–125. With permission

With further education and/or on-the-job training, one can gain a more specialized understanding of the theoretical principles underpinning the specific psychotherapeutic modalities (Binder & Betan, 2013). The specific therapeutic approaches may become the focus of the new psychotherapist's career, and, as presented in Fig. 16.2 may be located in one or both arms of the Y model. The comprehensive training required to practice modalities of psychotherapy as seen in the arms of the Y model can be further categorised into three parts: training, supervised practice, and personal therapeutic work (Psychotherapy and Counselling Federation of Australia, 2020).

Comprehensive training must recognize the range of modalities within psychotherapy and promote an understanding of both the similarities and differences between theories (Psychotherapy and Counselling Federation of Australia, 2020). Training should also include philosophical and theoretical perspectives as well as evidence-informed practice. Supervised hours should be completed by the student under a qualified supervisor to help further develop skills while working with clients using the application or therapeutic techniques and theories. An understanding of the goals, experiences, and perspectives of the client(s) being treated is foundational

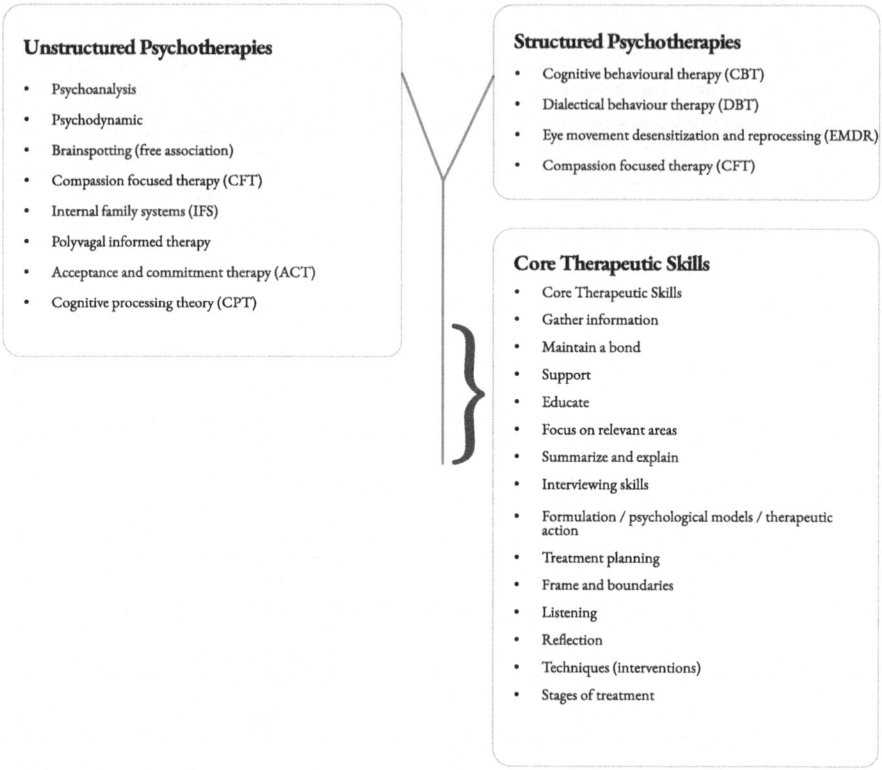

Fig. 16.2 Y-Model Restructured: Structured and Unstructured Therapies. Adapted from Goldberg, D. & Plakun, E. (2013). Teaching Psychodynamic Psychotherapy with the Y Model. *Psychodynamic Psychiatry, 31*(1), 111–125

to the practice of psychotherapy. Under supervision, the learner will develop the skills necessary to interact with and support clients effectively. Aspiring psychotherapists are also encouraged and, at times, required to participate in personal therapy (Psychotherapy and Counselling Federation of Australia, 2020). Psychotherapy heavily relies on self-development and exploration (Psychotherapy and Counselling Federation of Australia, 2020) and it is therefore important that clinicians be self-aware and engage in healing, growth, and change. The transformation and reflection that takes place in personal therapeutic work are self-determined by the client, however, guided by the practitioner that they chose to engage with (Psychotherapy and Counselling Federation of Australia, 2020). Training, supervision, and personal practice will be discussed more at length in upcoming chapters.

The development of a therapeutic relationship, known as the therapeutic alliance, cultivates trust between client and clinician so that they may have clear roles (Binder & Betan, 2013), work towards goals, and plan treatment (Hilsenroth et al., 2012). Together the practitioner and client can work collaboratively on decisions regarding health and treatment (Harris & Panozzo, 2019). The therapeutic alliance sets the foundation to support the clients' autonomy, collaborative treatment, and behaviours modeled by practitioners (Okamoto et al., 2019). Generally, therapeutic alliances are the sharing of personal thoughts and emotions with the goal of improving one's overall health (Okamoto et al., 2019). Developing a therapeutic alliance is fundamental for people accessing mental health support and ultimately leads to more positive outcomes (Hartley et al., 2020). Although in some cases they may be difficult to develop, therapeutic alliances offer a more person-centred and recovery-oriented treatment approach because they are rooted in human connection (Hartley et al., 2020). Within this relationship, core skills are used by practitioners to support the client(s), and may include general counselling skills (Hilsenroth et al., 2012) such as attentive behaviour, questioning, confrontation, focusing, and reflection (Binder & Betan, 2013). Concurrently, clinicians need to be aware of, and should strive for, culturally-sensitive therapeutic interventions (Binder & Betan 2013). For more information on cross-cultural considerations see Chap. 12.

Further, clinicians need an understanding of how to use specific theoretical foundations in order to formulate case conceptualization and treatment planning. Treatment planning considers the timeline, resources, and goals of the client while at the same time identifying interventions based on the trajectory of treatment sessions over time. Keeping in mind that individual sessions may deviate due to unexpected life circumstances and that flexibility is important. Treatment planning may also include diagnosis and case conceptualization prior to intervention implementation (Chap. 15). Throughout therapy sessions, the clinician and client may consider their own insight and emerging information to identify and assess interpersonal and intrapersonal patterns (Binder & Betan, 2013). A skilled clinician enables the client the opportunity to reflect on behaviours, thoughts, emotions, relationships, and situations that impact their lives in either the conscious or unconscious mind. Evaluation is continuously taking place with the ultimate goal of progression and termination of treatment. It is important to regularly assess treatment progress to ensure that the methods being used are effective for the clients' healing (Binder & Betan, 2013).

The approach used for assessment, case formulation or diagnosis, treatment planning, intervention, and termination is based on the theoretical foundations of the type of psychotherapy in which the clinician practices. It is therefore important to understand the many types of psychotherapies that exist, how they evolved from other forms of psychotherapy, the similarities and differences between the variety of modalities of psychotherapy, and how to identify which type of psychotherapy, or blend of psychotherapies, fit best for a particular clinician's interest and values. Once a clinician has decided upon the form of psychotherapy they wish to pursue, they will require a foundational course inclusive of training and supervision to ensure they are practicing with adequate skill. Upcoming chapters will review the training (Chap. 18) and supervision (Chap. 19) components at length. To help readers understand differing types of psychotherapy, a brief overview will now focus on the history of psychotherapy, how modern psychotherapy approaches were construed, and the types of evidenced-based psychotherapies available to explore and learn in more depth.

2 A Brief History of Psychotherapy

Before psychotherapy treatment was developed, mental illness was believed to be caused by evil spirits of dark magic by many cultures, societies, and religious groups throughout the world (Short, 2020). When the distinction was made which described sufferers of mental illness as "brothers ensnared in a treatable malady" (Short 2020), the distinction, although it helped, did not explain unintentional behaviour that sometimes occurs outside of conscious control in mentally healthy individuals (Short, 2020). To some, this new distinction of malady helped to identify the difference, but for others, it was still seen as intertwined with religious practices (Marks, 2017). The first to explore the connection between mental health and medicine were philosophers in Ancient Greece. Paracelsus (1493–1541) believed an emotional disconnect between a person and their world was the most common cause of poor mental wellness. Franz Anton Mesmer (1734–1815), who was an Austrian physician, treated patients using hypnosis and for this, was recognized as a founder of psychotherapy. Mesmer played an important role in understanding the effects of suggestion on the imagination and was a pivotal figure in the history of psychosomatic illness and psychotherapy (Lanska, 2007). Philippe Pinel (1745–1826) also disagreed with mainstream thinking, which blamed supernatural causes for mental health disorders, and is credited with seeking humane treatments for those living with mental illness and also for founding the field of psychiatry (Riese, 1951).

In the nineteenth century, Walter Cooper Dendy (1794–1871) studied dreams and introduced the term psycho-therapeia which came from the Greek words psyche, meaning "breath, spirit, soul and therapeia meaning healing and medical treatment" (Dendy, 1853). It was later when Josef Breuer (1842–1925) developed a talking cure for nervous disorders in collaboration with Sigmund Freud (1856–1939) that modern psychotherapy is cited as being truly born (Monroy, 2022). Studies on Hysteria (Freud & Breuer, 1895) are credited with formally founding psychoanalysis, the first type of psychotherapy ever developed. Sigmond Freud, along with his apprentices Carl Jung, Alfred Adler, Otto Rank, and Melanie Klein, are noted for developing the second type of psychotherapy which contributed to the development of psychodynamic psychotherapy (Taylor & Taylor, 2009). Karen Horney (1885–1952) was a neo-Freudian psychologist who identified three specific neurotic trends rooted in how an individual interacts with and perceives other people and is established as the first great psychoanalytic feminist (Paris, 1996). In the 1950s, Carl Rogers (1902–1987) continued the work of Freud's successors and created the approach known as person-centred therapy (Casemore & Tudway, 2012). Then, in the 1960s, Aaron T. Beck (1921–2021) expanded psychotherapy and developed cognitive therapy, now known as cognitive behavioural therapy (CBT) which is one of the most studied psychotherapies in the world. CBT has led to many other forms of modern therapies (Cavanna et al., 2023) which will be further discussed.

The historical context of psychotherapy is important to understand to appreciate the foundation and evolution of psychotherapy as well as the necessity for future advancement. It should be noted that there are many great contributions to the history of psychotherapy and for the brevity of this chapter only certain ones have been discussed. The reader is encouraged to educate themselves on multiple forms of psychotherapy and the contributions made by many. The upcoming section of this chapter will describe some of the types of psychotherapies that currently exist by separating them into two categories; structured psychotherapies and unstructured psychotherapies while using an adapted version of the Y model (Fig. 16.2) to help clarify these branches. These categories are not exhaustive or necessarily based on gold standard evidence, but rather were created to clarify the understanding of the types of therapies that currently exist to provide simplicity to the reader in their theoretical foundations. These categories are not meant to imply that a structured psychotherapy cannot be implemented in an unstructured way, or vice versa, nor that these therapy types cannot be combined. It is simply to provide a lens for the reader, who may be a novice in implementing psychotherapy, to aid in their understanding.

3 Structured and Unstructured Psychotherapies

Structured psychotherapy is an intervention that is systematic, short-term, and evidence-based (School Mental Health Ontario, 2023). The systematic approach used in structured psychotherapy often has protocol-based interventions, an approach where the majority of the treatment includes an outline that can be followed but can still be collaborative with the client. Although it is standard to follow a type of protocol with structured psychotherapy, the skilled clinician is often able to veer from or change the order of the protocol, depending on the needs of the client. Many modern psychotherapies utilized today would fall under this structured psychotherapy category and may include cognitive behavioral therapy (CBT), dialectical behavioural therapy (DBT), eye movement desensitization and reprocessing (EMDR) therapy, and compassion-focused therapy (CFT) (School Mental Health Ontario, 2023).

Unstructured psychotherapy, for the purpose of this chapter, may include approaches that are noted to be less collaborative (in that the client may not be aware of the steps the therapist is taking in the advancement of the therapeutic intervention), they may have few if any systematic steps, and may have underpinnings that are heavily based in theory rather than outline or protocol (Hong et al., 2021). Unstructured psychotherapy may be viewed as exploratory, often using free association methods whereby the clinician helps the client identify spontaneous, sometimes unconnected, conscious or unconscious themes in order to identify content that arises in the client's mind (Mueller, & Segal 2015). Psychotherapies that fall under this category might include: psychoanalysis, psychodynamic therapy, internal family systems, polyvagal-informed therapy, acceptance and commitment therapy, brainspotting therapy, and compassion-focused therapy (Mueller & Segal 2015). You will notice that compassion-focused therapy has been included in both structured and unstructured types of psychotherapy as it was born out of both forms and can naturally follow either a structured or unstructured approach (Hong et al., 2021).

Figure 16.2 demonstrates an adapted Y model distinguishing structured psychotherapies from unstructured psychotherapies to be more inclusive of newer and evolved forms of psychotherapy outside of CBT and psychodynamic alone as in the original Y model. Once a clinician is skilled in many different forms of psychotherapy, some may integrate multiple forms from either side of the Y model together in their practice. There are differing opinions regarding combining types of psychotherapy in one's practice, depending on the theoretical school of thought and/or a therapist's fidelity to a particular model.

To provide a brief overview, we have included in this chapter an overview of the following psychotherapies: cognitive behavioural therapy (CBT), dialectical behavioural therapy (DBT), eye movement desensitization and reprocessing (EMDR) therapy, compassion-focused therapy (CFT), internal family systems, polyvagal-informed therapy, acceptance and commitment therapy (ACT), cognitive processing therapy (CPT), psychoanalysis, psychodynamic, and brainspotting therapy (Fenn & Byrne 2013), but we recognize that this is not an exhaustive list.

4 Structured Psychotherapy Approaches

Cognitive behavioural therapy (CBT) uses goal setting to support clients in identifying and changing unhealthy thoughts and behaviours by considering the relationship between thoughts, emotions, and behaviours (Beck, 2011, 1964). This structured method can be utilised to treat various mental health concerns (Fenn & Byrne, 2013) and has been studied at length to validate its use across presentations (David et al., 2018). Treatment is tailored to fit the client's unique needs and goals (Roles, 2023). It works by targeting symptoms directly, reducing stress, and developing new thinking patterns and positive behavioural responses (Orvati Aziz et al., 2020). Practicing these goal-oriented skills is encouraged during sessions as well as for homework (Roles, 2023). CBT supports individuals in developing more adaptive cognitions and behaviours (Fenn & Byrne, 2013) through guided discovery and open collaboration (Beck, 2011).

Dialectical behavioural therapy (DBT) is a cognitive behavioural treatment that helps individuals build skills specific to emotional regulation, distress tolerance, mindfulness, and interpersonal effectiveness (Linehan, 2015). Originally developed as a treatment for clients with borderline personality disorder, it has since been studied and found to be successful with a variety of other psychiatric disorders such as PTSD, eating disorders, and depression (Granato et al., 2021). It is a structured therapy (Roles, 2023) that utilises strategies from behavioural therapy, dialectical philosophy, and mindfulness practices (Groves et al., 2012) to support clients in emotional and behavioural regulation (Roles, 2023). Behavioural analysis therapists can identify prominent interpersonal and environmental factors (Groves et al., 2012) that influence problematic behaviour as well as the functional consequences of the behaviour and build interventions to address these behaviours (Feigenbaum, 2007).

Eye movement desensitization and reprocessing (EMDR) is a therapy that examines eye movement and left–right stimulation to treat psychological concerns (Shapiro, 2018). This treatment can alleviate stress surrounding traumatic events, desensitization of triggering stimuli and development of desired behaviours (Shapiro, 2018). During sessions, clients briefly access traumatic memories with the support and guidance of a therapist (Roles, 2023). EMDR may be a suitable option for individuals who struggle to verbalize traumatic experiences.

5 Unstructured Psychotherapy Approaches

Psychoanalysis and psychodynamic therapy assist individuals in self-discovery by identifying the aspects of themselves they have yet to realise (Orvati Aziz et al., 2020). The primary assumption of psychoanalysis is the belief that all people possess unconscious thoughts, feelings, memories, and desires that are all in dynamic relation to one another (Gabbard, 2004). It considers the influence of the past on an individual's current behaviours allowing clients to explore unresolved emotions that continue to manifest in their daily life (Roles, 2023). Psychodynamic therapy focuses more on problem-solving and outcomes, on how previous life events are impacting current situations, and has a goal of alleviating current life problems (Gabbard, 2004). The treatment is considered to be beneficial as it supports lasting and sustainable results beyond symptom relief (Orvati Aziz et al., 2020).

Internal family systems (IFS) are based on psychoanalysis and seek to identify various "parts" that make up the Self. These subpersonalities interact internally with one another similar to that of individual people (Roles, 2023). Subpersonalities can often take on painful emotions like anger or shame becoming a part of the individual's sense of self. Through IFS clients explore and identify patterns and systems they have established to cope and survive in certain life experiences (Schwartz & Sweezy, 2019). By identifying and naming these parts, the client is better able to understand the role of each part and how they influence the overall system or self. The underlying belief of the theory is that clients have the innate ability to heal themselves and the therapist's role is to lead the discovery in order to achieve balance and harmony (Schwartz & Sweezy, 2019).

Polyvagal-informed therapy explores the neurophysiological responses to stressors (Porges, 2017). Through psychoeducation, the therapist leads the client in self-discovery exercises related to their neuroception followed by learning co-regulation techniques. Stephen Porges (2017) proposes that by learning to recognize signals and exercising the parasympathetic nervous system we can better live a safe and connected life (Porges, 2017).

Acceptance and commitment therapy (ACT) is an approach that combines radical acceptance of lived experiences and perceived emotions and seeks action and commitment to let go of control and take tangible steps towards positive change (Lee et al., 2021). This approach allows individuals to confront struggles, identify needs and improve behaviours (Roles, 2023).

Cognitive processing therapy (CPT) treats trauma by allowing clients to investigate their negative thoughts in order to make necessary changes (Resick et al., 2017). Thoughts and beliefs stemming from trauma are identified to allow rewriting of recurring narratives that are not aligned with the clients' goals (Resick et al., 2017).

Brainspotting focuses on managing psychological traumas and their associated symptoms (Masson et al., 2014). Using parts of psychodynamic therapies such as free association, brainspotting allows the client to reach the unconscious part of the mind (Grand, 2013). Brainspotting uses eye positioning that supports the psychological assimilation processes of traumatic memories and attunement with the clinician (Grand, 2013). Practitioners lead the individual towards an emotional or somatic activation that is associated with the concern allowing the individual to focus their attention on their inner experience in a safe environment (Masson et al., 2014). Somatic awareness, mindfulness, and the guided attunement and support of a therapist to process and release stored trauma are also utilized in this approach (Roles, 2023). Brainspotting can also be used alongside other brain-body-based treatments such as bilateral sound to achieve successful outcomes for clients (Grand, 2013).

Compassion-focused therapy (CFT) goes beyond empathy and accesses compassion with the intention to ease suffering to assess the origins behind an individual's symptoms and difficulties (Gilbert, 2009). This is done by encouraging and aiding clients in becoming more compassionate towards others and themselves (Roles, 2023). Individuals often develop safety strategies as a defence mechanism for situations they have endured and this can result in relating to the self in a critical way. Incorporating mindfulness, role play, chair work, visualization, and meditation, CFT supports individuals to recognize these critical approaches and work towards developing more compassionate experiences within the self (Gilbert 2009). Sessions explore self-talk, the origins of particular thoughts and tones, and in developing more compassionate internalized thoughts (Roles, 2023). CFT may also be integrated into more structured psychotherapy approaches to align with the identified needs of the client.

6 Learning Activity

Consider the following to help you reflect on your current level of competency (knowledge, skill, judgement), then create a learning plan to include further learning that will help you to build your capacity for delivering safe and ethical psychotherapy interventions.

1. In your own practice, why is it important to know and understand the history of psychotherapy?
2. How do you plan to ensure your practice is evidence-based?
3. What factors would impact your decision on the type of therapeutic approach you would choose for a given client?

4. How would a psychotherapist ensure adequate care when utilizing multiple approaches with a client?
5. How would a therapist ensure adequate care utilizing a single modality approach with a client?

7 Summary

- The variety of psychotherapies that exist far surpasses what we have reviewed in this chapter.
- This brief overview was created to give nurses an understanding of how far the practice of psychotherapy has come in a very short period of time, as well as to provide an overview of the vast interventions of psychotherapy that exist which can be utilized while conducting assessments, planning treatment, and providing interventions.
- The potential for ongoing learning as a nurse psychotherapist is endless.
- The future of psychotherapy will bring further advancements to the practice and better treatment interventions for clients.

References

Beck, J. (1964). *Cognitive Therapy: Basics and Beyond*. Guildford Press.

Beck, J. (2011). *Cognitive Behavior Therapy: Basics and Beyond* (2nd ed.). Guildford Press.

Binder, J. L., & Betan, E. J. (2013). *Core competencies in brief dynamic psychotherapy: Becoming a highly effective and competent brief dynamic psychotherapist*. Routledge.

Casemore, R., & Tudway, J. (2012). *Person-centred therapy and CBT: Siblings not rivals*. Sage.

Cavanna, A. E., Purpura, G., Riva, A., Nacinovich, R., & Seri, S. (2023). The Western origins of Mindfulness therapy in ancient Rome. *Neurological Sciences*, 1–9.

David, D., Cristea, I., & Hofmann, S. G. (2018). Why cognitive behavioral therapy Is the current gold standard of psychotherapy. *Frontiers in psychiatry, 9*, 4.

Dendy, W. C. (1853). *Psychē; A discourse on the birth and pilgrimage of thought*. Longman, Brown, Green, and Longmans.

Feigenbaum, J. (2007). Dialectical behaviour therapy: An increasing evidence base. *Journal of Mental Health, 16*(1), 51-68.

Fenn, K., & Byrne, M. (2013). The key principles of cognitive behavioural therapy. *InnovAiT, 6*(9), 579-585.

Freud, S. & Beurer (1895) Studies on Hysteria.

Gabbard, G. (2004). *Long-Term Psychodynamic Psychotherapy: A Basic Text*. American Psychiatric Publishing.

Gilbert, P. (2009). Introducing compassion-focused therapy. *Advances in Psychiatric Treatment, 15*(3), 199-208.

Goldberg, D. & Plakun, E. (2013). Teaching Psychodynamic Psychotherapy with the Y Model. Psychodynamic Psychiatry, *31*(1), 111-125.

Granato, H. F., Sewart, A. R., Vinograd, M., & McFarr, L. (2021). Dialectical behavior therapy. In A. Wenzel (Ed.), *Handbook of cognitive behavioral therapy: Overview and approaches.*, Vol. 1. (pp. 539–565). American Psychological Association. https://doi.org/10.1037/0000218-018

Grand, D. (2013). *Brainspotting: The revolutionary new therapy for rapid and effective change.* Sounds True Inc.

Groves, S., Backer, H. S., van den Bosch, W., & Miller, A. (2012). Dialectical behaviour therapy with adolescents. *Child and adolescent mental health, 17*(2), 65-75.

Harris, B. A., & Panozzo, G. (2019). Therapeutic alliance, relationship building, and communication strategies-for the schizophrenia population: An integrative review. *Archives of Psychiatric Nursing, 33*(1), 104-111.

Hartley, S., Raphael, J., Lovell, K., & Berry, K. (2020). Effective nurse–patient relationships in mental health care:A systematic review of interventions to improve the therapeutic alliance. *International Journal of Nursing Studies, 102*, 103490.

Hilsenroth, M. J., Cromer, T. D., & Ackerman, S. J. (2012). How to make practical use of therapeutic alliance research in your clinical work. In R. A. Levy, J. S. Ablon, & H. Kachele (Eds.). *Psychodynamic psychotherapy research: Evidence-based practice and practice-based evidence* (pp. 361–380).

Hong, C. T., Tan, S., & Huang, T. W. (2021). Psychotherapy for the treatment of anxiety and depression in patients with Parkinson disease: A meta-analysis of randomized controlled trials. *Journal of the American Medical Directors Association, 22*(11), 2289-2295.

Lambert, M. J., Bergin, A. E., & Garfield, S. L. (1994). The effectiveness of psychotherapy. *Encyclopedia of psychotherapy, 1*, 709-714.

Lanska, D. J., & Lanska, J. T. (2007). Franz Anton Mesmer and the rise and fall of animal magnetism: Dramatic cures, controversy, and ultimately a triumph for the scientific method. In *Brain, mind and medicine: Essays in eighteenth-century neuroscience* (pp. 301–320). Springer US.

Lee, E. B., Pierce, B. G., Twohig, M. P., & Levin, M. E. (2021). Acceptance and commitment therapy. In A. Wenzel (Ed.), *Handbook of cognitive behavioral therapy: Overview and approaches*, Vol. 1. (pp. 567–594). American Psychological Association. https://doi.org/10.1037/0000218-019

Linehan, M. (2015). *DBT Skills Training Manual.* (2nd Ed.). Guilford Press.

Marks, S. (2017). Psychotherapy in historical perspective. *History of the Human Sciences, 30*(2), 3-16.

Masson, J., Bernoussi, A., & Moukouta, C. S. (2017). Brainspotting therapy: About a Bataclan victim. *Global* Mueller, A. E., & Segal, D. L. (2014). Structured versus semistructured versus unstructured interviews. In R. Cautin & S. Lilienfeld (Eds.), *Encyclopedia of clinical psychology* (pp. 2732- 2738). Wiley-Blackwell

Monroy, E. O. (2022). Josef Breuer (1842–1925). *Journal of Neurology, 269*(12), 6688-6689.

Mueller, A., & Segal, D.L. (2015). *Structured versus Semistructured versus Unstructured Interviews.*

Okamoto, A., Dattilio, F. M., Dobson, K. S., & Kazantzis, N. (2019). The therapeutic relationship in cognitive–behavioral therapy: Essential features and common challenges. *Practice Innovations, 4*(2), 112.

Orvati Aziz, M., Mehrinejad, S. A., Hashemian, K., & Paivastegar, M. (2020). Integrative therapy (short-term psychodynamic psychotherapy & cognitive-behavioral therapy) and cognitive-behavioral therapy in the treatment of generalized anxiety disorder: A randomized controlled trial. *Complementary Therapies in Clinical Practice, 39*(Complete). https://doi.org/10.1016/j.ctcp.2020.101122

Paris, B. (1996). *Karen Horney: A Psychoanalyst's Search for Self-Understanding.* Yale University Press.

Porges, S. (2017). *The pocket guide to the polyvagal theory: The transformative power of feeling safe.* W. W. Norton & Company.

Psychotherapy and Counselling Federation of Australia. (2020, December 7). *Psychotherapy Training Standards.* https://www.pacfa.org.au/common/Uploaded%20files/Psychotherapy-Training-Standards-2020.pdf

Resick, P. Monsoon, C., & Chard, K. (2017). *Cognitive processing therapy for PTSD: A comprehensive manual.* Gillford Press.

Riese, W. (1951). Philippe Pinel (1745–1826): His views on human nature and disease. His medical thought. *The Journal of Nervous and Mental Disease, 114*(1), 313–323.

Roles, S. (2023). *Approaches to Therapy*. Psychotherapy. https://rolespsychotherapy.com/psychotherapy-services/

School Mental Health Ontario (2023, March 30). *Structured psychotherapy - school mental health ontario*. School mental health professionals. Author. https://smho-smso.ca/smh-professionals/structured-psychotherapy/

Schwartz, R. C., & Sweezy, M. (2019). *Internal Family Systems Therapy*. Guilford Publications.

Shapiro, F. (2018). *Eye Movement Desensitization and Reprocessing (EMDR) Therapy*. (3rd ed.). Guilford Press.

Short, D. (2020). *Beyond the margin and into positive depth psychology*. The Milton H. Erickson Institute of Phoenix. https://iamdrshort.com/New_Papers/Beyond%20the%20Margin%20and%20Into%20Positive%20Depth%20Psychology.pdf

Taylor, E., & Taylor, E. (2009). The Freudians. In E. Taylor (Ed.). *The Mystery of Personality: A History of Psychodynamic Theories* (pp. 75-100). Springer.

Chapter 17
Nursing Competencies: Evaluation and Outcome Measures in Psychotherapy

Sophia Woloschuk Gassanova and Kaitlin Marriner Brulotte

Abstract Establishment of clear outcome measures, along with timely evaluation of interventions, is critical to understanding what works for the client. This chapter will discuss the therapeutic alliance and its influence on the success of therapy, provide an overview of outcome measurement and change indicators, present strategies for analysis, and discuss effective data collection methods. Measurement tools available to evaluate the strength of the therapeutic alliance and the efficacy of common psychotherapeutic treatment modalities will be explored. Key principles and challenges of evaluating psychotherapy will be described, along with recommendations for nurse psychotherapists to evaluate the care they provide. Lastly, the importance of culture-specific evaluation measures will be discussed, followed by the reinforcement of key concepts via a case example.

Keywords Evaluating psychotherapy · Structured evaluation · Outcome evaluation · Progress monitoring

Learning objectives

After completing this chapter, the learner will:

1. Identify how the therapeutic alliance influences client progress throughout the duration of therapy.
2. Understand the rationale for, and components of, progress monitoring and routine outcome monitoring in psychotherapeutic treatment.
3. Recognize the cultural impact on the therapeutic alliance and outcome measurement methodology in psychotherapy.

S. Woloschuk Gassanova (✉)
Toronto, ON, USA
e-mail: sophia.woloschuk@gmail.com

K. M. Brulotte
Chelsea, QC, Canada
e-mail: kmbrulotte@gmail.com

S. Roles and K. Kalia (eds.), *The Nurses' Guide to Psychotherapy*,
https://doi.org/10.1007/978-981-97-4738-2_17

4. Identify strategies to address negative client feedback and the potential for ruptures in the therapeutic alliance.

1 Introduction

The establishment of clear progress and outcome monitoring methods and timely evaluations of the psychotherapeutic process are critical to the client's success. This chapter will discuss the evaluation of the therapeutic alliance, routine monitoring of client progress and outcomes, and the benefit that ongoing evaluation has on professional development and clinical excellence. Several assessment methods and reflective questions to support clinicians with ongoing evaluation methodologies will be introduced.

2 Therapeutic Alliance

The development of a strong therapeutic alliance (TA) between the nurse psychotherapist and client is central to the success of psychotherapy. TA measures the mutual engagement of the psychotherapist and client within the work of therapy, and it constitutes an important part of achieving success in treatment, regardless of which particular treatment modality is chosen (Stubbe 2018). Bordin's working alliance model consists of three main components: mutual agreement on therapy goals, collaboration on the decided tasks of therapy, and development of the bond between client and psychotherapist (Bordin 1979). Similar to Peplau's work as described in Chap. 3, Bordin's ideology highlighted the collaborative rapport between client and psychotherapist to be essential to the development of a strong TA, with common goals aimed at reduction in client suffering and self-destructive behavior (Ardito and Rabellino 2011). An optimal TA is achieved when the client and psychotherapist share beliefs about the goals of treatment and are aligned on what therapeutic methods are deemed relevant to achieve those goals (Ardito and Rabellino 2011). The client's trust in the psychotherapist's intentions and ability helps to enable the client to accept, follow, and believe in the treatment approach (Ardito and Rabellino 2011).

The main components of a strong TA include trust, collaboration, empathy, and positive regard (Ardito and Rabellino 2011). Feelings of trust promote client comfort, encouraging them to share and reflect upon their inner experiences without judgment, so they can collaboratively establish treatment goals and strategies for addressing presenting issues. Applying empathy enables the psychotherapist to look at the client's situation from their perspective, while positive regard maintains the psychotherapist's accepting, non-judgmental attitude regardless of what information the client shares. A strong TA is positively associated with better treatment outcomes in various types of psychotherapy and is one of the strongest predictors of treatment success (Barbisan et al. 2022). Feeling supported and understood is an essential element for clients to actively engage in the therapeutic process, share sensitive issues, and work towards establishing positive habits in their lives.

2.1 Strength-Based Communication

Traditionally, the focus of psychotherapy was to address client problems or weaknesses rather than aiming to capitalize on and develop strengths. Strength-based communication is foundational to the modern TA, involving the identification of, and building upon client strengths. The aim is for clients to leverage various strengths (communication, coping, lived experiences, etc.) to develop therapy goals, while the psychotherapist creates and maintains an encouraging and positive atmosphere, conducive to sustainable personal growth (Conoley and Scheel 2018). Effective strengths-based communication involves supporting the client in establishing self-directed goals that are within their control to positively impact their current situation. The client's negative emotions are acknowledged and given their own space and time, but the overall goal is to focus on the positive aspects of the lived experience (Conoley and Scheel 2018).

2.2 Strengthening Collaboration

Therapy goals are developed with consideration of the client's strengths and articulated concerns and preferences. Clients are active, autonomous participants in the therapeutic process. Research suggests that it is crucial for psychotherapists to keep patients involved throughout the therapy process by soliciting their ongoing input into treatment plans and goals as well as providing patients with systematic feedback (Tryon et al. 2018). Any assigned homework and skills development align with the client goals and interests, to ensure an increased likelihood of follow-through and active participation in sessions. The nurse psychotherapist remains flexible and strives to continuously adapt and re-evaluate the treatment approach to serve the client's needs.

2.3 Orienting Clients to the Information-Gathering Process

Orienting clients to the information-gathering process is a primary step in the establishment of the therapeutic relationship, which helps clients understand why the psychotherapist is interested in capturing progress-and outcome-related data. When commencing the TA, the nurse psychotherapist should explain how the information the client shares throughout therapy is collected and utilized, and why it supports the development of their treatment plan (College of Nurses of Ontario 2022). The psychotherapist's role is to ensure the client's understanding of which assessment tools will be utilized, and how results will inform outcome monitoring and next steps. The client is encouraged to express any questions or concerns they have about the information-gathering process, while the nurse psychotherapist remains receptive to feedback, addressing any fears or misconceptions that might arise. Client familiarity with the principles of privacy and confidentiality, as they apply to the therapeutic relationship and data-gathering strategies, ensure their understanding of the bounds of professional, ethical, and legal requirements and duty-to-report obligations (Jain and Roberts 2009). Ultimately, the client must understand that the value of the feedback they give their psychotherapist will positively influence their experience and outcomes.

2.4 Addressing Expectations of Therapy

At the commencement of therapy, the nurse psychotherapist must discuss and clarify the client's expectations of therapy to promote effective collaboration of goal setting through gathering information about the client's presenting concerns, context, and goals. During the initial session, the psychotherapist should try to promote positive client expectations towards treatment and the outcomes (Constantino 2012). The nurse psychotherapist should clarify their role by explaining what techniques, methods, and approaches clients can anticipate during sessions to help manage expectations. Collaboratively, the psychotherapist and client work to establish realistic goals, considering the therapeutic context, and expected timeframe. Routine progress towards identified goals and outcome monitoring will help both parties to ensure they are progressing on an effective track or determining if they need to redirect efforts.

2.5 Evaluation of Client Progress and the Benefits of Therapy

This section will explore some common patterns that can emerge throughout the course of therapy. In an ideal situation, the client would be making progress and actively working towards their goals; however, this is not always the case.

2.6 Deterioration or No Improvement

A timely and effective response from the nurse psychotherapist is crucial to ensuring the client's well-being, safety, and correction of the course of therapy. Psychotherapist strategies for addressing client deterioration or a therapeutic rupture include:

1. **Assessment and Evaluation** In order to effectively assess deterioration and potential crisis, the psychotherapist should stay focused on the present moment and what is relevant to the client's current situation, asking questions that are short and straightforward, all the while demonstrating empathy and reflective communication (Leiper and Kent 2001). The psychotherapist should discuss recent stressors, triggers, life events, or any changes to the client's circumstances which may require revisiting the client's diagnosis or case formulation and reassessing whether presenting issues have evolved since therapy commencement (Leiper and Kent 2001). In addition, analyzing client's outcome patterns can be helpful. The nurse psychotherapist might question; if the client is attending appointments, if they are completing homework assignments, if there are indications of progress towards the goal, or if the goal needs to be reestablished.
2. **Client safety and crisis intervention** If the client is at immediate risk of harm to self or others, safety is a priority. Appropriate actions by a psychotherapist would include contacting emergency services or involving other support systems as appropriate. In collaboration with the client, the development of a crisis plan that outlines steps to take in the event of a crisis will ensure that there is an effective plan in place, and that the client and psychotherapist have a mutual agreement as to how they will deal with a crisis situation (Ruchlewska et al. 2016). This plan should include coping strategies, emergency contacts, and available resources. The nurse psychotherapist should consider increasing the frequency of sessions or check-ins for closer monitoring of the client's condition.
3. **Non-judgment** Nurse psychotherapists should be initiating a non-judgmental and open conversation with the client about observed deterioration and express concern and readiness to support them at this challenging time.
4. **Continued collaboration** In collaboration with the client, the nurse psychotherapist will continuously be reassessing and modifying the current treatment plan to better suit the client's needs and this may involve changing approaches, go-to techniques, or frequency of sessions.
5. **Supervision** The nurse psychotherapist should engage in peer consultation or clinical supervision when necessary. If deterioration is beyond the scope of the psychotherapist's expertise, referrals to other mental health professionals specializing in the client's specific needs should be orchestrated. The nurse psychotherapist should also debrief and self-reflect to minimize counter-transference (Borders 2014).
6. **Focus on strengths** The nurse psychotherapist should incorporate positive reframing, strength-focused discussions, positive affirmations (as appropriate), psychotherapist feedback, and validation to enable activation of client strengths.
7. **Documentation** For accountability and continuity of care, keep up-to-date documentation of the client's clinical assessment, interventions, and any changes made to the treatment plan and evaluation (College of Nurses of Ontario 2008).

2.7 *Improvement*

In order to understand what may have contributed to positive change, the psychotherapist must first recognize the changes in the client's presentation and identify this to the client. Meaningful client improvements include positive changes to social, occupational, and individual functioning (Miller et al. 2020). Some improvements are noted by the psychotherapist, whereas many are self-identified by the client throughout the course of ongoing evaluation. Noticed change by the psychotherapist should lead to open conversation about changes the client has noticed about themselves, along with any reflections they would like to share. The nurse psychotherapist can then share their own observations and insights to help the client solidify and maintain positive changes.

3 Revisiting Goals and Outcomes: What is the Meaning of Progress?

When discussing outcomes with the client, it is important for psychotherapists to facilitate an understanding of the relationship between established therapy goals and monitoring outcomes. Progress can be noted in various ways, including those reported by the client, and those recognized by the psychotherapist. Established goals act as a roadmap toward a common destination that the psychotherapist and client are working towards. If the client reports feelings of dissatisfaction, it is important to return to the established goals to ensure the intentions and actions are aligned with the desired outcomes.

3.1 *Transition from Therapy*

Open discussions regarding the transition out of therapy should be embedded into therapeutic planning from the beginning of the counseling relationship. Clients may feel apprehensive and experience feelings of hesitance, discomfort, or resistance when facing changes to the therapeutic process and relationship; be it with a new psychotherapist, expected or unexpected changes to treatment goals and approaches, or an unplanned leave from therapy (Schlesinger 2013). Possible reasoning behind the client's apprehension to change might include fear of the unknown, worry about losing shown progress, resistance to change, an increase in vulnerability, or reliving previous negative transition experiences (Schlesinger 2013).

3.2 Building on Progress for the Future

As therapy comes to an end, or transitions into a less frequent format, it is important for the psychotherapist to make sure that the client experiences a sense of completeness and closure as described in Chap. 3 with the termination phase. Ideally, termination of therapy is discussed with the client ahead of time, giving both client and psychotherapist an opportunity to freely discuss their feelings and review the growth that occurred, while also discussing the client's self-care goals post-therapy (Knox et al. 2011; Marx and Gelso 1987; Quintana and Holahan 1992). To help clients continue building progress, psychotherapists should encourage clients to celebrate achievements, reflect on lessons learned, assist with identifying strengths, and setting realistic goals for the future. Emphasizing self-kindness and self-compassion as clients continue their growth journey in the face of life's challenges encourages clients to treat themselves with the same care and understanding as they would offer to a close friend. Providing follow-up resources can support clients to solidify their progress, along with referrals to virtual or in-person support groups as appropriate.

4 Professional Development and Clinical Excellence

4.1 Obtaining Feedback and Evaluating the Nurse Psychotherapist's Performance

Timely evaluation of the nurse psychotherapist's efforts is essential to understanding if they are making a positive difference. Effectiveness itself is not a straightforward concept to measure because of its subjective nature. Simon (2012) suggests that "effective therapists need to be passionately present, responsive, creative and flexible, because these are the qualities required to foster and maintain a therapeutic alliance" (Simon 2012, p. 8). Obtaining feedback from the client on the psychotherapist's performance is important at the session end and at the termination of the TA. Nurse psychotherapists must also self-reflect on the key aspects of their practice to consider if their perspective of their therapeutic approach is similar to what the client experienced.

Being an effective psychotherapist involves possessing a combination of qualities, approaches and skills that contribute to positive therapeutic outcomes and facilitate meaningful change in clients. Each psychotherapist possesses a unique combination of these qualities, however, there are some general principles that are present in all effective psychotherapists. An effective nurse psychotherapist should establish and maintain appropriate professional and ethical boundaries, possess strong communication, assessment, and diagnostic skills, and have a thorough understanding of psychological principles. Psychotherapist effectiveness is arguably measured most reliably by client outcomes, not through supervisor/peer reports since the latter tend to be neither reliable nor valid assessments (Sánchez-Bahíllo et al. 2014). Changes in a client's status do not necessarily mean changes in diagnosis, since patient outcomes are multidimensional and complex with multiple contributing factors (Sánchez-Bahíllo et al. 2014).

The field of psychotherapy is continuously evolving, and as such it is critical for nurse psychotherapists to remain informed about new research and treatment techniques to provide the best care possible. Nurse psychotherapists can also actively reflect on their own biases, reactions, and limitations in order to maintain an adaptable approach with each client. Finally, an effective psychotherapist possesses an improvement-driven mindset with a commitment to continuous growth and ethical practice. Psychotherapists who are focused on improving their practice learn from their mistakes, possess courage, and resolve to enhance their practice even when things are not going well.

4.2 Assessment of Therapeutic Alliance

A strong therapeutic alliance (TA) is central to the successful practice of psychotherapy. Multiple tools can help psychotherapists assess the quality of the TA, including the Working Alliance Inventory (WAI) (Horvath and Symonds 1991); the Penn Helping Alliance Scale (Morgan et al. 1982); and the Agnew Relationship Measure (ARM) (Stiles et al., 2022). WAI is one of the most widely used tools where clients use a Likert scale to rate statements about their perceptions of the TA, with different versions of WAI used for different therapeutic modalities. Other TA assessment tools include the Helping Alliance Questionnaire (HAq-II) (Lubrosky et al. 1996), the Group Questionnaire (GQ) specifically designed for group therapy (Burlingame et al. 2021, 2018) and the Outcome Questionnaire-45 (OQ-45) (Lambert et al. 1996).

In order to conduct a comprehensive evaluation of one's practice and of the TA with clients, it is beneficial for the psychotherapist to make use of self-evaluation tools as part of their regular practice. These tools gather the psychotherapist's perspective and are usually completed after each session. For example, the *Therapy Session Report (TSR)* scale measures various aspects of the interaction such as session content, relationship, participant motivation, and affective responses, and is measured by both the psychotherapist and client (Smith et al. 2003). Initial low TA scores are not necessarily bad news for therapy (Miller et al. 2020). Indeed, it is better to have an initially low TA score that improves over time as opposed to an initially high score that declines. It has been shown that lower initial alliance scores have the potential to lead to better outcomes as compared to instances where alliance is high to begin with but declines as treatment progresses (Miller et al. 2008; Owen et al. 2016).

4.3 Self-Reflection

Self-reflection is one important way a psychotherapist can progress on their professional growth journeys. Self-reflection allows psychotherapists to take a critical look at the effectiveness of their therapeutic skills, interventions, and techniques, leading to the gradual refinement of skills over time. Furthermore, regular self-reflection encourages psychotherapists to develop their decision-making and clinical judgment abilities, opening their eyes to different perspectives. For one to engage effectively in self-reflection, one must accept their emotions rather than aiming to suppress them (Greenberg 2007; Vyskocilova and Prasko 2013). Identifying and reflecting on personal biases helps nurse psychotherapists recognize and actively manage factors that could otherwise lead to the erosion of the TA. Self-reflection helps build self-awareness, which is crucial for nurse psychotherapists in gaining insights into and managing their own emotions during therapy. Self-reflection helps to prevent nurse psychotherapist burnout, contributes to ethically safe practice, promotes continuous learning, and strengthens the TA. Engagement in regular self-reflection has the potential to improve the psychotherapist's capacity to identify their own distress which decreases the negative influence on their client's well-being (Vasquez 1992; Vyskocilova and Prasko 2013). The novice psychotherapist may benefit from self-reflection techniques including reflective journaling, completion of psychotherapist-centered self-assessment questionnaires, video and audio recording of sessions, and participation in clinical supervision. The Taxonomy of Deliberate Practice Activities in Psychotherapy (Chow and Miller 2015) is useful for structured self-reflection, and is available in several versions, including one for clinical supervisors, making it suitable for novice psychotherapists. Additional strategies for self-reflection include writing down aspects of client interactions that were challenging, potential difficulties with showing empathy, and adhering to an earlier-agreed therapy session plan.

4.4 Addressing Negative Feedback

In some instances, feedback gathered during the evaluation will highlight some negative client experiences which can lead to rupture in TA if left unaddressed. Prompt negotiation of alliance rupture is crucial to therapeutic change (Safran et al. 2002; Hill and Knox 2009). It is critical for any potential alliance rupture to be promptly addressed, instead of disregarding the issue and hoping it will go away. Receiving negative feedback can be challenging but self-reflection can be instrumental in enabling the psychotherapist in recognizing the role they play in the client's negative experience. Overall, the use of confrontational language, making assumptions about clients' perceptions, and being rigid in one's approach, can all contribute to negative feedback. Receiving negative feedback may be challenging due to multiple factors, including the client's hesitation to provide feedback, the therapist's covert reactions, and considerable efforts associated with learning from the feedback received as the mere act of receiving feedback does not mean the psychotherapist will learn from it (Brattland et al. 2018a, 2008b). Upon receiving negative feedback, the psychotherapist should actively listen, ask for clarification as appropriate, and take care to manage their own emotional response to avoid coming across as dismissive or defensive. In case of a misunderstanding, the psychotherapist should explain their intentions, discuss solutions, and express their commitment to improvement, scheduling a follow-up with the client as appropriate. It may be beneficial to seek supervision or peer consultation in cases where feedback brings up complex issues for the psychotherapist.

For the novice psychotherapist, or the psychotherapist learning a new form of psychotherapy, obtaining structured and systematic feedback on their performance from peers and supervisors increases their awareness of their areas of strength and what might need improvement. Supervisors can act as both professional role models and mentors, offering support and guidance, providing constructive feedback, assisting with the navigation of complex clinical situations, presenting opportunities to explore ethical dilemmas, and overall monitoring of the supervisee's performance (Barnett and Molzon 2014). The supervisory relationship can be a source of emotional support, helping novice psychotherapists to work through emotionally challenging situations and acting as a sounding board to process thoughts and feelings that arise. Reflective practice is used in clinical supervision, with supervisees being encouraged to reflect on their performance to gain insights into their impact on client dynamics and potential biases that might impede quality care (Todd and Freshwater 1999). Receiving feedback is a skill best obtained when practiced repeatedly. See Chap. 19 for more information on clinical consultation and supervision.

4.5 Outcome Measurement in Psychotherapy

Evaluative data may be collected for research, knowledge, and therapeutic reasons. Collecting data to build upon knowledge is used to motivate individual practitioners and the profession to adapt to new knowledge, while gathering data for therapeutic reasons serves to better understand the client's desires and needs. Outcome measurement (OM) entails evaluating the client's outcomes and changes that took place between the beginning and the end of a process, in this case, between the start and end of a client's psychotherapy sessions (Evans and Carlyle 2021). Different audiences may have varied OM needs, thus having a clear understanding of what outcome is significant to the client, to the psychotherapist, or to the external audience is important (Evans and Carlyle 2021). Understanding which portion of therapy has worked towards what outcome(s) enhances the psychotherapist's ability to effectively guide the client towards more positive outcomes. This critical piece of evidence-based practice promotes informed decision-making while continuing to adapt to and refine psychotherapy directions based on the client's progress. Areas of outcome measurement for monitoring might include the therapist-client relationship, client motivation, social supports, and untoward life events (Lambert and Lo Coco 2013; Lambert et al. 2004).

Psychotherapists must first consider the specific outcomes they wish to measure, while considering the client's established goals, cultural context, and individual preferences. It is important for psychotherapists to select appropriate data collection methods in alignment with client needs, therapeutic goals, and within the specific context of the psychotherapy session; one must also keep in mind the limitation of using self-reports as evidence (Polkinghorne 2005). Data can be collected pre-treatment, during treatment and post-treatment using standardized methods and instruments including those to monitor progress and those to monitor outcomes. Monitoring progress involves the use of self-report questionnaires, behavioral observations, standardized assessment tools, and clinical rating scales to gather data about changes in specific behaviors, symptoms, or targeted goals over time. To adequately monitor progress and make treatment plan adjustments aligning with client needs, the nurse psychotherapist collects real-time data and responds promptly to unexpected changes or lack of progress (Meier 2014). Monitoring outcomes uses the combination of psychotherapist reflections, client's self-assessment, and standardized clinical measures to evaluate the overall impact of therapy at specific intervals of treatment (Meier 2014; Miller et al. 2020). This assessment is more detailed than tracking specific behaviors and symptoms, and assesses wider changes in the client's quality of life, well-being, and overall functioning. Monitoring outcomes assists with determining whether the therapeutic goals have been met and whether there have been meaningful improvements in the client's life due to psychotherapy.

The use of standardized data collection tools can help to ensure that the collected data is reliable and uniform, so that meaningful interpretation and analysis can occur. Some of the currently used standardized methods of data collection include:

1. **Self-report measures and questionnaires** These are structured sets of questions given to clients to complete before and/or after therapy sessions to gather insights into their subjective experience to help track their progress over time (Brattland et al. 2018a, 2018b). The tools selected will reflect the nature of the client's presenting problems. Some examples of tools are listed in Chaps. 14 and 15.
2. **Observational measures** Psychotherapists can use standardized assessment tools aimed at observing and rating specific interactions or behaviors during therapy sessions.
3. **Diagnostic assessment tools** Standardized criteria are used to assess and diagnose a client's potential mental health conditions. For examples of tools see Chaps. 14 and 15.
4. **Psychometric tests** These are standardized measures that look at specific psychological traits, characteristics, or abilities and include personality inventories, such as the Minnesota Multiphasic Personality Inventory (MMPI) (Butcher 2010), neuropsychological assessments, and intelligence tests, among others. Nurses must always assess their own limitations in competence as it relates to the administration and interpretation of different psychometric assessments.

Reliability refers to the assessment tool's consistent measurement of the outcomes that it is supposed to measure, whereas validity refers to how accurately it measures these outcomes (Evans and Carlyle 2021). Tools with shown validity and reliability can help reduce bias and enhance the quality of data. The availability of validated tools is constantly changing, with multiple digital and hard-copy options available. Psychotherapists can use various sources to find applicable tools, such as online databases, professional organizations, published research, and academic literature. Accessibility and cost of measurement tools are factors that must be considered. For example, some tools may require specific software or licensing fees, whereas others are available online for free. Accessibility of the tool in other languages, availability, and format might also impact which tools a nurse psychotherapist utilizes.

Ethical considerations of client privacy and confidentiality during the feedback-gathering process include obtaining informed consent prior to conducting any evaluation (College of Nurses of Ontario 2022). The nurse psychotherapist should explain the value of including progress and outcome monitoring related to the client's overall outcomes, but also indicate that the client has an option to refuse to incorporate this component into their therapy plan. When introducing measurement tools, nurse psychotherapists should share the rationale for the use of the tool and create an environment conducive to empowering client participation as sharing feedback is instrumental to obtaining quality results. Through modeling, the psychotherapist can subtly encourage sharing by demonstrating an attitude of openness, non-judgement, and willingness to hear both positive and negative feedback. Real-time feedback about the effectiveness of the therapeutic relationship and therapy progress can prevent client deterioration and avoid premature termination of therapy (Schuckard et al. 2017; Miller et al. 2020). Nurse psychotherapists may encounter limited meaningful feedback at first and are encouraged to continue with the process as the client gains trust (Brattland et al. 2018a, 2018b; Miller et al 2020).

4.6 Culture and Outcome Evaluation

Cultural sensitivity involves ongoing commitment from the psychotherapist to respect, learn from, and create a therapeutic environment that honors and values a variety of cultural experiences. When appropriate, the client's cultural background must be considered while evaluating the success of psychotherapy (Tseng 1999). Culturally sensitive evaluation tools help ensure that the assessment process is inclusive and respectful of diverse cultural populations. Characteristics of a culturally sensitive tool include questions that assess cultural identity, language needs, and experiences of discrimination and acculturation, if relevant. Tools that limit assumptions about cultural norms and allow flexible responses that encompass a variety of emotional expressions and cultural considerations are favorable. If the psychotherapist must choose a tool that does not consider culture, they must include this in their interpretation of results. If appropriate, the psychotherapist should consider collaboration with interpreters, or appropriate community members. See Chap. 12 for more on cross-cultural considerations.

5 Case Vignette

Katie, a 32-year-old female, was referred to Melanie (Registered Nurse) by her family doctor after being diagnosed with generalized anxiety disorder (GAD), accompanied by panic attacks and social anxiety. The therapeutic alliance has developed over time, with mutual respect and open communication. Katie demonstrated considerable progress during the first few months of structured CBT, learning to challenge unhelpful thought patterns, addressing social anxiety triggers, and learning relaxation techniques. There was a marked reduction in the frequency and severity of panic attacks, and evaluation questionnaires revealed an overall self-reported improvement. Despite the initial improvement, Katie's progress has plateaued over the past month. She stopped completing her take-home CBT exercises, appears less engaged during sessions, and has been canceling sessions citing scheduling conflicts.

5.1 Case Vignette Reflective Questions

1. What methods might the nurse psychotherapist use to assess the therapeutic alliance (TA)?
2. Which tools can the nurse psychotherapist apply to assess the factors that are potentially contributing to the stalled progression?
3. Which self-reflective exercises could the nurse psychotherapist complete to evaluate their perception of treatment progress and the TA status?
4. What questions can the nurse psychotherapist ask the client to evaluate the status of the TA?
5. How can the nurse psychotherapist address a rupture in the therapeutic alliance?

6 Summary

- This chapter introduced principles of the therapeutic alliance and strategies for evaluating client progress to increase the benefits of therapy across the spectrum of the therapeutic process.
- Effective approaches to routine client progress and outcome monitoring in practice, measurement tool selection strategies, and the principles of standardized data collection were highlighted.

- Continuously evaluating the therapeutic process increases the client's experience of desirable outcomes, develops the nurse psychotherapist's professional and clinical excellence, and collects valuable data contributing to the evolution of the profession in a culturally sensitive and trauma-informed manner.

References

Ardito, R. B., & Rabellino, D. (2011). Therapeutic alliance and outcome of psychotherapy: Historical excursus, measurements, and prospects for Research. *Frontiers in Psychology, 2,* article 270, 1–11. https://doi.org/10.3389/fpsyg.2011.00270.

Barbisan, G. K., de Pieri, L. Z., Gonçalves, L., Rebouças, C. D., & da Rocha, N. S. (2022). Positive association between therapeutic alliance and quality of life in psychodynamic psychotherapy, cognitive behavior therapy, and interpersonal therapy: The patient's perspective. *Frontiers in Psychiatry, 12,* article 613627, 1–9. https://doi.org/10.3389/fpsyt.2021.613627.

Barnett, J. E., & Molzon, C. H. (2014). Clinical supervision of psychotherapy: Essential ethics issues for supervisors and supervisees. *Journal of Clinical Psychology, 70*(11), 1051–1061.

Borders, D. (2014). Best practices in clinical supervision: Another step in delineating effective supervision practice. *American Journal of Psychotherapy.* 68(2), 151–162.

Bordin, E. S. (1979). The generalizability of the psychoanalytic concept of the working alliance. *Psychotherapy: Theory, Research & Practice, 16*(3), 252–260. https://doi.org/10.1037/h0085885.

Brattland, H, Hoiseth,J., Burkeland, O., Inderhaug, T., Binder, P., Iversen, V. (2018) Learning from clients: A qualitative investigation of psychotherapists' reactions to negative verbal feedback. *Psychotherapy Research, 28*(4), 545–559, https://doi.org/10.1080/10503307.2016.1246768.

Brattland, H., Koksvik, J. M., Burkeland, O., Gråwe, R. W., Ker, C., löcknLinaker, O. M., Ryum, T., Wampold, B., Lara-Cabrera, M.L., & Iversen, V. C. (2018). The effects of routine outcome monitoring (ROM) on therapy outcomes in the course of an implementation process: A randomized clinical trial. *Journal of Counseling Psychology, 65*(5), 641–652. https://doi.org/10.1037/cou0000286.

Burlingame, G., Whitcomb, K., Woodland, S., Olsen, J, Beecher,M, & Gleave, R. (2018). The effects of relationship and progress feedback in group psychotherapy using the Group Questionnaire and Outcome Questionnaire–45: A randomized clinical trial. *Psychotherapy, 55*(2), 116–131. https://doi.org/10.1037/pst0000133.

Burlingame, G., Allderedge, C.& Arnold,R. (2021). Alliance rupture Detection and Repair in Group Therapy: Using the Group Questionnaire-GQ. *International Journal of Group Psychotherapy, 71*(2), 338–370, https://doi.org/10.1080/00207284.2020.1844010.

Butcher, J.N. (2010). Minnesota Multiphasic Personality Inventory. In I.B. Weiner and W.E. Craighead (Eds.), The Corsini Encyclopedia of Psychology. https://doi.org/10.1002/9780470479216.corpsy0573·

Chow, D., & Miller, S. D. (2015). *Taxonomy of deliberate practice activities worksheets.* International Center for Clinical Excellence (ICCE).

College of Nurses of Ontario (2008). Practice Standard: Documentation. Author. https://www.cno.org/globalassets/docs/prac/41001_documentation.pdf.

College of Nurses of Ontario (2022). Confidentiality and Privacy–personal health information. Author. https://www.cno.org/globalassets/docs/prac/41069_privacy.pdf.

Conoley, C. W., & Scheel, M. J. (2018). *Goal focused positive psychotherapy: A strengths-based approach.* Oxford University Press.

Constantino, M.J. (2012). Believing is seeing: An evolving research program on patients' psychotherapy expectations. *Psychotherapy Research, 22*(2), 127–138.

Evans, C. & Carlyle, J. (2021). *Outcome measures and evaluation in counseling and psychotherapy (1st ed.)*. Sage Publication Ltd.

Greenberg, L. S. (2007). Emotion in the relationship in emotion focused therapy. In: P. Gilbert & R. L. Leahy (Eds.), *The Therapeutic Relationship in the Cognitive-Behavioural Psychotherapies* (pp. 43–62). Routledge.

Hill, C. & Knox, S. (2009). Processing the therapeutic relationship. *Psychotherapy Research, 19* (1), 13–29. https://doi.org/10.1080/10503300802621206.

Horvath, A. O., & Symonds, B. D. (1991). Relation between working alliance and outcome in psychotherapy: A meta-analysis. *Journal of Counseling Psychology, 38*(2), 139–149. https://doi.org/10.1037/0022-0167.38.2.139.

Jain, S., & Roberts, L. W. (2009). Ethics in psychotherapy: A focus on professional boundaries and confidentiality practices. *Psychiatric Clinics, 32*(2), 299–314.

Knox, S., Adrians, N., Everson, E., Hess, S., Hill, C., & Crook-Lyon, R. (2011). Clients' perspectives on therapy termination. *Psychother Res 21*(2):154–67. https://doi.org/10.1080/10503307.2010.534509. PMID: 21229469.

Lambert, M. J., Burlingame, G. M., Umphress, V., Hansen, N. B., Vermeersch, D. A., Clouse, G. C., & Yanchar, S. C. (1996). The reliability and validity of the outcome questionnaire. *Clinical Psychology & Psychotherapy, 3,* 249–258.

Lambert, M. J., and Gianluca Lo Coco. (2013). Simple methods for enhancing patient outcome in routine care: Measuring, monitoring, and feedback. *Research in Psychotherapy: Psychopathology, Process and Outcome, 16*(2), 93−101.

Lambert, M. J., Morton, J. J., Hatfield, D. R., Harmon, C., Hamilton, S., Shimokawa, K., et al. (2004). *Administration and scoring manual for the Outcome Questionnaire (OQ 45.2).* (3rd ed.). American Professional Credentialing Services LLC.

Leiper, R. & Kent, R. (2001). Working through setbacks in psychotherapy: crisis, impasse and relapse. *Sage..*

Luborsky, L., Barber, J.P., Siqueland, L., Johnson, S., Najavits, L.M., Frank, A., & Daley, D. (1996). The Revised Helping Alliance Questionnaire (HAq-II) : Psychometric Properties. *J Psychother Pract Res.* 5(3):260–71. PMID: 22700294; PMCID: PMC3330423.

Marx, J. A., & Gelso, C. J. (1987). Termination of individual counseling in a university counseling center. *Journal of Counseling Psychology, 34*(1), 3–9. https://doi.org/10.1037/0022-0167.34.1.3

Meier, S. T. (2014). Rediscovering the role of avoidance in psychotherapy progress and outcome. *Professional Psychology: Research and Practice, 45*(3), 212.

Miller, S., Hubble, M. & Duncan, B. (2008). Supershrinks: What's the secret of their success?. *Psychotherapy in Australia, (14)*, 14–22.

Miller, S. & Hubble, M. & Chow, D. (2020). Better results: Using deliberate practice to improve therapeutic effectiveness. American Psychological Association.

Morgan, R., Luborsky, L., Crits-Christoph, P., Curtis, H., & Solomon, J. (1982). Predicting the Outcomes of Psychotherapy by the Penn Helping Alliance Rating Method. *Arch Gen Psychiatry.* 39(*4*), 397–402. https://doi.org/10.1001/archpsyc.1982.04290040013002.

Owen, J., Miller, S.D., Seidel J., & Chow, D. (2016).The working alliance in treatment of military adolescents (2016). *Journal Of Consulting and Clinical Psychology, 84*(3), 200–210.

Polkinghorne, D. E. (2005). Language and meaning: Data collection in qualitative research. *Journal of Counseling Psychology, 52*(2), 137–145. https://doi.org/10.1037/0022-0167.52.2.137.

Quintana, S. M., & Holahan, W. (1992). Termination in short-term counseling: Comparison of successful and unsuccessful cases. *Journal of Counseling Psychology, 39*(3), 299–305. https://doi.org/10.1037/0022-0167.39.3.299

Ruchlewska, A., Kamperman, A.M., van der Gaag, M., Wierdsma, A., & Mulder, N. (2016). Working alliance in patients with severe mental illness who need a crisis intervention plan. *Community Ment Health J, 52,* 102–108. https://doi.org/10.1007/s10597-015-9839-7.

Safran, J. D., Muran, J. C., Samstag, L. W., & Stevens, C. (2002). Repairing alliance ruptures. In J. C. Norcross (Ed.), *Psychotherapy relationships that work: Therapist contributions and responsiveness to patients* (pp. 235–254). Oxford University Press.

Sánchez-Bahíllo, Á., Aragón-Alonso, A., Sánchez-Bahíllo, M., & Birtle, J. (2014). Therapist characteristics that predict the outcome of multipatient psychotherapy: Systematic review of empirical studies. *Journal of psychiatric research, 53*, 149–156.
Schlesinger, H.J.. (2013). *Endings and Beginnings: On terminating psychotherapy and psychoanalysis.* Routledge.
Schuckard, E., Miller, S. D., & Hubble, M. A. (2017). Feedback-informed treatment: Historical and empirical foundations. In D. Prescott, C. Maeschalck & S. Miller (Eds.), *Feedback-Informed Treatment in Clinical Practice: Reaching for Excellence* (pp. 13–35). American Psychological Association. https://doi.org/10.1037/0000039-002.
Simon, G. M. (2012). The role of the therapist: What effective therapists do. *Journal of marital and family therapy, 38*, 8–12.
Smith. S. R., Hilsenroth, M. J., Baity, M. R., & Knowles, E. S. (2003). Assessment of patient and therapist perspectives of process: A revision of the Vanderbilt Psychotherapy Process Scale. *Am J Psychother 57*(2), 195–205. https://doi.org/10.1176/appi.psychotherapy.2003.57.2.195. PMID: 12817550.
Stubbe, D. E. (2018). The therapeutic alliance: The fundamental element of psychotherapy. *Focus, 16*(4), 402–403. https://doi.org/10.1176/appi.focus.20180022.
Todd, G., & Freshwater, D. (1999). Reflective practice and guided discovery: Clinical supervision. *British Journal of Nursing, 8*(20), 1383–9. https://doi.org/10.12968/bjon.1999.8.20.1383.
Tryon, G. S., Birch, S. E., & Verkuilen, J. (2018). Meta-analyses of the relation of goal consensus and collaboration to psychotherapy outcome. *Psychotherapy, 55(4)*, 372-383. https://doi.org/10.1037/pst0000170.
Tseng, W. S. (1999). Culture and psychotherapy: Review and practical guidelines. *Transcultural psychiatry, 36*(2), 131–179.
Vasquez, M. (1992). Psychologist as clinical supervisor: Promoting ethical practice. *Professional Psychology: Research and Pracitice, 23*, 196–202.
Vyskocilova, J., & Prasko, J. (2013). Ethical reflection and psychotherapy. *Neuroendocrinology Letters, 34*(7), 590–600.

Chapter 18
Nursing Competencies: Training and Psychotherapy

Stacey Roles, Carly Valiente, Ingrid Rijo, and Natalie Castonguay

Abstract Training is a key component in obtaining competency to practice specific forms of psychotherapy. Nurses require knowledge, skill, and judgment to competently practice any type of psychotherapy. The therapeutic relationship is the foundation for psychotherapy and for this reason, a solid understanding of how to establish and maintain this rapport is pertinent. Secondly, core therapeutic micro-skills are important during or before the specialization into a specific stream of psychotherapy. These include active listening, interviewing skills, conceptualization, and evaluation in order to effectively engage and motivate the client in the therapeutic alliance and treatment plan. While different modalities of psychotherapy may have their own unique theories, approaches and models, all psychotherapies share a core understanding of knowledge and skill accompanying a specific goal to improve mental health and wellness. Case conceptualization that is developed through assessment, client preferences and best available evidence-based literature, will guide treatment interventions and outcomes. Receiving training in the many specific types of psychotherapies that exist is important to give clinicians a theoretical framework from which to practice. The critical components of these programs that one should consider while looking for education to broaden their nurse psychotherapy knowledge base will be reviewed in this chapter.

Keywords Psychotherapy training · Training programs · Foundational training · Core competencies · Nurse psychotherapy

---

S. Roles (✉) · C. Valiente · N. Castonguay
Roles & Associates Psychotherapy Services Inc. & CBT Training Centre of the North, Sudbury, ON, Canada
e-mail: stacey@rolespsychotherapy.com

C. Valiente
e-mail: carly@rolespsychotherapy.com

I. Rijo
Alliston, ON, Canada

S. Roles and K. Kalia (eds.), *The Nurses' Guide to Psychotherapy*,
https://doi.org/10.1007/978-981-97-4738-2_18

Learning Objectives

After completing this chapter, the learner will:

1. Understand the importance of training in building knowledge, skill, and judgement for the delivery of safe and ethical psychotherapy interventions.
2. Understand the concepts of therapeutic alliance, case conceptualization and evaluation, and their importance in establishing and maintaining effective treatment interventions and outcomes.
3. Demonstrate a solid understanding of the core principles underlying many forms of psychotherapy.

1 Introduction

Training is a key component in obtaining competency to practice in specific forms of psychotherapy. Nurses require knowledge, skill, and judgement to competently practice any type of psychotherapy. Nursing in Canada is a self-regulated profession and, as such, each province or territory grants the regulatory body the ability to set its own standards, policies and educational requirements (Stephany, 2020). In most jurisdictions in Canada, nurses are responsible for determining their needs for professional development and education in their chosen area of practice to provide safe and competent care (Stephany, 2020). The therapeutic relationship is the foundation of mental health nursing practice and nurses require an in-depth knowledge of what this entails (Registered Nurses' Association of Ontario [RNAO], 2006). As psychotherapy is a purposeful interaction, with clear intentions and goals, it is essential that the nurse reflects on their skills and ensures it adequately meets the needs and intended outcomes of the client (RNAO, 2006).

2 Training for the Delivery of Safe and Ethical Psychotherapy Care

Different modalities of psychotherapy may have their own unique theories, approaches, and models, however, all psychotherapies share a core understanding of knowledge and skill accompanying a specific goal to improve mental health and wellness. Case conceptualization that is developed through assessment, client preferences and best available evidence-based literature, will guide treatment interventions and outcomes (Chap. 15). Receiving training in the many types of psychotherapies that exist (Chap. 16) is important to give psychotherapists a theoretical framework from which to work from. Active listening, attending skills, and reflecting on thoughts and emotions may be used in many different types of psychotherapy (Veluri, 2015) and can be included in all training programs or taken as a foundational component.

Some general principles of training should include a recognition of the existence of different psychotherapies or modalities, and promote a respectful understanding of differences and similarities between approaches and theories. Training should also be evidence-based, or identify if there is a lack of evidence, potentially due to the newness of the therapy type. Further, supervision should be included as an integral part of the learners' experience and will be discussed in depth in Chap. 19. Training for the type of psychotherapy should include an expectation about the typical length of the course of psychotherapy based on the type being utilized and should be aligned with various presentations and populations of clients. These populations might include individuals, relationships, groups, or families. Training should explicitly explore the model being used inclusive of the clinical concepts to enable the learner to relate theory to practice (Psychotherapy and Counselling Federation of Australia, 2020). In addition to a sound curriculum regarding the psychotherapy type and relevant interventions, training should frame individuals' lived experiences including social, economic, trauma, and political contexts in relation to the type of psychotherapy being taught. The training should also include a critical understanding of cultural, racial, socio-economic, gendered, heteronormative, and disability bias in the theory and culture (Psychotherapy and Counselling Federation of Australia, 2020). When considering psychotherapy training, there are various factors that one should consider. Length and intensity or specialization of a training program in relation to the desired skillset one wishes to acquire should be carefully considered. Acquired competencies, which are the ability to achieve a specified level of proficiency in a practice resulting from both skill and judgement, should also be contemplated. One acquires these skills to practice psychotherapy through training, supervision, and experiential learning, thus, an integral part of the practice of psychotherapy includes sufficient and adequate training. Supervision and consultation following training will be discussed further in Chap. 19.

A core competency required to practice psychotherapy includes a foundational awareness of psychotherapeutic theory and research (Psychotherapy and Counselling Federation of Australia, 2020). Adequate training programs will include learning about both human psychological development and functioning, and the theoretical foundations that underpin the psychotherapeutic methods being used in the practice (College of Registered Psychotherapists of Ontario [CRPO], 2012). By having an understanding of the theory and research that supports psychotherapy, one is able to better use clinical judgment to inform their psychotherapeutic practice. This sound clinical judgment is an important competency in the delivery of psychotherapy as it reflects one's knowledge in determining when psychotherapy may or may not be indicated (Psychotherapy and Counselling Federation of Australia, 2020). It is important to cultivate an understanding of the benefits, limitations, and possible contraindications of any psychotherapy intervention (CRPO, 2012).

Once one has an understanding of psychotherapeutic theory and research, and has cultivated an understanding of both the benefits and limitations of psychotherapy for their clients, it is important for them to integrate theory and practice (Psychotherapy and Counselling Federation of Australia, 2020). Training will focus on integrating knowledge learned about psychotherapeutic theory and the knowledge of key concepts common to all psychotherapy practices (CRPO, 2012). As explained in Chap. 16, there are various psychotherapies that are practiced, and it is important for any training program to recognize that this range exists. Finally, it is important for training to cover an awareness of the self. It is highly recommended that the psychotherapist be taught to look for and recognize their impact on a client, and how their own belief systems and viewpoints may affect their work (CRPO, 2012). These beliefs can be unconscious or conscious, and they pose a risk of impacting objectivity. Therefore, it is important for training to help one recognize, learn about, and acknowledge their own beliefs in order to prevent them from influencing their professional role.

3 Core Principles of Psychotherapy in Training

While there is no universally accepted group of parameters that represent the core of all psychotherapies (Settanni et al., 2022), many forms of psychotherapy appear to share a set of knowledge, attitudes, and skills, even when they have uniquely distinct underlying theories, techniques, and goals for treatment (Goldberg & Plakun, 2013). Nurse psychotherapists should seek out additional education, supervision and mentorship as needed to ensure competency in these core fundamental psychotherapy principles, regardless of what psychotherapeutic model or approach they choose. The Y model of psychotherapy (Goldberg & Plakun, 2013), which was introduced in Chap. 16, outlines the core skills that should be addressed in or prior to engaging in psychotherapy training programs.

4 Therapeutic Alliance

When integrated with training, therapeutic alliance involves the effectiveness of instruction, modeling, practice and feedback from the trainer or trainees (Knox & Hill, 2021). Communication skills, including one's ability to engage in the explicit and nuanced exchange of vital information, thoughts, and feelings, is a core nursing and psychotherapeutic skill that drives the therapeutic relationship, process, and outcomes (Kourkouta & Papathanasiou, 2014). Hence, to be successful in their work, nurse psychotherapists must be educated and skilled in effective communication and interpersonal relations.

Therapeutic alliance is at the core of all nurse-client relationships (College of Nurses of Ontario [CNO], 2006; College of Registered Psychotherapists of Ontario, 2012). This therapeutic bond is the essential component of effective treatment (Goldberg & Plakun, 2013) and is recognized as a core competency across all approaches to psychotherapy. Albeit, specific models may have unique areas of focus, and ways of utilizing the therapeutic alliance in implementation and evaluation. In general, nurse psychotherapists demonstrate competence by building and maintaining rapport and expressing genuine interest and empathy towards the client throughout the entire psychotherapeutic process. Nurses can accomplish this by setting and maintaining professional boundaries, and identifying and addressing possible ruptures in the therapeutic alliance. Attuning to the unique individual clients' intellectual, physical, emotional, and spiritual needs as well as respecting cultural and social preferences helps to remove potential barriers to therapy and create an inclusive, respectful and supportive environment. See Chaps. 2 and 4 for more information on the therapeutic alliance, communication skills, theories, and other foundational concepts.

5 Case Conceptualization and Evaluation

Training programs must include education regarding the importance of case conceptualization and the evaluation of the effectiveness of treatment interventions in relation to client outcomes. Case conceptualization has been reviewed in Chap. 15 but is significant enough that it must also be included in this chapter on training. Case conceptualization is the premise by which we can dissect the significant history of the client, understand the life experiences that they have had, and continue to have, and determine how it impacts their current state and their future goals. Case conceptualization also enables clinicians to critically review barriers or obstacles to treatment and can help clinicians summarize needs when sending referrals or seeking out consultation. This succinct overview of the client's history, contributing factors to current problem areas, and treatment goals enable the clinician in delivering appropriate treatment interventions resulting in positive client outcomes and is a cornerstone for training clinicians in various forms of psychotherapy.

Assessment and case conceptualization are common to the different forms of psychotherapy and are pertinent in guiding any therapeutic process and treatment and should be included in training programs. All psychotherapies share the requirement of an initial and ongoing psychological formulation which becomes more specific according to the psychotherapeutic model and treatment being used (Goldberg & Plakun, 2013). Competence in assessment and case conceptualization is demonstrated when the clinician has the knowledge and skill to; effectively assess and interpret their clients' main areas of concern, identify any risk of self-harm, suicide and violent acts, enable treatment planning and allow for the recognition of the need for external professional consultations, or the involvement of other services (Settanni et al., 2022). Treatment planning is usually driven by case conceptualization or formulation and negotiates the best treatment method at the onset of therapy with the client. Training should identify that treatment planning is part of an ongoing evaluation, taking into account the clients' needs and preferences, such as their motivation, time and finances. While treatment methods will vary depending on the psychotherapy approach, any potential psychotherapeutic interventions, as well as the anticipated duration of individual sessions and therapy as a whole, should be clearly explained in order to co-create a clearly defined therapeutic plan with the client and to gain informed consent.

6 Reflective Activity

Consider the following to help you reflect on your current level of competency (knowledge, skill, judgement), then create a learning plan to include further learning that will help you build your capacity for delivering safe and ethical psychotherapy care.

6.1 Assessment and Case Conceptualization

How competent do I feel in:

- Assessing, describing, and interpreting the client's main areas of concern.
- Assessing the risk of self-harm, suicide and violent acts.
- Recognising my own or a client's need for external professional consultations, and the involvement of other services.
- Identifying specific therapeutic goals and their appropriate therapeutic interventions.

6.2 Therapeutic Rapport

How competent do I feel in:

- Delivering the skills needed to form and maintain a strong therapeutic alliance.
- Identifying and addressing potential ruptures in the therapeutic alliance that may ultimately interfere with therapeutic goals.
- Using effective communication, rapport building and empathy to maintain or repair the therapeutic relationship.
- Addressing and maintaining clear professional boundaries.
- Identifying and addressing ethical and cultural sensitivities, resources and barriers.

6.3 Implementation of Therapeutic Interventions

How competent do I feel in:

- My working knowledge and skill level of a variety of therapeutic interventions.
- Identifying the most relevant psychotherapeutic techniques, teaching them to the client, and guiding their implementation to achieve desired therapeutic goals.
- Evaluating and assessing their efficacy and recommending new interventions as needed to keep the psychotherapeutic process on track.
- Recognising and addressing barriers that may interfere with therapy, such as client resistance, breaks in the therapeutic alliance, and therapist errors or limitations.

7 Summary

- Psychotherapy is a proven effective, highly beneficial treatment for a wide range of mental health conditions such as anxiety, depression, disstress, trauma, pain, and personality disorders, among others (Emmelkamp et al., 2014).
- There is strong empirical support for the efficacy and effectiveness of evidence-based psychotherapies. Adequate training is vital to ensure clinical quality in their successful delivery and outcomes (Ecker et al., 2022).
- Psychotherapy is rooted in many different conceptual models and differing schools of thought (Emmelkamp et al., 2014).
- Nurse psychotherapists are responsible for; ensuring that they receive adequate training to be able to identify the most relevant psychotherapeutic techniques, disseminating these forms of psychotherapies clearly to the client, leading the implementation and interventions of said psychotherapy, and evaluating for desired therapeutic effect.
- Evaluation of training programs should include the assessment of trainees' ability to apply learned materials in clinical settings via role play, feedback forms, and perhaps most effectively through supervision and consultation as discussed in Chap. 19.

References

College of Nurses of Ontario. (2006). *Therapeutic Nurse-Client Relationship. Practice Standard.* Author. https://www.cno.org/globalassets/docs/prac/41033_therapeutic.pdf

College of Registered Psychotherapists of Ontario. (2012). Entry to Practice Competency Profile for Registered Psychotherapists. Author. https://www.crpo.ca/wp-content/uploads/2017/08/RP-Competency-Profile.pdf

Ecker, Anthony H., O'Leary, Kimberley, Fletcher, Terri L., Hundt, Natalie E., York-Ward, Kaki M., Kauth, Michael R, Kunik, Mark E., & Cully, Jeffrey A. (2022). Training and supporting mental health providers to implement evidence-based psychotherapies in frontline practice. *Translational Behavioral Medicine, 12*(1) Ibab084. https://doi.org/10.1093/tbm/ibab084

Emmelkamp, P. M., David, D., Beckers, T., Muris, P., Cuijpers, P., Lutz, W., Andersson, G., Araya, R., Banos Rivera, R.M., Barkham, M., Berking, M., Berger, T., Botella, C., Carlbring, P., Colom, F., Essau, C., Hermans, D., Hofmann SG, Knappe, S., …Vervliet B. (2014). Advancing psychotherapy and evidence-based psychological interventions. Int J Methods Psychiatr Res, 23(Suppl 1), 58–91. https://www.ncbi.nlm.nih.gov/pmc/articles/PMC6878277/

Goldberg, D. & Plakun, E. (2013). Teaching Psychodynamic Psychotherapy with the Y Model. *Psychodynamic Psychiatry, 31*(1), 111–125.

Knox, S., & Hill, C. E. (2021). Training and supervision in psychotherapy: What we know and where we need to go. In M. Barkham, W. Lutz, & L. G. Castonguay (Eds.), *Bergin and Garfield's handbook of psychotherapy and behavior change: 50th anniversary edition* (pp. 327–349). John Wiley & Sons, Inc.

Kourkouta, L. & Papathanasiou, I. V. (2014). Communication in nursing practice. *Materia socio-medica, 26*(1), 65–67. https://doi.org/10.5455/msm.2014.26.65-67

Psychotherapy and Counselling Federation of Australia (2020). *Psychotherapy training standards*. Author. https://www.pacfa.org.au/common/Uploaded%20files/Psychotherapy-Training-Standards-2020.pdf

Registered Nurses' Association of Ontario. (2006). *Establishing Therapeutic Relationships* (rev. suppl.). Author.

Settanni M, Bronzini M, Carzedda G, Godino, G., Manca, M., Martini, L., Provvedi, G., Quilghini, F., Zucconi, A.,& Francesetti, G. Introducing the QACP: development and preliminary validation of an instrument to measure psychotherapist's core competencies. *Res Psychother, 25*(2), 599. https://doi.org/10.4081/ripppo.2022.599

Stephany, K. (2020). *The Ethic of Care: A Moral Compass for Canadian Nursing Practice* (Revised Edition). Bentham Science Publishers Ltd.

Veluri, R. (2015). Psychotherapy Program Guide. NOSM University. http://learn.nosm.ca/moodle/mod/resource/view.php?id=14418

Chapter 19
Nursing Competencies: Supervision and Consultation

Stacey Roles, Carly Valiente, Natalie Castonguay, and Delaney Campbell

Abstract Supervision and consultation are key components of learning to practice psychotherapy competently. Supervision is critical as it allows for objective feedback while implementing the intervention, as well as continual learning and growth as a therapist. Supervision should continue throughout the nurse psychotherapists' career as they are constantly seeing new clients with different presentations, and gleaning new skills in various types of therapies. Supervision allows nurses to challenge themselves and to continuously become better therapists for the clients they treat. Consultation enables the therapist to ask questions about complex client presentations and can be an extremely valuable way to connect with peers and to seek advice from expert psychotherapists specialising in a particular modality. Naturally, many therapists shy away from supervision and consultation as their own anxiety or 'imposter syndrome' may get in the way. This chapter will discuss different types of supervision and consultation that exist, and the importance of this process for the nurse psychotherapist. In addition, the supervision process, roles and responsibilities of supervisors, the supervisory relationship, ethical, legal, and multicultural considerations unique to supervision will be explored. These include but are not limited to managing crisis situations, evaluation in supervision, and becoming an effective supervisor.

Keywords Supervision · Consultation · Imposter syndrome · Supervisory relationship

S. Roles (✉) · C. Valiente · N. Castonguay · D. Campbell
Roles & Associates Psychotherapy Services Inc. & CBT Training Centre of the North, Sudbury, ON, Canada
e-mail: stacey@rolespsychotherapy.com

S. Roles and K. Kalia (eds.), *The Nurses' Guide to Psychotherapy*,
https://doi.org/10.1007/978-981-97-4738-2_19

Learning Objectives

After completing this chapter, the learner will:

1. Explain the difference between supervision and consultation for nurses.
2. Understand the significance of supervision and consultation throughout a nurse psychotherapist's career.
3. Explain the importance of the supervision relationship and demonstrate the ability to outline a supervision or learning contract pertinent to the relationship and the identified goals.

1 Introduction

Consultation and supervision in psychotherapy are key components involved in learning to practice psychotherapy competently. Consultation allows for continual growth as a therapist while supervision is critical as it not only allows clinical advancement but also creates the opportunity for objective feedback regarding the implementation of the intervention. Clinical supervision is regarded as one of the most important components of psychotherapy training (Weck et al. 2017), however following undergraduate nursing education, supervision often becomes underutilised and deprioritised (Masamha et al. 2022).

2 Background

Nurse psychotherapists must strive to engage in ongoing supervision throughout their career. Supervision allows the ability to glean new skills in various types of psychotherapies while treating new clients with a variety of presentations. Supervision presents nurses with an opportunity to challenge themselves and to continuously improve their practice for the clients they treat. Consultation enables the therapist to ask questions about complex client presentations and can be an extremely valuable way of connecting with peers and seeking expert opinions from psychotherapists in a particular modality. Both consultation and supervision have a role in the continuing education of the nurse psychotherapist. Therefore, it is important for the nurse to adequately differentiate between the two in order to engage in the appropriate ongoing learning strategy.

3 Supervision

Supervision is a form of professional guidance, often provided by an experienced psychotherapist for the benefit of a less-experienced learner (Rousmaniere et al. 2017). Supervision can be broad and general, for example, a new nurse psychotherapist may seek guidance on general counselling skills such as active listening, open-ended questions, or ethical dilemmas. Supervision can also be modality-specific, such as a nurse looking for guidance in the treatment interventions of a client using cognitive behavioural therapy (CBT). During the supervision process, the supervisor can skillfully guide the nurse psychotherapist in learning the particulars of that modality to treat certain presentations so the supervisee can practice more effectively and ethically. For example, an expert in post traumatic stress disorder may supervise another clinician while they hone the skills within the modality needed to treat this clinical presentation. Supervision is an opportunity for novice clinicians to apply the knowledge acquired in formal training to real-life scenarios, while still accessing support for the inevitable questions that arise in early practice. In order to build these skills, supervision often has an observational component, either live, via audio and/or video recordings, or by using two-way mirrors. To ensure supervisees' optimal learning, methods that allow the direct evaluation of supervisees' competencies should be considered (Weck et al. 2017).

3.1 Supervisees' Perception of Supervision

Supervisees may understand that their participation in supervision is helpful for their professional responsibilities and agency mandates. The primary goals of supervision coincide with nursing core competencies as the nurse psychotherapist strives to work within the limits of their scope of practice and knowledge (College of Nurses of Ontario 2023). While engaging in supervision, the nurse psychotherapist is able to self-reflect while identifying individual learning needs to improve their competence. However, supervisees are also encouraged to understand the value of supervision in their professional and personal advancement. The most meaningful learning and skill development often occurs during the course of supervision, where clinicians can apply their newly acquired knowledge.

Naturally, many psychotherapists shy away from supervision as their own anxiety or 'imposter syndrome' may get in the way. Recognizing that supervision is part of the learning process as adjunctive to training is of the highest importance. Supervision is not meant to be punitive in nature, but rather a means to provide constructive feedback to solidify the learning process and adequately prepare the nurse psychotherapist to incorporate the learning outcomes into their practice. This understanding is crucial to the supervision process as there is a direct correlation between supervision and client outcomes (Keum & Wang 2021).

4 Consultation

Consultation, often synonymous with supervision itself, is a widely practiced method of offering professional guidance (Corey et al. 2020). In case consultation, the consultee offers a verbal account of their case(s), a brief summary of their client's social location and primary concerns, as well as specific questions or conflicts that have arisen. The consultant should seek a balance between time used for information gathering and guided direction. The consultant should gather enough information to understand the client's social location, primary concerns, barriers to success thus far, and help to guide the consultee in identifying the most appropriate therapeutic approach. The consultant's questions need not be limited to clinical questions, rather case consultation is an excellent opportunity for consultees to address issues (perceived or real) regarding their therapeutic alliance with the client, ethical issues, and transference and countertransference dilemmas, among others.

Though case consultation is dynamic in that it can be used in combination with a number of other methods of supervision, as will be outlined below, it can also be limited. If using a strict case consultation approach, the consultant cannot gain insight into the consultee's practical abilities in session (Corey et al. 2020). Thus, it is advised that case consultation is used intermittently or in tandem with one, or several, additional methods of intervention for supervision listed below.

5 Methods of Intervention

5.1 Co-Therapy

The supervisor employs a co-therapy approach when they work with the supervisee in session. Both clinicians work together with individual or group clients to deliver the decided-upon care plan. The supervisor and supervisee must discuss and plan their intervention prior to the session and engage in thorough debriefing after the session (Corey et al. 2020). Both clinicians are active in the provision, planning, and conceptualization of therapy. Used in combination with case consultation, this provides an opportunity for that particular method's shortcomings to be overcome. The supervisor can witness, first hand, the supervisee's clinical practical skills while modeling the intricacies of their chosen therapeutic approach (Corey et al. 2020).

5.2 Observation

Observation involves the supervisor observing the supervisee while they practice therapy (Corey et al., 2020). The supervisor can sit behind a two-way mirror, be in the same room as the supervisee and their client, or be on a live video monitor. This differs from co-therapy because the supervisor is not actively engaged in therapy, they are merely observing for the purpose of offering feedback to the supervisee. This, of course, is done with the consent of the client who is aware of the supervisor's passive participation. The supervisor may observe silently for the entire session, or interrupt occasionally to provide feedback (Corey et al. 2020). The supervisor, however, is offering that feedback to the supervisee, not interjecting to collaborate with the supervisee in their provision of therapy. This differs from audio and video recordings in that it is live as the supervisor observes while the supervisee is in session with their client, as opposed to after the session has been completed (Corey et al 2020).

5.3 Recordings

Recordings for supervision can be audio or audio–video. The supervisee obtains the client's consent before recording the session to share this recording with their supervisor before their supervision meeting. Both the supervisor and supervisee listen to this recording, take detailed notes, and develop meaningful feedback to review in session. This feedback can follow a specific structure, for example, the Cognitive Therapy Rating Scale (CTRS) used by the Academy of Cognitive Therapy (Young & Beck 1980), or it can be more general in its assessment of psychotherapy skills and techniques. Regardless, recordings are a helpful tool to be used in collaboration with case consultation, which has been previously discussed in this chapter. Recordings can overcome some of the scheduling issues, anxiety, and over-engagement of the supervisor that may arise in live observance, but of course, it decreases the opportunity for the supervisor to provide live feedback to influence the direction of the session.

5.4 Role Play

Role play involves the supervisor and supervisee(s) playing the roles of client and therapist. This is a method wherein the supervisor can model and witness specific clinical skills. Depending on the supervisee's skill level, they can either play the role of the therapist or the client. It is generally advisable for the supervisor to begin the exercise by playing the therapist, demonstrating the specific skill with the client (played by the supervisee). After this lesson, the supervisee can move to the role of therapist and practice the same demonstrated skill. This is helpful in combination with case consultation. For example, if a supervisor and supervisee decide that a client presenting with anxiety would benefit from CBT, they can engage in role-play of an exposure hierarchy before the supervisee introduces this therapy intervention to the client in session. Role play is also helpful in practicing psychoeducation, wherein a supervisor can ask the learner to share information about a specific diagnosis or modality of therapy that is relevant to the client being discussed.

5.5 Modelling

Modelling, otherwise known as demonstration, is a practice wherein the supervisor exemplifies a clinical or administrative skill in the presence of their supervisee. The supervisee may bring a specific question forward, such as using transference as an intervention in psychodynamic psychotherapy. Alternatively, the supervisor can create scenarios that they believe the supervisee will need to practice, such as reporting a concern to child protective services. Both options enhance the supervisee's exposure to various elements of practice including those related to clinical, ethical, and administrative situations (Corey et al. 2020).

6 Supervisee and Supervisor Competencies

Clinical supervision is a training element that provides direct feedback regarding supervisees' competencies (Weck et al. 2017). The focus of supervision includes both the advancement of the supervisee's learning and the application of the learned skill to their clinical practice. It has been noted that supervision yields largely positive outcomes for supervisees (Martin et al. 2021). Finding a supervisor who is competent in the identified method or model of psychotherapy, as well as having been trained and supervised as a supervisor in that method, will help to ensure fidelity to the model being applied. It is therefore important to find a supervisor who is not only a competent clinician, but also a competent supervisor in the modality being used.

Through their training as supervisors, it is crucial that they learn the degree of separation that must occur while supervising a supervisee. The supervisor must understand and be able to apply the concept that the client the supervisee is treating is not the supervisor's client. Rather, the supervisee they are supervising is the supervisor's client. Just as a therapist's goal is in the pursuit of enabling their clients to become their own therapists, supervisors want their supervisees to become their own supervisors. This shift enables them to critically reflect on clinical questions and cases as they arise by asking themselves the questions their supervisor would have previously asked them. By encouraging growth and transferability in their practice, the supervisee is able to move along the novice to expert continuum. Self-sufficiency of the supervisee is the goal of the supervisory relationship. Factors that may contribute to such outcomes include the strength of the supervisory alliance, the supervisors' use of both basic and advanced supervision skills, and the supervisor's ability to provide effective feedback to the supervisee (Knox & Hill 2021). A supervision contract is pertinent in outlining each individual's expectations of the experience and includes goals for professional advancement.

7 Supervision Models

The supervision approach should parallel the type of psychotherapy that the supervisee is implementing with their client. For example, a supervisor in CBT would not only help the supervisee to role-play and model the CBT experience by identifying the client's thoughts, emotions, behaviours, core beliefs, and rules and assumptions, but would also help the supervisee to understand their own thoughts, emotions, behaviours, core beliefs, and rules and assumptions in relation to themselves as a therapist (Sudak et al. 2016). The relational model of supervision, the nature of the supervisor's view of their own knowledge and authority, the range of the material taken up in supervision, and the supervisor's mode of participation will all contribute and impact the supervisor's role as an objective expert (Sarnat 2016).

According to Corey (2020), there are several available models to use in supervision. The developmental model, the integrated developmental model, and the psychotherapy-based model will be discussed. **The developmental model** is based on the belief that supervision is a process that grows and adapts to the supervisee's knowledge and abilities (Corey 2020). The supervisor must be flexible and take into account the supervisee's skill, knowledge, and experience in each situation presented. **The integrated development model**, created by Stoltenberg and colleagues, might be the most common developmental model (Corey 2020). This model is comprised of three levels that supervisees work through and incorporates the supervisee's level of confidence, experience and skills in a specific area and further identifies the role and needs required from their supervisor in order to progress. In the first level, supervision is structured and aimed at providing guidance, the second level allows for more autonomy as confidence builds, and the third level begins to resemble a consultation with informal case discussions (Corey 2020). It is important to note that a therapist may be practicing at different levels at the same time depending on the skill being applied. **In psychotherapy-based models**, an experienced supervisor utilizes specific modalities within their supervision approach. For example, a supervisor who prioritizes a psychodynamic approach might focus on transference and countertransference in role-play with their supervisee. A supervisor who is skilled in cognitive behavioural therapy would structure their supervision in line with CBT while utilizing methods such as check in, agenda setting, and assigning homework. Similar to the integrated development model, the psychotherapy-based model integrates various methodologies and theories. This model is adaptive to a variety of supervisee needs, however, it does require the supervisor to have extensive experience with several modalities.

8 The Supervisory Relationship

8.1 Boundaries and Ethics in a Supervisory Relationship

Practising psychotherapy in an ethical manner requires an ongoing commitment to standards of practice. The nurse psychotherapist may be challenged by ethical dilemmas as they endeavour to provide effective treatment to their patients. In order to remain up to date with ethics and standards of practice, it is important to participate in continuing education, as well as both supervision and consultation practices (Thomas, 2010). Practitioners' objectivity can be challenged at times, and supervision can help the practitioner challenge their own personal biases to take intentional steps to mitigate their impact. For more information on ethics and nursing psychotherapy, see Chap. 13.

It is important to note that supervision is not psychotherapy for the supervisee, though there may be therapeutic benefits. For example, if a supervisee is learning how to assess and treat a client for a specific symptom, which they may also experience themselves, the supervisee may benefit personally from this learning. The benefit to the supervisee's client is that the supervisee may have a better understanding of how to help treat the symptoms experienced. The supervisor and supervisee, however, must maintain the supervisory boundary without crossing over into psychotherapy themselves. Self-reflection and open discussion within the foundation of a strong rapport can help support boundaries within a supervision contract. Avoiding dual relationships so that there is no interference with the quality and objectivity of the supervision experience is paramount.

The guidelines for clinical supervision in health services psychology are built on the following assumptions:

- Requires formal education and training;
- Prioritises the care of the client/patient and the protection of the public;
- Focuses on the acquisition of competence by and the professional development of the supervisee;
- Requires supervisor competence in the foundations and functional competency domains being supervised;
- Is anchored in the current evidence base related to supervision and the competencies being supervised;
- Occurs within a respectful and collaborative supervisory relationship that includes facilitative and evaluative components and is established, maintained, and repaired as necessary;
- Entails responsibilities on the part of the supervisor and supervisee;
- Intentionally infuses and integrates the dimensions of diversity in all aspects of professional practice;
- Is influenced by both professional and personal factors, including values, attitudes, beliefs, and interpersonal biases;
- Is conducted in adherence to ethical and legal standards;

- Uses a developmental and strength-based approach;
- Requires reflective practice and self-assessment by the supervisor and supervisee;
- Incorporates bidirectional feedback between the supervisor and supervisee;
- Includes evaluation of the acquisition of expected competencies by the supervisee;
- Serves a gatekeeping function for the profession;
- Is distinct from consultation, personal psychotherapy and mentoring. (American Psychological Association 2014, p. 5)

Further, interprofessional supervision and collaboration is of importance. Teaching supervisees how to work appropriately within various professional domains (Rousmaniere et al. 2017) is paramount to the growth of the therapist and the profession. Through effective, intra-professional and collaborative practice, nurse psychotherapists can optimise their scopes of practice, enhance the health of others, and engage in person-centred care (Canadian Nurses Association 2020). As stated by the College of Nurses of Ontario (2023), nurses must assess the learning needs of supervisees, regardless of the discipline that they are teaching or supervising and, should determine whether supervisees have the proper knowledge, skill and judgement to provide safe care. Through inter professional collaboration and integration, nurses and other professionals who practice psychotherapy can learn from one another. For more information on interprofessional collaboration see Chap. 20.

8.2 Methods of Supervision

Supervision can be delivered in a number of formats including dyadic supervision, also known as individual supervision, triadic supervision, and group supervision (Borders 2014; Corey 2020). Dyadic supervision consists of the supervisor and supervisee meeting on a one-to-one basis and is required of many graduate-level programs because of the detailed attention it places on the supervisee's competency (Borders 2014; Corey 2020). Alternatively, triadic supervision consists of the supervisor meeting with two supervisees at a time, and group supervision consists of the supervisor meeting with three or more supervisees at a time. Group supervision has many benefits, one of which includes providing an opportunity for a diversity of perspectives. In this section, we will explore the types of supervision in greater detail.

Dyadic supervision, consisting of the supervisor and supervisee, is the most common form of supervision and can be integral to the development of the supervisee's clinical skills (Bakes, 2005). Dyadic supervision can take different forms including the use of video or audio recordings, and detailed case conceptualizations (Corey, 2020). Direct observation, such as video and audio recordings, allows the supervisor to review the supervisee's work and allows for an accurate evaluation of the supervisee's skill set and required areas of improvement, ultimately making supervision an effective learning experience. Dyadic supervision can also include time spent having discussions that examine case information and the psychotherapeutic approaches being used (Corey, 2020). Due to the one-on-one nature of dyadic supervision, supervisees may feel more inclined to express vulnerabilities regarding their shortcomings in their practice as opposed to when in a group format (Corey 2020).

Another form of supervision is triadic supervision, which is characterized by one supervisor meeting with two supervisees simultaneously. This form of supervision has become recognized as an acceptable alternative to individual supervision (Corey 2020). During these sessions, the supervisor can follow various models or structures for conducting supervision. These may include a split-focus format where each supervisee receives roughly half the time during each session, or a single-focus format where the supervisor will alternate weeks where each supervisee receives all of the allotted time (Bakes, 2005). Triadic supervision can be helpful for supervisees because it creates opportunities for peer learning and reflection which is not be present during dyadic supervision. Although triadic supervision is considered to be a more cost-effective approach and conserves time for the supervisor, it may increase the demand on the supervisor due to having to balance interactions, approaches, and feedback between two supervisees (Corey 2020).

Group supervision is a valuable experience for supervisees as it gives them the opportunity to develop their own skills while being witness to the learning of other novice therapists. In addition to facilitating the session, focusing on specific content, and offering feedback, the supervisor must work to create a group atmosphere whereby the supervisees feel comfortable to participate (Corey, 2020). In a group supervision setting, supervisees tend to acquire a sense of connection to their peers which would be absent in dyadic supervision. This peer learning can be especially beneficial because supervisees are exposed to a more covert process of learning by simultaneously experiencing the skill development of other supervisees (Corey 2020). It is not uncommon for supervisees to experience self-defeating thoughts during their learning where they question their own skill set and competence. By interacting with their peers, supervisees are guided by their supervisors to challenge these beliefs and gain more confidence in their ability (Bakes, 2005). Similar to triadic supervision, group supervision can include the challenge of balancing both individual and group needs. However, those who are part of group supervision will benefit from alternative perspectives and valuable insights due to the nature of group supervision that may otherwise be absent. At times, the group may not necessarily be limited to a specific profession and, thus, the supervisees may bring an interdisciplinary lens to learning.

9 The Role of Feedback in Professional Development

Within the above methods of supervision, there is a need for feedback in the professional development process. There is also a need to tailor feedback depending on the type of psychotherapy the supervisee is learning. Providing corrective or constructive feedback and guidance in a style that is congruent and accessible to the learner is of utmost importance to their learning and advancement from novice to expert. It is often beneficial for the clinician to offer their own feedback including both positive and constructive ideas about the session being discussed. During triad or group supervision, it is also pertinent for others to offer constructive and positive feedback. Feedback can be formal or informal, and can also be formative or summative. Formal feedback often involves systematically offering concrete, objective and scheduled input about the progress and interventions that the clinician is executing (Sudak et al. 2016). Informal feedback is typically unexpected or unscheduled, and might be at the request of the clinician or supervisor on an ad-hoc basis (Sudak et al. 2016).

Formative feedback is presented throughout the course of the supervision experience while summative feedback is at key points in the supervision, for example, at midterm or final evaluations. Formative feedback may include noting a specific item that was well executed followed by an important skill example of how the trainee can execute the intervention differently (Sudak et al. 2016). This may include a demonstration of the modified skill with a request to re-demonstrate the skill and offer corrections as needed. Providing positive feedback around the demonstrated skill and assigning homework can be essential to enhance the supervisees' learning. Summative feedback includes keeping and reviewing records of all supervision sessions so that a summary is possible at pertinent scheduled times. Summative feedback can help to promote specific behavioural changes in supervisees, can increase learning motivation, and can enhance a supervisee's knowledge (ACT, 2018; Beck 2011; Sudak et al. 2016).

Offering emotional encouragement through any form of feedback can boost the learner's morale and mitigate the emotional challenges inherent in learning how to practice any form of therapy (Duckworth et al., 2011). Emotional encouragement can include engaging with the personal responses of the supervisee and supervisor in either supervision sessions or in client sessions. These discussions can involve unearthing the particular responses involving emotions experienced in therapy, as well as assumptions, core beliefs, and values that may have arisen.

10 Selecting a Supervisor

It is important to select a supervisor that aligns with one's learning style, and this should be determined in the early stages of supervision. For example, some supervisees strongly prefer role-play, others recorded examples, while others learn best by doing. In any full course of supervision, it can be helpful to use a variety of learning strategies, including but not limited to those mentioned previously. Furthermore, it is important for the supervisor to understand the supervisee's strengths and weaknesses as a learner, and approach supervision accordingly. The supervisory relationship may be strengthened by the use of exploring questions, such as asking the supervisee to share past experiences with previous supervisors. These experiences can include ways in which the previous supervisor helped them learn and ways in which they didn't feel supported, clinically or otherwise. Perhaps a previous supervisor was helpful by presenting as warm and welcoming, and also committed to the concept of 'no bad questions'. On the other hand, perhaps a previous supervisor took on a 'sink or swim' approach that the clinician found more stressful than helpful. There are no objective right or wrong approaches; however, it is important to find a supervisor who is interested in understanding the unique qualities of the supervisee and their preferences.

11 Reflective Practice

Reflective practice is the ability to connect theoretical knowledge with practice, and to reflect on ourselves, our actions and our behaviours in order to identify areas of strength and improvement and become better self-directed learners (College of Registered Nurses of Manitoba 2022). Nurses are required to engage in reflective practice to ensure safe and competent care. Patel and Metersky (2022) identified the outcomes of a reflective practice in nursing to be a circular process beginning with reflection, leading to a renewed understanding of an experience, followed by a change in practice by integrating new learnings, resulting in personal and professional growth, and improved client outcomes. It is imperative that nurse psychotherapists adopt reflective practices in their personal and professional lives. Therapists who engage in reflective practice tend to have increased confidence, leading to decreased anxiety in their ability to practice competently (Patel & Metersky 2022). As nurses gain more experience and confidence by engaging in reflective practice, their insight may enable a broader awareness of the social impact and larger influences one can have beyond the therapeutic relationship. Thompson and Pascal (2012) propose the concept of critical reflective practice, which takes into consideration a larger social context and goes beyond the therapist's experience and connections. Some points to consider when engaging in critical reflection can include the role of language, the emotional dimension of reflection, the importance of power dynamics, and the issue of timing.

11.1 Models of Reflective Practice

There are several models of reflective practice and nurse psychotherapists are encouraged to become familiar and incorporate at least one into their practice. Although this list is not intended to be exhaustive, some models are summarized below.

Rolfe's Reflective Cycle and **Driscoll's Model of Reflection** was intended for use by nurses in a continuous, cyclical methodology to reveal actionable outcomes to improve patient care and nurses' knowledge. It asks three questions:

1. What? A series of questions to describe the situation and the nurses' perspective.
2. So what? Evaluate and analyze the entirety of the situation.
3. Now what? A movement to action by reviewing the first two questions and conceptualizing potential change (Business Bliss Consultants FZE 2018b&f).

Pender's Health Promotion Model is based on a humanist approach and the belief that the role of a nurse is to accompany clients on their path to optimal well-being. The model highlights three concepts: individual characteristics/experiences, behaviour-specific cognitions, and behaviour outcomes. By reflecting on the bi-directional therapeutic relationship and the impact the nurse psychotherapist has on client health promotion, the therapist is better positioned to target their own education to meet the needs of their clients with the goal of inspiring health-promoting behavioural change (Business Bliss Consultants FZE 2018e).

Atkins and Murphy's Model of Reflection is another model designed for nursing practice and includes four steps that serve to challenge the therapist's approach and patterns in therapy (Business Bliss Consultants FZE 2018a, para. 3). It includes the following:

1. Self-awareness of uncomfortable feelings and thoughts.
2. The ability to describe.
3. The ability to critically analyze events or experiences using logical thinking.
4. The ability to evaluate learning, events or experiences.
5. The ability to identify any learning that has occurred.

Kolb's Learning Cycle includes reflective practice within a larger professional development model. It is composed of four steps: concrete experience, reflective observation, abstract conceptualization and active experimentation. This model prioritizes experiential learning and reflection which may be more time consuming but can hold great benefit (Business Bliss Consultants FZE 2018d).

Gibb's Reflective Cycle is an older model originally aimed to provide reflective practice for nurses, and is now used transprofessionally. Similar to Rolfe's and Driscoll's model, this framework is cyclical and includes six core elements: description, feelings, evaluation, analysis, conclusion, and action plan. The goal of the model is to provide an opportunity to apply changes in a thoughtful and purposeful manner (Business Bliss Consultants FZE 2018c).

Models of reflective practice are not limited to nursing or health care and there are several others inspired by social services, psychology or education that can be equally insightful to a nurse psychotherapist. The reader is encouraged to find a reflective model that meets their individual learning needs.

12 Risk Management in Supervision

A large part of managing risk in any situation is to ensure clear, and detailed communication. In supervision, a contract between supervisor and supervisee ensures both parties' interests are protected and expectations are identified in a clear manner. Due to the ever-changing nature and variances in laws, statutes and policies, consulting and retaining the appropriate professional support from legal and other experts is advisable.

Some considerations when developing a contract can include, but are not limited to:

- Scope of work to be done during supervision;
- Liability limitations and insurance requirements;
- Documentation of sessions;
- When to seek outside consultations including differing areas of expertise and education;
- Consent forms, with a focus on client, practice and supervision;
- Evaluation plans, including the frequency, method, and outline;
- Current and potential conflicts of interest as well as the process to follow if conflicts arise;
- Limits of confidentiality and duty to report.

Outlining responsibilities for both the supervisee and supervisor can also be included in a contract or memorandum of understanding. Clear role definition is an essential piece of supervision and prevents favouritism, confusion, and allows for realistic expectations (Corey, 2020).

Supervisee responsibilities can include:

- Outlining desired learning outcomes;
- Choosing an appropriate supervisor;
- Adequately preparing for each session;
- Protecting and prioritizing supervision time;
- Keeping an open mind in receiving constructive feedback;
- Providing consistent and honest feedback to the supervisor;
- Actively participating in reflective practice;
- Being open to self-disclosure where appropriate;
- Creating action plans and implementing them;
- Maintaining accountability and appropriately documenting (Bond & Holland 2011).

Supervisor responsibilities should include at a minimum:

- Ensuring protected time for supervision sessions;
- Upholding core nursing values of reliability, confidentiality, accountability, and honesty;
- Maintaining appropriate boundaries where dual relationships are avoided;
- Challenging supervisees;
- Evaluating supervisee competencies and safety;
- Investing in outside supervision as a supervisor;
- Keeping appropriate documentation (Bond & Holland 2011).

13 Evaluating Supervision

The purpose of evaluating supervision is to ensure a positive impact on client outcomes, therapist competency, and efficacy (O'Donovan et al. 2011). There are several methods and models of supervision, therefore there are various ways to evaluate supervision. Bi-directional evaluation ensures that clear communication between both parties is maintained and can highlight gaps and possible conflicts, which can indicate the need to refer out or end a supervisory relationship. Ultimately, the goal of supervision is to empower the supervisee to 'self-supervise' later on in their career (Corey et al. 2020). Self-evaluation contributes to a supervisee's professional development by exercising self-reflection on one's abilities, competencies, strengths, and areas requiring improvement (Corey et al. 2020; Borders 2014). Supervisors can model self-evaluation in supervision sessions and an openness to life-long learning.

Traditional evaluation methods can also be used within the context of supervision. Supervisors evaluating supervisees can use standardised tools which may be readily available online. The use of outcome measures, whether self-reported or clinician-rated, are important evaluation tools for both the clinician, to evaluate client progress and for the supervisor, to ensure supervision has a positive effect on client outcomes (Cuijpers et al. 2010). Supervisor evaluations, on the other hand, are less commonly used. Corey et al. (2020) identify some of the qualities that might be considered in the evaluation of a supervisor. These include:

- Abilities in communication and ethics;
- Knowledge in cultural competencies, legal issues, and clinical and professional theory;
- Effective support and supervision of clinical cases;
- Availability and punctuality.

Evaluations are an important tool for professional development and also play a vital role in nurse psychotherapists' accountability and continuous educational requirements of the profession. Bidirectional evaluations of both the supervisor and the supervisee are encouraged, however, due to the lack of evidence-based supervisor evaluations, the onus may be on the supervisee and supervisor to develop and implement an evaluation tool that best meets their needs.

14 Case Vignette

Adam is an experienced mental health nurse who has decided to sign up for a cognitive behavioural therapy (CBT) training course. He has heard a lot about CBT but has never taken any formal training in CBT. After completing the course, he is offered the option of supervision with a qualified CBT supervisor. Adam feels he does not need structured supervision because he has many years of experience in mental health and states that he can 'check-in' with other CBT providers on his team if he has any questions.

14.1 Case Vignette Reflective Questions

1. How would you describe the difference between supervision, consultation and what Adam is suggesting he do above?
2. When would it be appropriate to engage in either supervision, consultation or reflection with colleagues?
3. What is the potential harm of not engaging in the appropriate level of support when learning a new form of psychotherapy?
4. What would you consider to be important qualities, knowledge and characteristics of both a supervisor and a consultant?

15 Summary

- Supervision allows for the solidification of the training process, enabling the supervisees to apply what they've learned in clinical practice with guidance, continuous assessment, and support.
- There are many different supervision and consultation approaches that exist.
- Choosing the right supervisor with the correct training, as well as setting a supervision contract with goals pertinent to both the supervisor and supervisee, are crucial to the learning process.
- Evaluation in supervision and continuous feedback are important to the learning process in helping the nurse move from novice to expert in differing types of psychotherapy.

References

American Psychological Association. (2014). *Guidelines for clinical supervision in health services psychology.* Author. http://www.apa.org/about/policy/guidelins-supervision.pdf

Beck, J. (2011). *Cognitive behavior therapy: Basics and beyond* (2nd ed.) Guilford Publications.

Borders, D. (2014). Best practices in clinical supervision: Another step in delineating effective supervision practice. *American Journal of Psychotherapy.* 68(2), 151-162.

Bond, M., & Holland, S. (2011). *Skills of clinical supervision for nurses.* McGraw-Hil Education.

Business Bliss Consultants FZE. (2018a). *Atkins and Murphy Model of Reflection.* Author. .https://nursinganswers.net/reflective-guides/driscoll-model-of-reflection.php?vref=1

Business Bliss Consultants FZE. (2018b). *Driscoll's Model of Reflection.* Author. https://nursinganswers.net/reflective-guides/driscoll-model-of-reflection.php?vref=1

Business Bliss Consultants FZE. (2018c). *Gibbs' Reflective Cycle.* Author. https://nursinganswers.net/reflective-guides/gibbs-reflective-cycle.php?vref=1

Business Bliss Consultants FZE. (2018d). *Kolb's Learning Cycle.* https://nursinganswers.net/reflective-guides/kolbs-learning-cycle.php?vref=1

Business Bliss Consultants FZE. (2018e). *Pender's Health Promotion Model.* Author. https://nursinganswers.net/reflective-guides/penders-model.php?vref=1

Business Bliss Consultants FZE. (2018f). *Rolfe's Reflective Model.* Author. https://nursinganswers.net/reflective-guides/rolfe-reflective-cycle.php?vref=1

Canadian Nurses Association. (2020, March). *Intra-professional collaboration. Position statement.* Author. https://hl-prod-ca-oc-download.s3-ca-central-1.amazonaws.com/CNA/2f975e7e-4a40-45ca-863c-5ebf0a138d5e/UploadedImages/documents/CNA-Position-Statement_Intra-Professional-Collaboration.pdf

College of Nurses of Ontario. (2023). *Code of conduct. Practice standards.* Author. https://www.cno.org/globalassets/docs/prac/49040_code-of-conduct.pdf

College of Registered Nurses of Manitoba. (2022, February 9). *Practice expectation spotlight: Self-reflection.* Author. https://www.crnm.mb.ca/2021/05/28/practice-expectation-spotlight-self-reflection/

Corey, G., Haynes, R., Moulton, P., & Muratori, M. (2020). *Clinical supervision in the helping professions: A practical guide* (3rd ed.). American Counseling Association.

Cuijpers, P., Li, J., Hofmann, S. G., & Andersson, G. (2010). *Self-reported versus clinician-rated symptoms of depression as outcome measures in psychotherapy research on depression: A meta-analysis. Clinical Psychology Review, 30*(6), 768–778. https://doi.org/10.1016/j.cpr.2010.06.001

Keum, Brian & Wang, Lei. (2021). Supervision and psychotherapy process and outcome: A meta-analytic review. *Translational Issues in Psychological Science, 7*(1), 89-108. https://doi.org/10.1037/tps0000272

Knox, S., & Hill, C. E. (2021). Training and supervision in psychotherapy: What we know and where we need to go. In M. Barkham, W. Lutz, & L. G. Castonguay (Eds.), *Bergin and Garfield's handbook of psychotherapy and behavior change: 50th anniversary edition* (pp. 327–349). John Wiley & Sons, Inc..

Martin P, Lizarondo L, Kumar S, & Snowdon D. (2021, November 19). Impact of clinical supervision on healthcare organisational outcomes: A mixed methods systematic review. *PLoS One,* 2021 Nov 19;16(11):e0260156. https://doi.org/10.1371/journal.pone.0260156. PMID: 34797897; PMCID: PMC8604366.

Masamha, R., Alfred, L., Harris, R., Bassett, S., Burden, S. & Gilmore, A. (2022). 'Barriers to overcoming the barriers': A scoping review exploring 30 years of clinical supervision literature. *Journal of Advanced Nursing, 78,* 2678–2692. https://doi.org/10.1111/jan.15283

O'Donovan, A., Halford, W.K. & Walters, B. (2011), Towards best practice supervision of clinical psychology trainees. *Australian Psychologist, 46,* 101–112. https://0-doi-org.aupac.lib.athabascau.ca/https://doi.org/10.1111/j.1742-9544.2011.00033.x

Patel, K. M., & Metersky, K. (2022). Reflective practice in nursing: A concept analysis. *International Journal of Nursing Knowledge*, 33, 180–187. https://doi.org/10.1111/2047-3095.12350

Rousmaniere, T., Goodyear, R. K., Miller, S. D., & Wampold, B. E. (Eds.). (2017). *The cycle of excellence: Using deliberate practice to improve supervision and training.* Wiley-Blackwell. https://doi.org/10.1002/9781119165590

Sarnat, J. (2016). *Supervision essentials for psychodynamic psychotherapies.* American Psychological Association. Washington, DC.

Sudak, D., Codd, R., Ludgate, J., Sokok, L., Fox, M., Reiser, R., & Milne, D. (2016). *Teaching and supervising cognitive behavioral therapy.* John Wiley & Sons.

Thompson, N., & Pascal, J. (2012, January 1). Developing critically reflective practice. *Reflective Practice, 13*(2), 311–325.

Weck, F., Kaufmann, Y., & Witthöft, M. (2017). Topics and techniques in clinical supervision in psychotherapy training. *The Cognitive Behaviour Therapist, 10*, E3. https://doi.org/10.1017/S1754470X17000046

Young, J., & Beck, A. (1980). Cognitive Therapy Scale (CTS) [Database record].

Part III
Future State of Nurse Psychotherapy—Advancing

Chapter 20
Interprofessional Approaches to Practice

Vivian Oystrick and Stacey Roles

Abstract The practice of interdisciplinarity in psychology involves applying the process of disciplinary integration to addressing complex biopsychosocial problems. It requires the acquisition of a broad scope of disciplinary knowledge and a willingness to consider any knowledge that may contribute to successfully understanding the problem in as much depth as possible. In the context of psychotherapy, the goal is to form a more comprehensive understanding of the mental health disorder and to take a more holistic approach to treating it. An integrated or interprofessional approach to psychotherapy requires examining a combination of skills and perspectives from psychology, social work, sociology, nursing, and other health disciplines. To this end, an interdisciplinary approach is also central to the development of policy and practices that support an integrated approach to assessment and intervention, and to ensuring that knowledge is shared among relevant services and systems. In this chapter, we discuss the importance of interdisciplinary care and strategies for taking an interprofessional and integrated approach to psychotherapy. Learners will be encouraged to think critically about how taking an interdisciplinary approach to treating mental health disorders can best meet the needs of clients and improve collaborative working relationships across sectors.

Keywords Interprofessional · Interdisciplinary · Psychotherapy · Integrated approaches · Holistic care

V. Oystrick (✉)
Cambrian College, Sudbury, ON, Canada
e-mail: vivian.oystrick@cambriancollege.ca

S. Roles
Roles & Associates Psychotherapy Services Inc. & CBT Training Centre of the North, Sudbury, ON, Canada

S. Roles and K. Kalia (eds.), *The Nurses' Guide to Psychotherapy*,
https://doi.org/10.1007/978-981-97-4738-2_20

Learning Objectives

After completing this chapter, the learner will:

1. Understand the benefits and barriers to interprofessional and integrated approaches to practice.
2. Explain the difference between interdisciplinary and interprofessional practice as well as the factors leading to successful interprofessional practice at the interactional, organizational, and systemic levels.
3. Demonstrate an ability to think critically about the complex needs of a client and how best to support an interprofessional approach to client care.

1 Theoretical Background of Interdisciplinarity

There are numerous terms that have been used in the literature to describe collaborative practice between professionals. They include the terms interdisciplinary, interprofessional, multidisciplinary, and collaborations (Nancarrow et al. 2013). Although these terms are often used interchangeably, they warrant some distinction. This chapter will provide some historical context on the origin of these terms and how they came to be applied in research and practice today.

In the academic context, the term "discipline" refers to a specific body of knowledge, such as history, psychology, or physics. Each discipline has its own subject matter, assumptions, concepts, theories, and methods (Repko 2008). In their book, *Practicing Interdisciplinarity*, Peter Weignart and Nico Stehr state that "disciplines are not only intellectual but also social structures, made up of human beings with vested interests based on time investments, acquired reputations, and established social networks that shape and bias their views on the relative importance of their knowledge" (2000, p. xi). Therefore, a practice that takes a monodisciplinary approach relies on only one discipline to solve a societal problem; it draws solely on the concepts and constructs associated with that particular body of knowledge. Turner (2017) states that, in the old sense, disciplines began with the creation of rituals of certification and exclusion of knowledge. In the new sense, they are the product of the university's organization, in relation to their research, teaching, knowledge production, and knowledge reproduction. Disciplines arose out of a need for an academic division of labor and a need to divide the vast intellectual terrain into differing fields of inquiry (Jacobs 2017).

While interdisciplinarity is often used as a synonym for innovative research (Jacobs 2017), early interdisciplinary developments can be traced back to the 1930 and 1940s, in the philosophy of science context (Frodeman and Klein 2017). As theories and scholarship moved beyond a positivist paradigm in multiple disciplines, new fields of study started to emerge, forming a new generalism (Frodeman and Klein 2017). This new way of thinking gave rise to alternative forms of scholarship and teaching and facilitated new uses and openings for the humanities (Klein 2005). Today, an interdisciplinary approach gives consideration to the ways that the integration of distinctive disciplinary approaches or methodologies can enhance the understanding of societal problems. The "inter" part of interdisciplinarity refers to being "derived from two or more" and the state of being "between disciplines" (Repko 2005). Klein (2017) states that although many regard interdisciplinarity as synonymous with collaboration, it is not. Though relying on teamwork to solve complex social problems creates connections across disciplines, interdisciplinary work requires greater attention to the interaction between cognitive and social integration.

In the broadest sense of the term, Moran (2008) takes interdisciplinarity to signify any form of questioning between two disciplines aimed at creating a deeper understanding. Interdisciplinarity is often confused with multidisciplinary which draws on multiple perspectives from multiple disciplines but makes no attempt to integrate the insights produced by these perspectives into an interdisciplinary understanding of the topic (Repko 2008). The processes differ in that multidisciplinary appreciate and consider disparate disciplinary perspectives and approaches, whereas interdisciplinarity attempts to cross disciplinary boundaries where the theories, concepts, and methods are appropriate to solving a problem. It requires a willingness to alternate methods of inquiry and recognizes the usefulness of disparate disciplinary tools to help solve the problem. Although they both seek to overcome disciplinary silos, they do so in different ways (Repko 2008). This is an important distinction. Many real-world problems cannot be understood through the lens of one discipline; rather, advancing our understanding and crafting viable solutions requires insight and integration from multiple disciplines (Boix-Mansilla and Gardner 2003).

According to the literature, "interdisciplinarity" provides a collaborative and cooperative alternative to the traditional siloed way of disciplines, however despite the emergent trend in academic settings to introduce interdisciplinary programs, there remains a number of questions around the issues of where and how interdisciplinary work is done (Shailer 2005). For the purpose of this chapter, we will use the term "interprofessional" to describe an approach to practice that integrates skills and knowledge from multiple professionals from different disciplines, who come together with the common goal of improving patient outcomes (Bridges et al. 2011).

2 Barriers and Facilitators to Interprofessional Practice

As social problems are becoming more complex there is a greater need for professionals to create partnerships through interprofessional practices (Korazim-Kőrösy et al. 2014). Interprofessional practices are becoming integral to health care and have the potential to optimize patient care (Sargeant et al. 2008). In fact, the American Public Health Association states that interprofessional practice is a key element of public health, and to be effective agencies, and professional disciplines must work together well (Korazim-Kőrösy et al. 2014).

However, despite the acknowledgement of such by healthcare professionals, managers, and political decision-makers, there is very little empirical evidence to identify the characteristics of organizations that effectively encourage the development of interprofessional healthcare teams (San Martín-Rodríguez et al. 2005). By way of a scoping review, San Martinez-Rodriquez et al. (2005) identified several elements that influence interprofessional practice and how it is consolidated in healthcare teams. These elements included: (1) interactional factors (interpersonal relationships between team members), (2) organizational factors (conditions within the organization), and (3) systemic factors (conditions outside of the organization). Their literature review revealed that interprofessional practice is an interpersonal process, and at the interactional level requires a willingness to collaborate, trust in each other, have mutual respect and communication. At the systemic level, social factors such as power indifferences impact how collaborative practices develop and power differences based on gender stereotypes and disparate social status create barriers to interprofessional collaboration (San Martín-Rodríguez et al. 2005).

Similarly, a scoping review of the literature conducted by Rawlinson et al. (2021) identified the system, organizational, inter-individual, and individual barriers and facilitators of interprofessional practice in primary care settings. Through the scoping review, they discovered that most barriers and facilitators were reported at the organizational and inter-individual levels. Common barriers referred to lack of time and training, lack of clear roles, fears relating to professional identity, and poor communication. Principal facilitators included tools to improve communication, co-location and recognition of other professionals' skills and contributions. At the system's level, the barriers most often reported concerned financial barriers, and lack of long-term funding along with a lack of leadership and lack of support for the expansion of roles. At the organizational level, limitations in human resources, lack of training, and lack of time were identified. At the inter-individual level, the imbalance of power between professionals due to hierarchies between disciplines was mentioned. Also mentioned was the lack of clarity regarding functions, scope of practice, and fear of loss of professional identity in newly defined roles. At the individual level, professionals were concerned about the benefits of collaboration for the patients. The most reported facilitators at the individual level related to: (1) available funding, supportive policies, incentives and compensations for professionals at the system level; (2) reorganizing practices and team structure, co-location, tools for care processes, and providing training and sufficient human resources at the organizational level; (3) the quality of communication, the respect and cohesion between professionals and a shared power at the inter-individual level; and (4) a positive attitude toward interprofessional practice at the individual level (Rawlinson et al. 2021).

3 An Interprofessional Framework

Much of the research in the area of interprofessional collaboration or practice builds on previous research conducted by D'Amour and Oandasan (2005) which proposed a new framework for the development of cohesive and integrated healthcare practice among professionals in response to client's needs. One of the objectives of D'Amour & Oandasan was to distinguish the concept of interprofessionality from interdisciplinarity. As discussed earlier on in this chapter, interdisciplinarity concerns the development of new knowledge in response to fragmented disciplinary knowledge. The concept of interprofessionality as defined by D'Amour and Oandasan (2005) concerns the development of cohesive practice among different professionals from either the same organization or from different organizations and the factors influencing it. D'Amour and Oandasan state the following about interprofessionality:

> It is the process by which professionals reflect on and develop ways of practicing that provides an integrated and cohesive answer to the needs of the client/family/population. Interprofessionality comes from the preoccupation of professionals to reconcile their differences and their sometimes opposing views and it involves continuous interaction and knowledge sharing between professionals organized, to solve or explore a variety of education and care issues all while seeking to optimize the patient's participation. (2005, p. 9)

Another objective of their research was to bridge the gap between interprofessional education and interprofessional practice and to establish linkages between determinants and processes of collaboration across the micro, meso, and macro levels. Figure 19.1 illustrates their framework of Interprofessional Education for Collaborative Patient-Centered Practice" (IECPCP). The model has two circles: the first for education and the second for practice. The circles show the process through which health professionals structure their collaboration. Interprofessional education offers learning environments where learners can be exposed to educational experiences and trained as competent collaborative practitioners. The idea being that practice is linked with education, and if more students are afforded this educational opportunity to learn how to be collaborative practitioners, then more collaborative practice settings will be developed. However, the competencies shared by collaborative practitioners are still being defined (D'Amour and Oandasan 2005). Where educational systems are unable to sufficiently meet the workforce demands, organizations must be able to provide Interdisciplinary Team Training (IDT), as an essential component to an integrated care system (Farrell et al. 2018).

In a study conducted by Nancarrow et al. (2013), the characteristics and competencies that support effective interdisciplinary teamwork were explored by way of a scoping review. The scoping review included input from 253 staff from 11 community rehabilitation and intermediate care teams in the UK. The content analysis resulted in the development of 10 themes related to the characteristics of a good interdisciplinary team. They were further reformulated as competency statements for an effective interdisciplinary team. The following are the 10 competencies identified by Nancarrow et al. (2013):

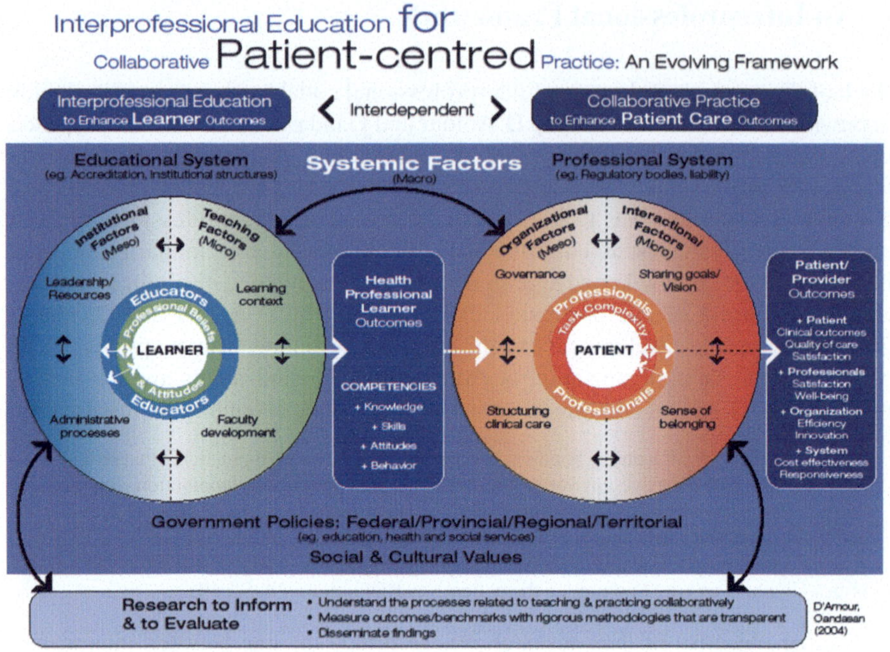

Fig. 19.1 Interprofessional education for collaborative patient-centered practice. From D'Amour and Oandasan (2005). With permission

1. Identifies a leader who establishes a clear direction and vision for the team, while listening and providing support and supervision to the team members.
2. Incorporates a set of values that clearly provide direction for the team's service provision; these values should be visible and consistently portrayed.
3. Demonstrates a team culture and interdisciplinary atmosphere of trust where contributions are valued, and consensus is fostered.
4. Ensures appropriate processes and infrastructures are in place to uphold the vision of the service (for example, referral criteria, communications infrastructure).
5. Provides quality patient-focused services with documented outcomes; utilizes feedback to improve the quality of care.
6. Utilizes communication strategies that promote intra-team communication, collaborative decision-making, and effective team processes.
7. Provides sufficient team staffing to integrate an appropriate mix of skills, competencies, and personalities to meet the needs of patients and enhance smooth functioning.
8. Facilitates recruitment of staff who demonstrate interdisciplinary competencies including team functioning, collaborative leadership, communication, and sufficient professional knowledge and experience.
9. Promotes role interdependence while respecting individual roles and autonomy.
10. Facilitates personal development through appropriate training, rewards, recognition, and opportunities for career development. (pp. 5–8)

In a study that explored the experiences of new nurses in interprofessional healthcare teams in mental health, participants identified interpersonal and organizational factors that contributed to their transition to the team. They identified that being on a team that is open and nonjudgmental to their questions is central to feeling supported and valued, and that establishing credibility and building trust was central to the success of transitioning into an interprofessional healthcare team in a mental health organization. Trust was deemed essential for interprofessional practice as it allowed members of the team to feel safe in knowing their knowledge, expertise, and decision-making capabilities were valued and appreciated (Schwartz et al. 2011). Understanding the competencies required for an effective interprofessional team is critical to the development and sustainability of these teams in practice, as well as, retaining mental health nurses in the field. There is little research that explores nurses' experiences in interprofessional practice and even less work within the mental health context.

4 Interprofessional Approach to Mental Health Care

In recent years, interprofessional approaches to mental health have been emerging as best practice in hospitals, government agencies, and primary care facilities (Greidanus et al. 2020). The need for interprofessional approaches to practice was exacerbated by the COVID-19 pandemic when the prevalence of anxiety and depression increased significantly in the context of overwhelmed healthcare systems (Przybylko et al. 2021). There was never a greater need for interdisciplinary approaches that could offer therapeutic strategies that meet mental health needs through holistic care that addressed mental, social, physical, and spiritual healthcare issues (Przybylko et al. 2021). Despite the need and recognition that this approach would lead to better outcomes for patients, there are few evidence-based strategies within the literature for bringing mental health and health disciplines together to improve mental health and well-being (Przybylko et al. 2021).

In a scoping review conducted by Greidanus et al. (2020), the role of professional counselling and clinical counselling psychology in collaborative models of mental health care were explored. The study was conducted to address a gap in practice knowledge to support collaborative practice models for certified counsellors and/or psychologists, indicating that much of the focus has been on collaboration among mental health professionals more broadly (e.g., psychiatric nurses and social workers). A total of 40 studies were included in the review and results suggested that collaborative practice in mental health care provides value for clients. Collaborative practice considerations included (1) ethical considerations; (2) professional scope of practice and competencies; and (3) common codes of conduct. Similar barriers to collaboration were identified as mentioned earlier in the chapter e.g., territorial issues, philosophical differences, lack of time, and standards of confidentiality. Regarding implications for practice, the authors stated that collaborative practice in counselling needs clear leadership in terms of practice guidelines for shared documentation and that consultation should be incorporated into education as a core competency.

Although little is offered on how to operationalize interprofessional care models with measurable outcomes, psychiatric mental health care nurses and nurse psychotherapists are well-positioned to be influential in the development of models that can potentially eliminate treatment barriers and promote well-being (Ellis and Alexander 2016). As stated by Ellis and Alexander (2016), nurses are the gatekeepers of today's healthcare system, and have the opportunities to collaborate, integrate, and expand services by integrating education, practice, research, and policy shifts, by way of their engagement with their professional counterparts. Beyond collaboration, integrating care requires "an interdisciplinary, nonhierarchical blending of conventional, complementary, and alternative approaches that relies on a seamless continuum of decision-making, person-centered approaches, and structural support" (Ellis and Alexander 2016, p. 4). Research suggests that the optimal role for mental health nurses and nurse psychotherapists is to integrate their knowledge and skills with other allied health professionals to expand mental health services that facilitate growth on a much larger scale (Tsiachristas et al. 2011).

5 Reflective Questions

1. How do interprofessional and integrated approaches to psychotherapy differ from traditional, single-discipline approaches, and what advantages do they offer in promoting holistic patient care?
2. Reflect on your own role as a nurse psychotherapist. How might an interprofessional or integrated approach enhance your ability to provide comprehensive care to your clients or patients?
3. What are some common challenges or barriers that professionals face when attempting to implement interprofessional or integrated psychotherapy approaches, and how can these challenges be overcome?
4. Consider the benefits of information-sharing and communication among mental health professionals from various disciplines. How can improved communication lead to better patient outcomes?
5. Reflect on the ethical considerations discussed in the chapter related to interprofessional and integrated psychotherapy. How can professionals navigate issues such as confidentiality, informed consent, and professional boundaries within a team-based approach?
6. Think about the importance of cultural competence and diversity awareness in interprofessional and integrated psychotherapy. How can practitioners ensure that their approach is inclusive and sensitive to the diverse backgrounds and experiences of their clients?
7. Consider the potential benefits and challenges of incorporating technology and telehealth into interprofessional and integrated psychotherapy. How might these tools enhance or disrupt collaborative efforts among professionals?

8. Finally, consider any personal biases or assumptions you may have had about working collaboratively with professionals from other disciplines. Have your views evolved after reading this chapter, and if so, in what ways?

6 Case Vignette

Background: Sarah is a 35-year-old woman who recently lost her job as a software engineer due to company downsizing. She lives with her husband, John, and their two children, ages 8 and 10. Sarah has been experiencing symptoms of depression, including low energy, feelings of hopelessness, and difficulty sleeping. She also reports increased irritability and frequent crying spells. Sarah's husband, John, has noticed these changes and is concerned about her mental health.

Interprofessional Team:

Family Doctor–Dr. Daniel Miller

Psychiatrist–Dr. Emily Reynolds

Registered Nurse Psychotherapist–Lisa Carter, RN

Social Worker–Michael Anderson, MSW

Scenario:

Sarah has sought help from her family doctor, Dr. Daniel Miller, after experiencing these symptoms for several months. Dr. Miller has conducted a thorough physical examination and ruled out any underlying medical conditions. Concerned about Sarah's mental health, Dr. Miller decided to initiate an interprofessional approach to her care.

Dr. Daniel Miller, Family Doctor, assists with coordinating care and referrals among the various healthcare providers, prescribing medication as needed and providing follow-up to Sarah during the treatment process. Dr. Miller refers Sarah to a psychiatrist, Dr. Emily Reynolds, for a comprehensive psychiatric evaluation to determine the severity of her depression and potential medication management. Dr. Miller also refers Sarah to Lisa Carter, an RN Psychotherapist, who will provide individual therapy sessions to help Sarah explore her thoughts and feelings, develop coping strategies, and work on improving her emotional well-being. Lisa Carter identifies the need for family support and requests that Michael Anderson, a social worker, join the interprofessional approach to aid in assessing the family dynamics and providing support and resources to Sarah's husband, John, and their children. Michael also works with Sarah on developing a holistic care plan that addresses the social and environmental factors contributing to her depression.

6.1 Case Vignette Reflective Questions

1. How can the interprofessional team collaborate effectively to provide comprehensive care for Sarah's mental health needs while also considering the well-being of her family?
2. How can the nurse psychotherapist best work within this interprofessional team to best meet Sarah's goals around her depression?
3. How might the social worker address the family's concerns and provide them with resources and support to cope with Sarah's depression?
4. What ethical considerations should the team be mindful of, such as patient confidentiality and informed consent, as they work together to develop and implement Sarah's care plan?
5. How can the interprofessional team involve Sarah and her family in the decision-making process to ensure that the care plan is patient-centered and aligns with their goals and preferences?
6. What strategies can the team use to monitor Sarah's progress and adjust the treatment plan as needed to achieve the best possible outcomes for her mental health?
7. How might cultural competence and sensitivity be important in this case, considering Sarah's background and the potential impact on her treatment and recovery?

7 Summary

- There is a growing need for interprofessional approaches to practices as the potential benefits for both patients and practitioners/organizations are well documented in the literature.
- Improved quality of care and decreased cost of care delivery are two of the potential benefits that motivate researchers and professionals to move towards interprofessional care.
- Barriers and facilitators to implementing interprofessional practice approaches at the interpersonal, organizational, and systemic levels, are also well documented by researchers.
- Although there is consensus that the development of interprofessional practice competencies must begin in education for nurses and other health professionals, education continues to primarily take place in silos with discipline-specific curriculum.
- Psychotherapy training and education in undergraduate curricula have the ability to break down these silos and exist with consistency permeating silos across multiple disciplines.
- A willingness from allied health professionals to engage in interprofessional collaboration is a starting point for true interprofessional/interdisciplinary care.

- Factors such as inadequate communication, lack of respect and trust, unequal power, and role confusion can create significant barriers at the interpersonal level.
- A lack of time and core structures allowing for interprofessional practice create very real challenges in the workforce.
- Despite these challenges, nurse psychotherapists are well-positioned to encourage and support interprofessional practice and to address the structural and organizational challenges that are slowing our progress toward interprofessional care.

References

Boix-Mansilla, V., & Gardner, H. (2003). Assessing interdisciplinary work at the frontier. An empirical exploration of 'symptoms of quality.' *Interdisciplines: Rethinking Interdisciplinarity, Paper, 6*(6), 1.

Bridges, Diane R., Davidson, R. A., Soule Odegard, P., Maki, I. V., & Tomkowiak, J. (2011). Interprofessional collaboration: Three best practice models of interprofessional education. *Medical Education Online, 16*(1), 6035. https://doi.org/10.3402/meo.v16i0.6035.

D'Amour, D., & Oandasan, I. (2005). Interprofessionality as the field of interprofessional practice and interprofessional education: An emerging concept. *Journal of Interprofessional Care, 19 Suppl 1*, 8–20. https://doi.org/10.1080/13561820500081604.

Ellis, H., & Alexander, V. (2016). Eradicating barriers to mental health care through integrated service models: Contemporary perspectives for psychiatric-mental health nurses. *Archives of Psychiatric Nursing, 30*(3), 432–438. https://doi.org/10.1016/j.apnu.2016.01.004.

Farrell, T. W., Luptak, M. K., Supiano, K. P., Pacala, J. T., & Lisser, R. (2018). State of the science: Interprofessional approaches to aging, dementia, and mental health. *Journal of the American Geriatrics Society, 66*, S40–S47. https://doi.org/10.1111/jgs.15309.

Frodeman, R., & Klein, J. T. (2017). Interdisciplining Humanities. In R. Frodeman, J. Klein, & R. C.S. Pacheeco (Eds.). *The Oxford Handbook of Interdisciplinarity* (pp. 144–156). Oxford University Press.

Greidanus, E., Warren, C., Harris, G. E., & Umetsubo, Y. (2020). Collaborative practice in counselling: A scoping review. *Journal of Interprofessional Care, 34*(3), 353–361. https://doi.org/10.1080/13561820.2019.1637334.

Jacobs, J. A. (2017). The need for disciplines in the modern research university. In R. Frodeman, J. Klein, & R. C. S. Pacheeco (Eds.).*The Oxford Handbook of Interdisciplinarity* (pp. 35–39). Oxford University Press. https://doi.org/10.1093/oxfordhb/9780198733522.013.4.

Klein, J. T. (2005). *Humanities, culture, and interdisciplinarity: The changing American academy*. SUNY Press.

Klein, J. T. (2017). Typologies of Interdisciplinarity. In R. Frodeman, J. Klein, & R. C.S. Pacheeco (Eds.).*The Oxford Handbook of Interdisciplinarity* (pp. 21–34). Oxford University Press. https://doi.org/10.1093/oxfordhb/9780198733522.013.3.

Korazim-Kőrösy, Y., Mizrahi, T., Bayne-Smith, M., & Garcia, M. L. (2014). Professional determinants in community collaborations: Interdisciplinary comparative perspectives on roles and experiences among six disciplines. *Journal of Community Practice, 22*(1/2), 229–255. https://doi.org/10.1080/10705422.2014.901267.

Moran, J. (2008). *Interdisciplinarity*. Taylor & Francis.

Nancarrow, S. A., Booth, A., Ariss, S., Smith, T., Enderby, P., & Roots, A. (2013). Ten principles of good interdisciplinary team work. *Human Resources for Health, 11*, 19. https://doi.org/10.1186/1478-4491-11-19.

Przybylko, G., Morton, D. P., & Renfrew, M. E. (2021). Addressing the COVID-19 mental health crisis: A perspective on using interdisciplinary universal interventions. *Frontiers in Psychology, 12*. https://www.frontiersin.org/articles/10.3389/fpsyg.2021.644337.

Rawlinson, C., Carron, T., Cohidon, C., Arditi, C., Hong, Q. N., Pluye, P., Peytremann-Bridevaux, I., & Gilles, I. (2021). An overview of reviews on interprofessional collaboration in primary care: Barriers and facilitators. *International Journal of Integrated Care, 21*(2), 32. https://doi.org/10.5334/ijic.5589.

Repko, A. F. (2005). *Interdisciplinary practice: A student guide to research and writing*. Pearson.

Repko, A. F. (2008). *Interdisciplinary research: Process and theory*. Sage.

San Martín-Rodríguez, L., Beaulieu, M.-D., D'Amour, D., & Ferrada-Videla, M. (2005). The determinants of successful collaboration: A review of theoretical and empirical studies. *Journal of Interprofessional Care, 19 Suppl 1*, 132–147. https://doi.org/10.1080/13561820500082677.

Sargeant, J., Loney, E., & Murphy, G. (2008). Effective interprofessional teams: "Contact is not enough" to build a team. *The Journal of Continuing Education in the Health Professions, 28*(4), 228–234. https://doi.org/10.1002/chp.189.

Schwartz, L., Wright, D., & Lavoie-Tremblay, M. (2011). New nurses' experience of their role within interprofessional health care teams in mental health. *Archives of Psychiatric Nursing, 25*(3), 153–163. https://doi.org/10.1016/j.apnu.2010.08.001.

Shailer, K. (2005). *Interdisciplinarity in a disciplinary universe: A review of key issues*. Ontario College of Art & Design. http://www.cou.on.ca.

Stehr, N., & Weingart, P. (2000). *Practising interdisciplinarity*. University of Toronto Press.

Tsiachristas, A., Hipple-Walters, B., Lemmens, K. M. M., Nieboer, A. P., & Rutten-van Mölken, M. P. M. H. (2011). Towards integrated care for chronic conditions: Dutch policy developments to overcome the (financial) barriers. *Health Policy, 101*(2), 122–132. https://doi.org/10.1016/j.healthpol.2010.10.013.

Turner, S. (2017). Knowledge Formations: An Analytic Framework. In R. Frodeman, J. Klein, & R. C.S. Pacheeco (Eds.), *The Oxford Handbook of Interdisciplinarity* (2nd ed.) (pp. 9–20). Oxford University Press.

Chapter 21
Nurse Psychotherapists as Autonomous Mental Health Providers: Advocating for Change

Sabrina Merali and Irmajean Bajnok

Abstract In Canada, as in other jurisdictions, the complexity of the healthcare system, care delivery, emerging healthcare needs, and demographics impacted by aging populations and immigration policies are influencing the need for advanced education and expanded roles for nurses. The scope of practice and educational pre-licensure requirements for nurses has incrementally evolved and expanded. While driven by healthcare needs, scope of practice changes, like any change, are impacted by many factors—stakeholder acceptance, safety considerations, felt need, and political will. Expanded scope of practice has thus been authorized by regulators and governments, only after intense advocacy related policy initiatives that reinforce the need for such a service, the cost quality benefits of such a service, and the ability of nurses to provide the service have been demonstrated. In Ontario, this was the case for the authorization of nurses to be included in those able to perform the controlled act of psychotherapy. This chapter explores key elements that are part of a successful advocacy strategy to enable autonomous roles in nursing, in this case, nurse psychotherapy. These elements include visionary leadership, strategic advocacy, education, regulation and standards. Nurses themselves often lead such advocacy initiatives through specialty interest groups, and/or their professional associations.

Keywords Advocacy · Autonomous practice · Insurance coverage · Collaboration · Leadership competencies

S. Merali (✉)
Registered Nurses' Association of Ontario (RNAO), Toronto, ON, Canada
e-mail: smerali@rnao.ca

I. Bajnok
Wounds Canada, North York, ON, Canada
e-mail: irmajean.bajnok@woundscanada.ca

S. Roles and K. Kalia (eds.), *The Nurses' Guide to Psychotherapy*,
https://doi.org/10.1007/978-981-97-4738-2_21

Learning Objectives

After completing this chapter, the learner will:

1. Analyze the role of advocacy for nurse psychotherapists.
2. Reflect on the leadership competencies necessary in achieving new scope of practice change and roles for nurses.
3. Identify the role of education and standards in enabling scope of practice changes.
4. Examine the autonomous nurse role within the context of Canada's publicly funded health system and the health insurance framework.
5. Showcase/demonstrate concepts through a review of an exemplar of how the RN psychotherapy role was embedded in regulation in a Canadian jurisdiction.

1 Introduction

The breadth of the work of Registered Nurses (RN) in all sectors of healthcare and all areas of health and illness is not often understood by members of the public, other health professions, and health-related partners (Almost 2021; Registered Nurses' Association of Ontario [RNAO] 2023; RNAO 2017). The nursing role and scope are well supported by the requirement of a nursing baccalaureate as entry to practice throughout Canada with the exception of Quebec. This entry-to-practice requirement, in place for almost two decades, was necessitated by the increasingly complex health system and the focus of the nursing role across the health continuum, as delineated in the Canadian Council of Registered Nurse Regulators (CCRNR) Entry-Level Competencies for the Practice of Registered Nurses (Canadian Council of RN Regulators 2018). The practice experience and expectations in nursing are extensive—fully reinforcing nursing as a practice discipline. Given this background, in many jurisdictions RNs have been authorized by the nursing regulatory body to take on increasing scopes of practice (Canadian Institute for Health Information 2022). In some cases, this expanded scope of practice has been sanctioned by regulators and governments only after intense advocacy and related policy initiatives that reinforce the need for such a service, its cost-quality benefits, and the ability of RNs to provide the service. In Ontario, this was the case for the authorization of nurse psychotherapy.

In 2018, the College of Nurses of Ontario, responding to intense advocacy by the Registered Nurses' Association of Ontario (RNAO), the professional association for RNs, NPs, and nursing students, introduced regulations to authorize both RNs and RPNs to provide the controlled act of psychotherapy. These regulations were approved by the government in December 2019 (Government of Ontario 2019). This chapter will explore key elements that are part of successful advocacy to enable autonomous roles in nursing, in this case, nurse psychotherapy. These elements include visionary leadership, strategic advocacy, education, and standards.

RNAO has a long history of speaking out for nursing and speaking out for health care (RNAO 2021). It is recognized as an extremely successful voluntary professional organization with close to 52,000 members, over 40% of the number of RNs and NPs registered in Ontario. RNAO provides an unmatched library of resources to enable evidence-based practice including: evidence-based guides for nurses in their practice through the world-renowned Best Practice Guidelines, programs and supports for organizations to assist nurses to implement and sustain best practices, and tools to measure organization, practitioner, and client outcomes of evidence-based practice. In addition, RNAO has, through its almost 100 years of existence, honed a successful approach to influencing healthy public policy. This dual mission of the association has enabled RNAO, as a visionary leader, to successfully advocate for initiatives that advance nursing practice and benefits persons, their communities, and the health system.

RNAO uses key advocacy domains outlined in RNAO's Framework for Advancing Healthy Public Policy Planning Template (Grinspun et al. 2018), adapted from Grinspun (2007), to garner stakeholder attention and engagement through letters, submissions, proposals, reports, and the media. This framework for advancing healthy public policy guided RNAO's work in advocating for RN psychotherapy as outlined in the Ontario RN Psychotherapy Exemplar in Appendix A. Use of the framework was augmented by the four elements of the advocacy strategy; visionary leadership, strategic advocacy, education, and standards highlighted next in this chapter.

2 Visionary Leadership

Visionary leadership is a key component of successfully achieving an expanded scope of practice for nurses. Visionary leadership entails initiating and managing the change processes, and creating momentum (social movement), for the change. It is not enough that nurses understand the need for scope expansion, it is imperative that the public, and key decision-makers be brought on board to be aware of the need for the change, its impact, and why it is important that it be adopted. For example, advocating for an expanded scope of practice and autonomy for nurses would require sharing the healthcare need and overall value for the health of the public to gain their support.

3 Strategic Advocacy

According to the World Health Organization's (2005) definition, advocacy combines individual and social actions to gain political and community support for a specific goal. Advocacy implies speaking for someone or something, and in the context of the health system, it relates to creating conditions that promote health. Some of the components of successful strategic advocacy include clear messaging, appropriate timing, client-centred approaches, passion, and persistence.

All of these components help frame the why, who, when, how, and where the advocacy action is carried out. RNAO's *Leading Change Toolkit* (RNAO and Healthcare Excellence Canada, 2021) outlines distinct approaches to gaining momentum in advocacy action. *Clear messaging* defines the why, the target of the advocacy (who has decision-making authority), and who is the beneficiary. The messaging must be soundly understood by both those advocating for the change and the target audience and must be based on evidence and shared in a consistent manner. In selecting targets it is important to work first with networks built over time, where there is respect and acknowledgement of past credible advocacy work. Throughout its almost 100-year history, RNAO garners such relationships and networks, that continues to support its advocacy initiatives.

Numerous advocacy initiatives have failed because of poor timing. Framing the focus of the advocacy as a needed and evidence-based solution to a current issue in healthcare provides greater possibilities for success. In the case of RN psychotherapy, in the post-COVID context, there was a strong opportunity to link RN scope of practice to address the myriad of gaps in mental health care at the jurisdiction and national levels (Canadian Nurses Association 2024; Canadian Mental Health Association 2023). Successful advocacy messaging in nursing always *puts the client first*. Self-serving advocacy is often viewed with suspicion, therefore,it behooves healthcare advocates to shape their messaging to demonstrate how decisions affecting practitioners will benefit clients, families, and populations. Building the social movement to mobilize change is fuelled by knowledge and evidence as well as *passion and persistence*. Strategic advocacy takes time to build and sustain the social movement for change; therefore, advocates leading change need patience and unwavering passion to keep the vision alive and advancing. RNAO has employed these key components in the journey to support RN psychotherapy.

3.1 Advocacy and Context of the Role

In the case of nurse psychotherapy in Ontario, RNAO garnered full support from RNs who were currently engaged in or preparing to be engaged in psychotherapy work as part of their nursing practice. This included affirming their commitment to speak out and share stories, describe its impact, and reinforce the value-added so that clients, the government, the regulatory college, and other health partners, were informed. Given nursing is a regulated health profession, changes in the scope of practice require changes in jurisdictional nursing regulations that must be approved by the nursing regulatory body and the government, and then communicated widely to ensure awareness and acceptance of the new scope of practice for nurses. RNAO's advocacy also involved working closely with the nursing regulatory body and government decision-makers (See Table 1).

Table 1 RNAO's framework for advancing healthy public policy planning template

Pillars	Stages/domains of action	Examples of evidence used in RNAO policy work
Evidence	Statistics	Amendments to the regulated health professions act
	Policy papers	RNAO nursing career pathways, 2023 (Policy reports I RNAO.ca) RNAO nursing through crisis, 2022 (Policy reports I RNAO.ca) RNAO Mind the safety gap in health system transformation-2016 I RNAO.ca
	Best practice guidelines	Assessment and Intervention for perinatal depression, 2018 Crisis intervention for adults using a trauma-informed approach: initial four weeks of management, 2017 Engaging clients who use substances, 2015 Person and family centred care, 2015
Advocacy	Knowledge mobilization	Letters to CNO re initiation and continuation of nurse psychotherapy
	Communication and grassroots mobilization	Letters to MOH: re: nurse initiation of psychotherapy Meetings with CNO and MOH re nurse psychotherapy
	Advocacy resolutions	Action alerts for members regarding CNO regulation changes Media: social media
	Coalition building Mass media and social media	Annual general meeting (AGM): resolutions regarding nurse psychotherapy (RNAO mental health and substance use best practices program I RNAO.ca)
	Direct advocacy with politicians and civil servants	RNAO mental health nurses interest group (MHNIG) resolution to advocate for accessibility to psychotherapy through billing insurances (2018) RNAO, MHNIG, and the nurse psychotherapy association, the groups have jointly developed, and provided to the CNO, practice standards for adoption by CNO (Nurse Psychotherapist Association of Ontario 2022)

4 Importance of Education, Regulation and Standards in Autonomous Practice

RNs, as all regulated professionals across jurisdictions in Canada, have a breadth of practice that is dictated and governed by standards, however, because nursing is a self-regulated profession, the regulation is by nurses through a jurisdictional nursing regulatory body (Almost 2021). The expectation is that regulated health professionals practice in areas where they feel confident and possess the knowledge, skills, and judgment to do so. In some cases, regulatory bodies or other specialty groups develop standards to guide the extended scope of practice. Such standards provide practitioners with support in determining their skill level in the area, and/or achieving the expected level of competency to practice the expanded scope skills.

Nurse psychotherapy as a controlled act is a skill that must be supported by additional knowledge in the area and opportunities to acquire skills and judgment through supervised practice. In nursing, the basic baccalaureate programs provide RNs with a foundation of mental health enabling them to be adept at counselling and, with experience, some acts of psychotherapy, not unlike many of the other regulated colleges who can perform the controlled act of psychotherapy. In Ontario, the controlled act of psychotherapy has a specific definition, and requires additional knowledge and practice.

The CNO (2023) describes levels of counselling and psychotherapy. All nurses engage in interventions such as health teaching, motivating, giving information and instruction, counselling, and providing evidence to support decision-making. Some nurses provide psychotherapy and only those nurses with specific knowledge skills and judgment are performing the controlled act of psychotherapy, as described above.

Nurse psychotherapy specialty groups and RNAO's Mental Health Nurses Interest Group (MHNIG) developed standards that are generally followed by nurses who call themselves *Nurse Psychotherapists* (Nurse Psychotherapy Association of Ontario 2022; RNAO and Nurse Psychotherapy Association of Ontario 2022).

As is the case for all nurses, those practicing psychotherapy must keep abreast of new knowledge, and maintain a skill level in working with a variety of clients and families. The hallmark of a professional nurse is their attention to the maintenance of competence through education, reflective practice, and supervision, which must be demonstrated annually on re-registration.

In many jurisdictions, some sectors have policies that restrict nurses from engaging in non-traditional roles, in an autonomous way. For example, in Ontario, through the Public Hospitals Act (1990), employers sanction the scope of practice of nurses in their settings and may not allow RNs to practice psychotherapy as part of their role. RN psychotherapy in Ontario is therefore implemented largely in community settings not under the jurisdiction of the Public Hospitals Act. Many RN psychotherapists turn to working in independent practice roles requiring business acumen and a clear understanding of practice and regulatory limitations.

In most jurisdictions, there are no funding models for clients to receive publicly funded care and service from nurses in independent practice in non-traditional roles that are within their scope of practice. Funding models enabling not-for-profit publicly funded access to these services are not available which is a challenge in relation to mental health services where the excessive needs could be met by available nurse psychotherapists. Clearly, further advocacy is needed to advance not-for-profit funding models for nursing practice roles that increase access to much-needed mental health services.

Some nurses practicing psychotherapy in Ontario, as independent practitioners provide this service to clients funded through their health insurance benefits. However, many insurance carriers may not be aware of the nurses' ability to provide psychotherapy, and/or are not supportive of nurses in this psychotherapy role. Some insurance companies identify that they are looking for clearer indication of the legitimacy of the RN psychotherapy role. Advocacy and public awareness regarding the role and competency of the nurse psychotherapist must include insurance carriers to help mitigate this access barrier to the public.

5 Present State and Next Steps Related to Expanded Scope of RN Practice

Acknowledgement of the nurse psychotherapy role by insurance companies and others has been an ongoing advocacy initiative that has existed in Ontario for over a decade. It is clearly not over, and requires continued vigilance, incorporation of new partners, and enduring advocacy.

At this time in Ontario, RNAO along with the RNAO MHNIG, the Canadian Federation of Mental Health Nurses and other nurse psychotherapy stakeholder groups are collaborating to move the needle on acceptance of nurse psychotherapists. The goal is that nurses are fully acknowledged as a health profession regulated by the CNO who have the authority to provide psychotherapy on the continuum extending from counselling, to the controlled act of psychotherapy.

Current plans include developing a public awareness campaign regarding the need for mental health and psychotherapy interventions, identifying the limited access to publicly funded services, and highlighting the critical role nurses can play in closing the gaps related to access to psychotherapy. Through mobilization and full acceptance of the role, nurse psychotherapists can make a positive impact on the mental health of the population.

6 Reflective Questions

1. How do you, or could you, advocate for your role as a nurse psychotherapist?
2. What are the next steps that could be taken in your setting to better spotlight the role of nurses in psychotherapy?
3. How can you use the example of Ontario to help make changes in your jurisdiction?
4. What evidence could be used to support greater acceptance and understanding of nurse psychotherapy in your setting?
5. Consider what needs to change at the local, organizational, and jurisdictional levels to better integrate the role of nurse psychotherapists.

7 Summary

- Building and advancing expanded roles for nurses will not happen without visionary leadership, sharp advocacy skills, showcasing new roles as timely population health solutions, and incorporating education and standards to foster role competence and acceptance.
- Consistently and passionately actioning these advocacy strategies to engage a wide range of partners in generating a social movement for the change will, over time, result in success.

Appendix A

Exemplar Showcasing Ontario's Experience of Advocating for RN Psychotherapy

This exemplar showcases the Ontario experience of advocating for RN psychotherapy over a period of almost two decades. The lessons learned can be used by other jurisdictions to advance changes to enable this much needed role for the Canadian public and fully utilize the skills of registered nurses. The exemplar will address the situation from the following perspectives:

- Change in Regulation;
- CNO actions on controlled act for nurse psychotherapy;
- RNAO response to advocate for RNs to initiate and practice psychotherapy;
- Need for standards;
- Advocacy: The way forward.

Psychotherapy: Change in the Regulated Health Professions Act

Years 2001 to 2005

In March 2001, the Health Professions Regulatory Advisory Council (HPRAC) undertook a review of the Regulated Health Professions Act (RHPA) and made recommendations to amend the RHPA to list psychotherapy as a controlled act. The committee defined psychotherapy as "an intense client-therapist relationship which often involves the examination of deeply emotional experiences, destructive behaviour patterns and serious mental health issues" (Health Professions Regulatory Advisory Council 2006) recognizing that, if administered properly, psychotherapy can be performed by trained and skilled professionals, including Registered Nurses

(RN). Psychotherapy is a highly complex form of treatment that requires corresponding expertise and skilled application of knowledge. RNs, the single largest group of healthcare professionals in the province, can have a huge impact on the lives of people who require psychotherapy, if authorized to perform this vital service.

Upon the release of the recommendation from HPRAC, RNAO publicly declared its support of the recommendation and the fundamental concepts that underlie the legislation–protection of the public and self-regulation. "Psychotherapy Recommendation #6: RNAO recommends that the performance of psychotherapy be regulated utilizing the most appropriate legislative strategy and that RNs with the required qualifications have the regulatory authority to practice it" (RNAO 2005). In their 2005 submission to HPRAC, RNAO indicated there is serious risk of harm to clients from psychotherapy. As a result, it is in the public interest to regulate this practice so that potential harm to the public is minimized. Any regulation of psychotherapy must take into account the diverse needs of marginalized communities and maintain access to services for those communities. RNAO advocated that RNs and NPs should have the authority to perform these acts within the nursing scope of practice based on their knowledge, skill, and experience. This would ensure timely access to care, reduce the need for delegation, and support the progression of care management in a timely way.

In April 2006, HPRAC's final report to the Ministry of Health and Long-Term Care, provided recommendations to mandate regulation of psychotherapy and psychotherapists under the RHPA, citing that a controlled act would "provide the highest level of regulation and public protection. HPRAC recommended an "enforceable scope of practice" and defined psychotherapy as "the provision of a psychological intervention or interventions delivered through a therapeutic relationship for the treatment of cognitive, emotional or behavioural disturbances" (RNAO 2006). HPRAC further advised that the regulatory colleges develop, implement and enforce their own minimum qualifications and standards of practice specific to psychotherapy. "If they fail to do so, their members would be required to adhere to standards of College of Psychotherapists." (RNAO 2006).

RNAO applauded this decision to regulate psychotherapy as it supports a number of important objectives including: protecting the public from harm; ensuring access to psychotherapeutic services for the population; providing for existing professional colleges to set standards and educational requirements for psychotherapy; and, eliminating dual registration for professionals with the new College of Psychotherapy as well as their own colleges (RNAO 2006). RNAO's advocacy also recommended that the definition of psychotherapy be amended to include the vital role of psychotherapy in health promotion and disease prevention areas. RNAO's advocacy requested an amendment to the proposed Sect. 8 (1) of the Psychotherapy Act enabling other professionals who can perform the act-physicians, occupational therapists and social workers- also regulated under the Psychotherapy Act to use the title "psychotherapist" or "registered mental health therapist" (RNAO 2007).

In June 2007, Bill 171, which supported a Psychotherapy Act received royal assent. This means that the practice of psychotherapy was subject to the terms, conditions and limitations of the health professionals' certificate of registration. In

2009, the Regulated Health Professions Statute Law Amendment Act amended the RHPA to create the legislative framework enabling these changes. Further changes to the Nursing Act as well as the RHPA were made and provided instructions on the use of the title "psychotherapist" to qualified members of the specified colleges, including the College of Nurses of Ontario, as well as the inclusion of the controlled act of psychotherapy within their scope of practice. Thus, in 2009, psychotherapy was authorized as part of the scope of practice of RNs and Nurse Practitioners (NP).

The College of Nurses of Ontario: Nurse Psychotherapy–the Controlled Act

The CNO Decision Re: The Need for an Order for Nurses to Perform Psychotherapy

In March 2014, the CNO carried a motion that required RNs and Registered Practical Nurses (RPN) to obtain an order to perform the controlled act of psychotherapy. This meant that RNs and RPNs no longer had the autonomy to perform psychotherapy to those who required it, but rather needed the order of a physician or NP to initiate it. RNAO advocacy efforts were in favour of nurses having the authority to continue to make an autonomous, independent decision to initiate psychotherapy without a physician's order. When probed on this decision, CNO stated that "the theoretical and clinical components required to safely perform the controlled act of psychotherapy are not included in basic nursing programs at this time" and stated that the perceived vague definition of psychotherapy in legislation and the assertion that psychotherapy is a high-risk activity demonstrates the need for nurses to be cautious and to receive an order. The CNO failed to demonstrate how they arrived at these conclusions.

RNAO raised objections to CNOs request, stating that RNs needed to be consulted in these decisions. Furthermore, RNAO reinforced that RNs understand their responsibilities as professionals and could hone their knowledge, skills, and judgment to effectively and safely practice psychotherapy, should they be lacking skills in this area (RNAO 2014a). RNAO stressed that the nurse must be competent and accountable to initiate psychotherapy or assess and refer the individual for more appropriate treatment and/or to another health care provider. It is always the responsibility of a regulated health professional to know the limits of their abilities and work collaboratively with other members of the interprofessional team in providing appropriate client-centred care (RNAO 2014b).

The CNO's requirement that nurses obtain an order to initiate psychotherapy provided a lot of concerns. (1) Nurses who were already initiating psychotherapy were worried about the limits of their practice. (2) The CNO decision would disrupt and threaten the continuity of care of clients already in a psychotherapeutic relationship with an RN since requiring an order could delay access to mental health services, especially in rural and remote communities. (3) Some nurses, fearful of inadvertently engaging in the controlled act of psychotherapy without an order, may self-limit their nursing practice, further limiting access to care. (4) Nurses with specialized skills and training, felt devalued, deskilled, and demoralized about the lack of recognition for their expertise. This compounded the severe mental health access issues for the public (RNAO 2014b).

Standards and Regulations to Support Nurse Psychotherapy

It is interesting to note that HPRAC never made any recommendations regarding the need for a physician's order to initiate psychotherapy, rather they indicated "that the Colleges of regulated professionals who practice psychotherapy (the Colleges of Psychologists, Social Workers and Social Service Workers, Nurses, and Physicians and Surgeons) develop, implement and enforce their own minimum qualifications and standards of practice specific to psychotherapy" (RNAO 2014b). Given this, RNAO, alongside the RNAO Mental Health Nursing Interest Group (MHNIG), advocated for the CNO to focus its attention on the development of standards of practice and regulations for psychotherapy for nurses, including recognition of the educational preparation and expertise required. Furthermore, the MHNIG offered to collaborate with the CNO in developing standards and regulations by outlining the knowledge, skill, and experience required to perform the controlled act of psychotherapy (RNAO 2014). To date, the CNO has not proceeded to develop standards citing this as an entry-level nursing competency that can be further addressed by nursing specialty groups in this area. The lack of recognized standards remains a challenge for nurse psychotherapists in their quest for full integration as part of a transformed health system.

RNAO Advocacy Response to Allow RNs to Initiate and Continue Psychotherapy

Despite advocacy efforts, from 2014 to 2018, the CNO remained steadfast on its decision, that RNs and RPNs would require an order for any controlled act unless there is a CNO regulation for initiation in place. Based on surveys and focus groups with nurses who were performing psychotherapy, the CNO determined many of the nurses were performing interventions that would not fall under the legislative definition of psychotherapy. Therefore, the CNO concluded an order to perform these activities was not required. The CNO also ascertained clients with "such a serious health issue" requiring psychotherapy would benefit from care provided by an MD or NP, not an RN or RPN.

RNAO continued to advocate for a CNO regulation to authorize RN initiation of psychotherapy, given the competency of nurses and the need for access to psychotherapy services. RNAO requested meetings with the CNO and the CNO council to discuss the alarming impacts of this decision on public safety. In March

2015, a meeting was held with CNO, however, the college held steadfast on their decision, citing a lack of evidence.

In 2016, RNAO continued to advocate for nurses through letter-writing campaigns, as well as meeting with John Fraiser (then Parliamentary assistant to the Minister of Health) to reinforce the need for access to psychotherapy and the active role RNs can play in treating mental health conditions. Advocacy efforts also stressed the need for clarity around why other regulated professions such as occupational therapists, social workers and social services workers, psychotherapists, psychologists, nurse practitioners and physicians, could initiate psychotherapy while RNs were limited in their scope of practice. RNAO's incessant advocacy stressed that CNO is abdicating responsibility for an element of nursing practice that a subset of nurses already have the competency to perform.

There was considerable activity among all partners in 2017:

- RNAO released an action alert to urge CNO to allow RNs to continue to initiate the controlled act of psychotherapy independently, given that the Ontario government was going to proclaim this new controlled act on December 31, 2017
- Then Minister of Health, Eric Hoskins, wrote to the CNO president requesting CNO authorize RNs to initiate this controlled act
- HPRAC sought feedback from partners about the controlled act of psychotherapy.
- Throughout this period, RNAO continued to provide recommendations including:
  - The need for a clear definition that incorporates a wellness approach to psychotherapy;
  - Approval for members of the six colleges to use the term 'psychotherapist' without having dual membership with the College of Registered Psychotherapists;
  - Authority for registrants of the six colleges to initiate the controlled act of psychotherapy without seeking permission from another provider.

At the end of 2017, psychotherapy was proclaimed a controlled act, and health providers from the six disciplines were granted a two-year exemption period to allow professionals to become regulated with one of the six colleges. The September 2018 CNO council meeting was presented with an analysis of the level of risk associated with RNs and RPNs performing the controlled act of psychotherapy without an order. At this time the Council directed that a draft regulation be written for government approval to authorize RNs and RPNs to independently perform (e.g., without an order) the controlled act of psychotherapy as of January 1, 2020, after the exemption period. At the end of 2018, the College developed and sought feedback about proposed regulatory changes to the controlled act. The proposed changes would have allowed RNs and RPNs to independently initiate the controlled act of psychotherapy without an order, where not prohibited by legislation.

RNAO publicly supported the proposed regulation change and launched an Action Alert campaign to mobilize members to respond to the proposed regulation changes. In March 2019, the CNO approved the amendments to the regulation authorizing RNs and RPNs to perform the controlled act of psychotherapy without an order, unless prohibited by other legislation such as the Public Hospitals Act. This came into effect January, 1, 2020, following the two-year exemption period ending December 31, 2019.

Given the changes from the CNO, RNAOs advocacy efforts pivoted to now focus on removing the legislative impediments to RN initiation and delivery of psychotherapy. Amendments to legislation, including but not limited to the Public Hospitals Act and the Health Promotion and Protection Act, would ensure that RNs are able to practice to their full scope across all healthcare settings (e.g. hospital settings, remote nursing stations and community settings attached to hospitals). RNAO alongside the MHNIG, met with the Health Workforce Regulatory Oversight Department of the Ontario Ministry of Health and discussed barriers present in legislation for this scope. By Oct 2019, the Ministry requested consultation on the regulatory changes. RNAO was pleased to learn from the Ministry of Health later that year, that psychotherapy is not considered a "treatment" under the Public Hospitals Act and thus the Public Hospitals Act is not a barrier to RN psychotherapy in hospitals.

The Road Ahead: Advocacy Efforts to Support the Spread and Scale up of Psychotherapy

Great successes were made through advocacy efforts of the RNAO and its partners to ensure that the controlled act of psychotherapy is widely accepted to be within the scope of nursing, where nurses can initiate and continue this practice. However, our advocacy efforts don't stop here. RNAO and its partners need to continue to focus on the spread and scale of nurse psychotherapy, to further provide mental health support to Canadians who need it. Current wait lists and access to psychotherapy are long and limited; nurses, who are well trusted and instrumental in the lives of clients, are well situated to support the provision of psychotherapy to those who need it. Through the use of nurse psychotherapists, Canadians will have increased access to this needed resource, therefore decreasing the burden on the healthcare system. To ensure this practice is available to those who need it, RNAO and its partners pivoted their advocacy efforts to support nurse psychotherapists.

Some of these advocacy efforts, as discussed in this chapter, focus on developing standards of practice to clarify the role and guide nurse psychotherapists and public education for key partners including insurance carriers to enhance awareness and acceptance of nurse psychotherapists. This education is so that insurance providers will be able to fund nurses to provide this vital service to their clients. Incorporating RN psychotherapists as vital care providers can aid in addressing the burgeoning mental health needs across Canada.

Practice Standards

RNAOs long-standing advocacy in the area of psychotherapy, since 2014, has always included an element of the need for clear and consistent practice standards. Standards, as defined by the CNO "... outline the expectations for nurses that contribute to public protection. They inform nurses of their accountabilities and the public of what to expect of nurses" (CNO 2023, p. 1).

The development of standards for the act of psychotherapy will provide the nurse guidance with regard to the scope of practice and skill level, while also providing adequate protection for the public. The five other regulatory colleges–social workers and social service workers, occupational therapists, physicians and surgeons, psychologists and psychotherapists–whose members are authorized to provide psychotherapy, have clearly defined practice standards. However, there was an absence of CNO standards to support nurses who practice psychotherapy to govern their practice. Under the leadership of RNAO's Mental Health Nurses Interest Group and the Nurse Psychotherapy Association of Ontario, a jointly developed comprehensive set of guides for nurse psychotherapists was created. The purpose of these peer-reviewed standards is to 'ensure the safe, effective, and ethical delivery of psychotherapy services' and outlines the minimum expectations for nurses to provide competent and safe psychotherapy. The standards outline areas related to professionalism, scope of practice, title of the nurse psychotherapist, competence, supervision, consent, quality assurance, tele-practice, documentation, professional boundaries, discontinuation of service and responsible business management. These standards were presented to the CNO with a recommendation for adoption (Nurse Psychotherapist Association of Ontario 2022).

Insurance Coverage

RNAOs advocacy efforts have also ensured that accessibility to psychotherapy is available to all Ontarians who need it. An area of concern is with insurance providers. Currently, if a nurse independently offers psychotherapy, insurance companies oftentimes do not recognize nurse psychotherapy and therefore may deny benefit coverage for clients who are engaged in therapy. Insurance companies, including the Workplace Safety and Insurance Act (WSIB), Motor Vehicle Accident (MBA) and private insurance companies (Sunlife, Manulife, Great West Life) oftentimes do not allow for billing by any other regulated psychotherapy professionals except psychologists, registered psychotherapists, or social workers. This lack of acknowledgement of nurse psychotherapists from insurance providers, further limits access to funded mental health services making publicly funded wait lists long, private nurse psychotherapy services next to nonexistent and increased out-of-pocket costs for recipients of services.

In 2019, the MHNIG submitted a resolution to the RNAO Annual General Meeting calling for RNAOs advocacy efforts to support RNs and NPs who would be authorized to perform the controlled act of psychotherapy. This resolution has led to meetings with ministry officials, including the Minister of Health as well as insurance companies to advocate for the inclusion of nurse psychotherapy as a billable service.

How Can I Get Involved?

Supporting advocacy efforts to have nurse psychotherapists recognized for their vital work is critically important. Advocacy supports, such as talking about the vital role of nurse psychotherapists, joining letter-writing campaigns (i.e. action alerts) to provide your support, as well as talking to your local members of parliament, can help to create the change we need. For more information, please visit: RNAO Mental Health and Substance Use Best Practices Program I RNAO.ca.

References

Almost, J. (2021). *Regulated nursing in Canada: The landscape in 2021.* Canadian Nurses Association. https://www.cna-aiic.ca/en/nursing/regulated-nursing-in-canada.

Canadian Institute for Health Information. (2022). *Legislated scopes of practice across Canada: Registered nurses.* Author. https://www.cihi.ca/en/legislated-scopes-of-practice-across-canada-registered-nurses.

Canadian Mental Health Association. (2023). *Investing in Community: Submission to the Standing Committee on Finance in Advance of the 2024 Federal Budget.* Author. https://cmha.ca/brochure/investing-in-community/#:~:text=The%202023%20federal%20budget%20included,specialists%20into%20health%20service%20teams.

Canadian Nurses Association. (2024). *Mental Health.* Author. https://www.cna-aiic.ca/en/policy-advocacy/advocacy-priorities/mental-health.

College of Nurses of Ontario (2023). *Psychotherapy and the controlled act component of psychotherapy.* Author. https://www.cno.org/en/learn-about-standards-guidelines/educational-tools/ask-practice/aGrinspunnswers-to-your-questions-about-psychotherapy/.

College of Nurses of Ontario (2023). *Psychotherapy and the controlled act component of psychotherapy.* Author. https://www.cno.org/en/learn-about-standards-guidelines/educational-tools/ask-practice/answers-to-your-questions-about-psychotherapy/.

Canadian Council of RN Regulators (2018). *Entry-Level Competencies (ELCs) for the Practice of Registered Nurses (2018).* Author. https://www.ccrnr.ca/assets/ccrnr-rn-entry-level-competencies---2019.pdf.

Government of Ontario. (2019). *Ontario's Regulatory Registry. Iinitiation of Psychotherapy by Registered Nurses and Registered Practical Nurses.* https://www.ontariocanada.com/registry/view.do?postingId=30587&language=en.

Grinspun, D., Botros, M., Mulrooney, L.A., Mo, J, Sibbald, R.G. & Penny, T. (2018). Scaling deep to improve people's health: From evidence-based practice to evidence-based policy. In G. Grinspun and I. Bajnok (Eds.), *Transforming nursing through knowledge: Best practices for guideline development, implementation science, and evaluation* (pp.466-494). Sigma.

Grinspun, D. (2007, November). *Using evidence, politics, communications and media to shape health policy: A framework for action*{PowerPoint slides). Oral presentation at University of Ottawa, master's level nursing course, Policy, Political Action, and Change. Ottawa, ON.

Nurse Psychotherapy Association of Ontario. (2022). *Nurse Psychotherapy Standards of Practice*. Author. https://docs.google.com/document/d/1xrrGN-QtRfZbiUiH8KH4ATh09jZJsZtNtOsGbGZ3TGQ/edit.

Public Hospitals Act, R.S.O. 1990. https://www.ontario.ca/laws/statute/90p40.

Registered Nurses of Ontario. (2021). *RNAO InFocus. Registered Nurses, Clinical Nurse Specialists and RNAO*. Author. https://rnao.ca/in-focus/rns-cns-and-rnao.

Registered Nurses' Association of Ontario and Nurse Psychotherapy Association of Ontario. (2022). *Psychotherapy practice of the Nurse Psychotherapist*. Registered Nurses' Association of Ontario.

Registered Nurses' Association of Ontario. (October, 2005). *Review of the Legislative Framework: Submission to the Health Professions Regulatory Advisory Council*. Author. https://rnao.ca/sites/rnao-ca/files/storage/related/1535_RNAO_Submission_HPRAC.pdf.

Registered Nurses' Association of Ontario. (2006, June 29). *Letter and HPRAC Recommendation Feedback Form*. Author, https://rnao.ca/sites/rnao-ca/files/storage/related/1223_RNAO_Response_to_HPRAC_New_Directions.pdf.

Registered Nurses' Association of Ontario. (2007). *RNAO Submission on Bill 171: Health System Improvements Act to Standing Committee on Social Policy*. Author. https://rnao.ca/sites/rnao-ca/files/storage/related/3164_RNAO_-_Submission_on_Bill_171.pdf.

Registered Nurses' Association of Ontario. (2014a, September 3). *Letter to the College of Nurses of Ontario regarding Requiring an Order to Perform Psychotherapy*. Author. https://rnao.ca/sites/rnao-ca/files/RNAO_Letter_to_CNO_-_re_Requiring_an_order_to_perform_psychotherapy_-_Se_.pdf.

Registered Nurses' Association of Ontario. (2014b, November 19). *Letter to College of Nurses of Ontario regarding RNAO Recommendation to Rescind Requirement for Order to Perform Psychotherapy*. Author. https://rnao.ca/sites/rnao-ca/files/RNAO_to_CNO_psychotherapy_FINAL_nov_19_2014_1.pdf.

Registered Nurses' Association of Ontario. (2017). *70 Years of RN Effectiveness*. Author. https://rnao.ca/sites/rnao-ca/files/Backgrounder-_RN_effectiveness.pdf.

Registered Nurses' Association of Ontario. (2023). *Nursing Career Pathways*. Author. https://rnao.ca/media/3828/download.

Registered Nurses' Association of Ontario and Healthcare Excellence Canada. (2021). *Leading change toolkit* (3rd ed.). Author. https://rnao.ca/leading-change-toolkit.

World Health Organization (2005). "Introduction to Toolkit". From Health Service Planning and Policy-Making: A Toolkit for Nurses and Midwives. World Health Organization.

College of Nurses of Ontario (2023). Psychotherapy and the controlled act component of psychotherapy. Author. https://www.cno.org/en/learn-about-standards-guidelines/educational-tools/ask-practice/aGrinspunnswers-to-yourquestions-about-psychotherapy/

Chapter 22
Final Remarks

Stacey Roles and Kamini Kalia

Nurses possess a breadth of knowledge which they apply through a holistic lens in diverse settings. This book aspires to acknowledge and apply the educational foundations of the art and science of nursing towards the intervention of nurse psychotherapy.

In part one, this book sets the stage for *becoming* a nurse psychotherapist and examines the history of nurse psychotherapy through the foundational theories and concepts that underpin our profession. The chapters explore these concepts through the phases of the therapeutic relationship and from a trauma-informed lens from which nurse psychotherapists practice. Much of the psychotherapeutic knowledge discussed and skills explored are introduced and start to develop within pre-licensure education for entry to practice, however, must be further developed through clinical practice and additional education during or post-licensure.

Part two delves into *being* a nurse psychotherapist, exploring the current state of nurse psychotherapy and how nurses deliver psychotherapy in the present. The chapters describe nurses working in the public and private sectors and how they do so with and without digital technologies. Population needs including individual and group psychotherapy, vulnerable populations, cross-cultural considerations, as well as ethics and risk management are reviewed. This section also examines nurse psychotherapy in relation to the nursing process, assessment, case formulation, and types of psychotherapy, in addition to evaluation and outcome measures in psychotherapy.

Essential competencies and methods of continuous learning are explored in training as well as in supervision and by consultation with colleagues to advance

S. Roles (✉)
Roles & Associates Psychotherapy Services Inc. & CBT Training Centre of the North, Sudbury, ON, Canada
e-mail: stacey@rolespsychotherapy.com

K. Kalia
Mississauga, ON, Canada

S. Roles and K. Kalia (eds.), *The Nurses' Guide to Psychotherapy*,
https://doi.org/10.1007/978-981-97-4738-2_22

the nurse psychotherapist and the care they provide to clients. Nursing, as a self-regulated profession, has a responsibility to maintain the quality assurance of its members. Post-graduate education, participating in ongoing clinical supervision, and evaluation of one's psychotherapy services are critical to ensure safe, ethical, unbiased, and competent nurse psychotherapy practice. Each individual must continuously assess areas for further development or enhancement to strengthen the delivery of psychotherapy practice.

Lastly, in part three, the final chapters describe *advancing* nurse psychotherapy. The future state of psychotherapy, and the means by which we can get there, through current and ongoing interprofessional approaches to practice, and continuous advocacy for nurse psychotherapists as autonomous mental health providers are reviewed.

Nurses have influenced the ways in which healthcare has transformed, from the days of Florence Nightingale and Hildegard Peplau, to the constant changes in the landscape of interprofessional teams and practice autonomy, including nurse prescribing. Nurses continue to meet the needs of those in the most vulnerable situations and populations and those in the most rural and remote areas of the world. Nurses have been practicing psychotherapy for decades and the hope is that this book will encourage nurses to acknowledge, pursue, invest, and continue to advance the state of nurse psychotherapy.

SPRINGER NATURE

GPSR Compliance

The European Union's (EU) General Product Safety Regulation (GPSR) is a set of rules that requires consumer products to be safe and our obligations to ensure this.

If you have any concerns about our products, you can contact us on ProductSafety@springernature.com

In case Publisher is established outside the EU, the EU authorized representative is:

Springer Nature Customer Service Center GmbH
Europaplatz 3
69115 Heidelberg, Germany

The manufacturer's authorised representative in the EU is Springer Nature Customer Service Centre GmbH, Europaplatz 3, 69115 Heidelberg, Germany. If you have any concerns regarding our products, please contact ProductSafety@springernature.com

Printed and bound by CPI Group (UK) Ltd, Croydon, CR0 4YY
01/10/2026
02225858-0009